NEUROANATOMY
BASIC AND APPLIED

M.J.T. FitzGerald MD, PhD, DSc

Professor and Chairman, Department of Anatomy, University College,
Galway, Ireland; Formerly Associate Professor, Department of
Biological Structure, University of Washington School of Medicine,
Seattle, Washington; Formerly Associate Professor, Department of
Anatomy, St Louis University School of Medicine, St Louis, Missouri

Illustrated by the author

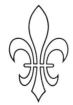

Baillière Tindall London Philadelphia Toronto
Sydney Tokyo

Ballière Tindall   24–28 Oval Road
W.B. Saunders   London NW1 7DX

The Curtis Center, Independence
Square West, Philadelphia,
PA 19106-3399, USA

55 Horner Avenue
Toronto, Ontario M8Z 4X6, Canada

Harcourt Brace Jovanovich Group
(Australia) Pty Ltd.,
30–52 Smidmore St,
Marrickville, NSW 2204, Australia

Harcourt Brace Jovanovich (Japan) Inc.,
Ichibancho Central Building,
22–1 Ichibancho
Chiyoda-ku, Tokyo 102, Japan

First published 1985
Reprinted 1985 and 1990

This book is printed on acid-free paper ∞

Typeset by Scribe Design, Gillingham, Kent
Printed in Great Britain at The Alden Press, Oxford

British Library Cataloguing in Publication Data

FitzGerald, M.J.T.
    Neuroanatomy: basic and applied.
    1. Neuroanatomy
    I. Title
    611′.8   QM451

ISBN 0-7020-1064-2

Contents

Preface

This book is an account of the functional anatomy of the nervous system, intended for students of medicine and psychology. It is designed to provide a basis for later studies of clinical disorders, and for the treatment of these disorders by surgery or by drugs.

The emphasis throughout is on function, with numerous examples of the ways in which functional disturbances reveal themselves at clinical level. Most chapters end with a section on applied anatomy in order to demonstrate the immediate clinical relevance of what has gone before. Both the basic and the applied anatomy sections include material related to general medical, surgical, and obstetric practice, as well as to clinical neurology.

Because of the functional orientation, the gross anatomy of the brain is not treated in detail. Medical students will dissect the brain as a separate exercise, and they will become familiar with specialized diagnostic techniques in their senior years. These curtailments have made it possible to dwell upon synaptic activity at greater length.

With a few exceptions, my illustrations are simple. Most are placed beside the relevant text. Photomicrographs are not included: medical students should already possess an adequate store in their histology texts.

Space requirements have made it necessary to condense the material, without detailed discussion of the evidence for many statements. This has inevitably given the book a dogmatic tone, but the bibliographies list sources of further information on controversial details. The emphasis in the bibliographies is on articles comprising or containing reviews of human or other primate material.

I should be grateful for comments about the work from colleagues, and from junior and senior students.

Elementary textbooks of neuroanatomy abound. My purpose has been to go beyond the elementary, in order to reflect present thinking about how the nervous system operates. Day-to-day encounters with students of medicine and psychology have convinced me of the need for an intermediate-level book to bridge the large gap that exists between the elementary texts and specialist monographs.

Acknowledgements

May I start at home? My wife, son, and two daughters have given me great support. My wife, Maeve, is a medical doctor and a professional histologist. Her comments on the text and illustrations have been immensely helpful. Peter is an experimental psychologist: he taught me a little about information processing and a great deal about artwork. Claire is a clinical psychologist with special interest in asymmetries between the two cerebral hemispheres; she also collated the bibliographies. Finally, Mary Pat has given me the viewpoint of a preclinical medical student.

Within my department, I acknowledge the suggestions of Drs Justin Brophy, Philomena Comerford and Noel O'Neill. Mary O'Donnell patiently typed several drafts of the text over the past three years.

Irish colleagues who commented on earlier drafts include Drs Alec Blayney, Kevin Breathnach, Dom Colbert, John Fraher, Roddy Kernan, Brian Leonard, John Moran, Jim Murray, Jim O'Donnell, and John Sheehan.

From Great Britain, I am grateful for the comments of Drs Martin Berry (Guy's Hospital Medical School, London), John Gosling (Victoria University of Manchester Medical School), Anthony Hoyes (St Mary's Hospital Medical School, London), John Patten (Regional Neurological Unit, Guildford, Surrey, and author of *Neurological Differential Diagnosis*, published by Harold Starke and Springer-Verlag in 1977), and Patrick Wall (Cerebral Functions Group, Department of Anatomy, University College, London).

From Europe, I am particularly grateful for CT scans (Appendix) provided by Drs Hans-Joachim Kretschmann and Wolfgang Weinrich, authors of *Neuroanatomie der kraniellen Computertomographie*, published by Georg Thieme Verlag in 1984 (an English translation is in press).

From the United States of America, I acknowledge the comments of Drs Richard Coggeshall (University of Texas at Galveston), Roger Miller (Pueblo, Colorado), Bryce Munger (Milton S. Hershey Medical Center, Pennsylvania State University), Alan Peters (Boston University Medical Center), and John Sundsten (University of Washington School of Medicine, Seattle).

I have had valuable talks with Dr Jairo Osorno (currently at the University of South Africa, at Pretoria).

Finally, I acknowledge the advice and firm support of my publishers – in particular David Dickens, David Cross, Barend ter Haar, and Ted Hillman.

January 1985   *M.J.T. FitzGerald*

I
NEUROCYTOLOGY

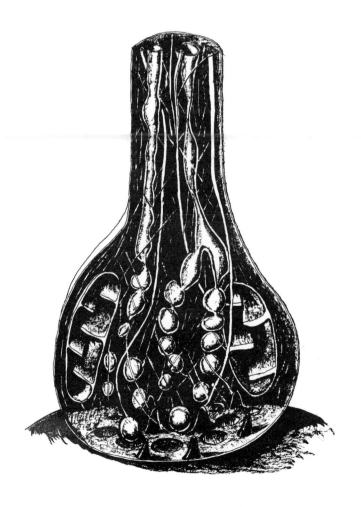

1
Neurons

Nerve cells are called *neurons*. Neurons consist of a cell body, or *soma*, and protoplasmic extensions, called *neurites*, which contact other neurons. Neurites conducting impulses toward the soma are called *dendrites*; the *axon* conducts impulses away from the soma.

Types of neuron (Fig. 1-1)

Multipolar neurons make up almost the entire neuronal population of the CNS (brain and spinal cord). They are also found in autonomic ganglia. *Bipolar* neurons carry impulses from special sense epithelia. *Unipolar* neurons are found in peripheral sensory nerves in general; a single stem process divides into a peripheral neurite, innervating, for example, the skin, and a central neurite, which enters the CNS.

Division of labor (Fig. 1-2)

The soma synthesizes the protoplasm, including organelles, for extrusion into dendrites and axon. Transmitter substances are synthesized in the soma and transported by the axoplasm to the terminal knobs (boutons).

The plasma membranes of dendrites and somas contain *receptors*–protein molecules which are activated by transmitters from other neurons. The activated receptors cause the resting potential (electrical charge) of the dendrites and soma to be altered (raised or lowered). The altered potential is conveyed to the *initial segment* (first $30\,\mu m$) of the axon, where nerve impulses are initiated. The impulses are conducted to the nerve endings by the axolemma.

Organelles (Fig. 1-3)

The cytoplasm of the soma is the *perikaryon* (Gr. around the nucleus). It contains clumps of granular endoplasmic reticulum known as *chromophil substance* or *Nissl bodies*. Nissl bodies extend into the larger dendrites, but are absent from the *axon hillock*–the region from which the axon emerges–and from the axon itself.

The perikaryon and neurites contain neurofilaments, microtubules and a microfilament network (Fig. 1-4). The *neurofilaments* resemble the intermediate filaments of other cells but have a distinctive structure. The *microtubules* have the same structure as those of other cells. The *microfilament network* permeates the protoplasm, forming a matrix in which all of the other cell components are suspended. This network is not unique to neurons.

The soma also contains Golgi complexes around the nucleus, lysosomes, mitochondria (some of which are exported into the axon), and smooth endoplasmic

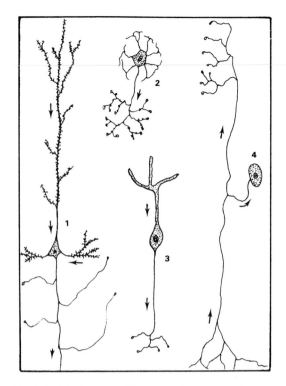

Fig. 1-1 1, Multipolar pyramidal neuron from the cerebral cortex. 2, Multipolar neuron from an autonomic ganglion. 3, Bipolar neuron from the retina. 4, Unipolar neuron from a spinal (posterior nerve root) ganglion. Arrows indicate direction of impulse conduction.

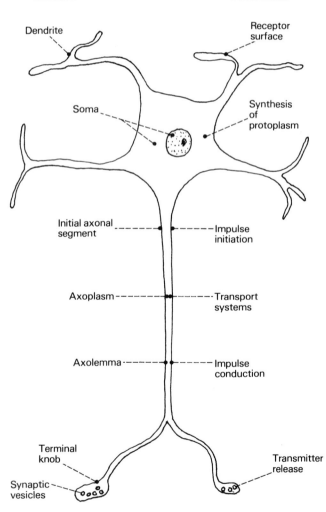

Fig. 1-2 Structure/function relationships in neurons.

reticulum (SER). The SER extends into the axon and reaches the terminal knobs.

Intracellular transport

Transport of cytoplasmic materials occurs in all cells. In neurons it differs in degree because of the length of the axon – as much as a meter in some neurons.

Transport occurs in all of the neurites, but has mainly been studied in axons. Transport is both *orthograde*, from soma to nerve endings, and *retrograde*, from nerve endings to soma.

Orthograde transport

Orthograde transport is of two kinds: fast (300–400 mm/day) and slow (0.3–4 mm/day). Structures undergoing *fast* orthograde transport include the SER and neurotransmitter substances – the transmitter itself in some cases, precursor molecules (including enzymes) in others. SER is incorporated into the axolemma, which undergoes continuous renewal in this way. SER also provides a steady supply of synaptic vesicles by breaking up in the terminal knobs.

The main bulk of the axoplasm undergoes *slow* transport, as do neurofilaments, microtubules and the microfilament network embedded in the axoplasm.

Mitochondria are exceptional in that they travel in intermittent spurts. Some can be found within sacs of SER, which contribute the outer mitochondrial membrane as they emerge into the axoplasm (Fig. 1-4).

Retrograde transport

Worn out mitochondria and segments of plasma membrane are returned rapidly to the soma for degradation by lysosomes. There is also pinocytotic uptake of molecules from target cells at synaptic contacts. The pinocytotic vesicles are incorporated into Golgi complexes in the soma. The uptake of target cell 'markers' (type-specific surface molecules) is important for target cell recognition during development. It is also necessary for the viability of the adult neuron, which will shrink or even die if the axon is cut proximal to its first branches.

Transport mechanisms

The microtubules and neurofilaments are involved in producing fast transport in both directions. A ratchet action involving proteins projecting outward from the microtubules has been invoked. Separate orthograde and retrograde channels may be present in the intervals between the microtubules and neurofilaments. The microfilament network contains actin and myosin, which may afford contractile assistance.

The mechanism of slow transport is unknown. It is not merely a matter of the axoplasm being pushed along by the continuous synthesis of fresh axoplasm in the soma, because if an axon is cut slow transport continues in the severed (distal) part of the axon for several hours.

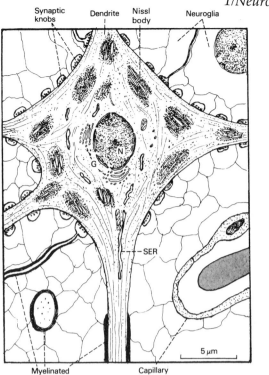

Fig. 1-3 Multipolar neuron in anterior gray horn of spinal cord. G, Golgi complexes; N, nucleus; SER, smooth endoplasmic reticulum.

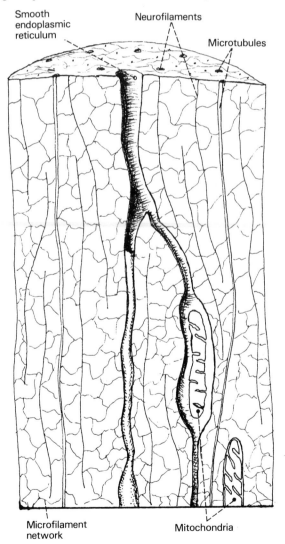

Fig. 1-4 Internal structure of an axon.

Nuclei and ganglia

A discrete group of nerve cell bodies in the CNS is called a *nucleus*; in the peripheral nervous system it is known as a *ganglion*. Sensory ganglia are found in the posterior roots of the spinal nerves (Fig. 1-5). Autonomic ganglia are cell stations in the peripheral autonomic system.

Afferent, efferent and internuncial neurons (Fig. 1-5)

Afferent neurons convey impulses toward the CNS. Peripheral sensory nerves are called *primary* or *first-order* afferents. (*Secondary* afferents are contained within the CNS; they receive synaptic contacts from primary afferents and their axons travel to the brain.) *Efferent (effector)* neurons conduct impulses away from the CNS, for instance to skeletal or smooth muscle. *Internuncial* (intercalated) neurons link afferent to efferent neurons.

These terms are often used in a purely local sense; for example afferent neurons enter the cerebellum and efferent neurons leave it to reach other parts of the brain. 'Internuncial' is applied to short connecting neurons throughout the CNS.

All primary afferent neurons are excitatory. So, too, are virtually all efferent neurons leaving the CNS.

SYNAPSES

Synapses are specialized areas of contact between neurons or between a neuron and a skeletal muscle fiber. The vast majority of mammalian synapses are *chemical*: the effect of one neuron upon another is mediated by a neurotransmitter substance. At *electrical* synapses the neurons are merely linked by gap junctions (see later).

Chemical synapses

In the CNS, the commonest synapses are either *axosomatic* or *axodendritic*. The dendritic trees of many neurons have short (2 μm) projections called *spines* (as on the pyramidal neuron in Fig. 1-1). Each spine receives at least one bouton, forming an *axospinous* synapse (Fig. 1-6).

Most axonal boutons are *en passant* (Fr. passing by): axonal branches weave through the dendritic trees of target neurons, making synaptic contacts on one side as they travel. Only the final bouton is *terminal*. (The synapses in Fig. 1-6 are terminal.)

Structure of synapses

The synaptic knob (bouton) contains all components of the axon, including many mitochondria. In addition, it contains *synaptic vesicles*. In most boutons forming excitatory synapses the transmitter substance is contained in vesicles which appear clear and round after fixation. In most inhibitory ones many of the vesicles appear clear and oval.

The *presynaptic membrane* has proteinaceous material on its inner surface, raised at regular intervals to form

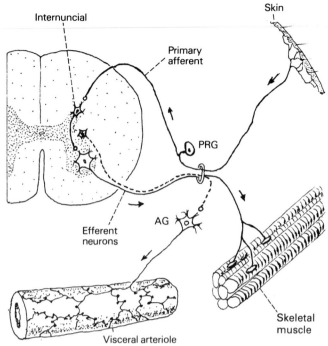

Fig. 1-5 Afferent, internuncial and efferent neurons. AG, autonomic ganglion cell; PRG, posterior root ganglion. Arrows indicate direction of impulse conduction.

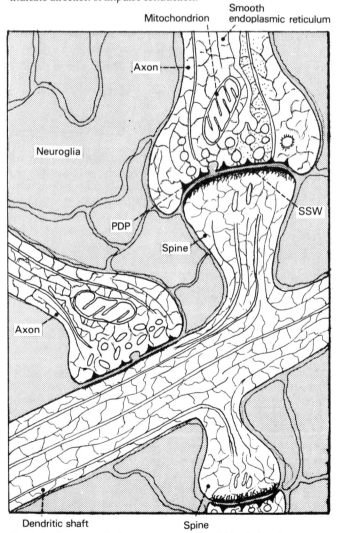

Fig. 1-6 A symmetrical synapse upon a dendritic shaft and two asymmetrical synapses upon dendritic spines. PDP, presynaptic dense projection; SSW, subsynaptic web.

presynaptic dense projections. At the *vesicle-attachment sites* between the projections the synaptic vesicles undergo exocytosis into the synaptic cleft. Microtubules attached to the projections may guide the vesicles to the attachment sites and microfilaments may contract to pull the vesicles into position. The contraction would follow the entry of Ca^{2+} ions into the bouton during depolarization.

The *synaptic cleft* is continuous with the extracellular space. It is 20–30 nm wide and contains electron-dense material.

The *postsynaptic membrane* (also called subsynaptic) has a proteinaceous layer on its cytoplasmic aspect, continuous with a *subsynaptic web*. Where the web is thick the synapse is called *asymmetrical*, where it is thin, *symmetrical*. In most locations excitatory synapses are asymmetrical and inhibitory ones are symmetrical.

Fig. 1-6 shows the structure of excitatory and inhibitory synapses in the cerebral cortex. Both are invested with neuroglial cell processes, which do *not* enter the synaptic clefts. The excitatory synapses shown are asymmetrical and the boutons contain only round vesicles; the inhibitory one is symmetrical and the bouton contains oval vesicles. However, it is not the *structure* that determines the nature of a synapse: rather it is the activity of the *receptor proteins* embedded in the postsynaptic membrane (Fig. 1-7). An excitatory transmitter is one that activates receptors which in turn activate ion channels in the neighboring postsynaptic membrane, so as to lower the electrical potential of the neuron toward the threshold for impulse initiation. An inhibitory transmitter activates receptors of a different kind: these cause the electrical potential to be raised. Excitatory transmitters are said to have a *depolarizing* action on the target neuron. Inhibitory transmitters have a *hyperpolarizing* effect. The electrical charges are passed from the synaptic sites to the initial segment of the axon in decremental waves known as *electrotonus*.

Nerve impulses (action potentials) are generated at the initial segment of the axon. However, where dendritic trees are very large, action potentials may be generated at some synaptic contacts; the action potentials are converted to electrotonus close to the soma.

The commonest excitatory transmitter in the CNS is glutamate. The commonest inhibitory one is γ-aminobutyric acid (GABA).

Sources of synaptic vesicles (Fig. 1-8)

Synaptic vesicles are derived from three sources: (1) rapid transport all the way from Golgi complexes in the perikaryon, (2) budding of the SER within synaptic boutons, and (3) endocytosis of presynaptic membrane. At some synapses the transmitter is recaptured during endocytosis and recycled together with recaptured membrane.

Notes on dendritic spines

Spines are numerous on the dendrites of pyramidal cells and spiny stellate cells in the cerebral cortex, on Purkinje cell dendrites in the cerebellum, and on many

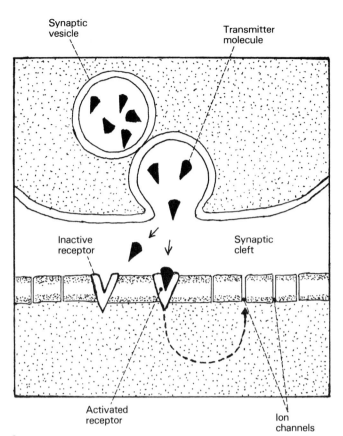

Fig. 1-7 Diagram of synapse (elements not to scale) to indicate the sequence of events following transmitter release.

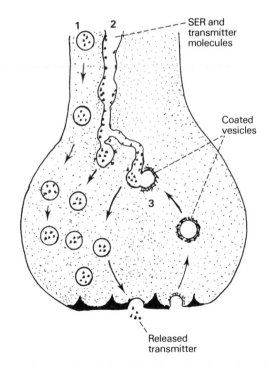

Fig. 1-8 Sources of synaptic vesicles. Recaptured membrane is initially coated. At some synapses transmitter molecules are also recaptured.

neurons in the basal ganglia, thalamus and posterior gray horn of the spinal cord. They may have several functions, with different emphases in different areas. In the cortex of the hippocampus they are highly *plastic*, new spines being formed or deleted in a matter of minutes – a feature likely to be significant in the laying down of memory traces. The thickness of the neck of a spine is related to the effectiveness of spine synapses: a concentration of actin filaments in spine cytoplasm indicates that neck thickness is readily modifiable. Spines have also been invoked to account for dendritic action potentials in pyramidal cells of the cerebral cortex and in the Purkinje cells of the cerebellum. Finally, the extrusion of K^+ ions from active dendrites may cause the nearby neuroglial cells to release nutrients to the neuron.

Less common synapses

Axo-axonic synapses are formed by axons which are applied to axons of other neurons. All axo-axonic synapses studied so far seem to be inhibitory. Two varieties are recognized. 'Initial' axo-axonic synapses occur on the initial segment of the target axon, where they have a powerful inhibitory effect. They are commonly found on pyramidal cells in the cerebral cortex (Fig. 1-9). 'Terminal' axo-axonic synapses are applied to excitatory synaptic knobs. The effect produced here is known as *presynaptic inhibition*. The meaning of the term 'presynaptic' may be clear from Fig. 1-10, where a primary afferent synapses upon a secondary afferent projecting to the brain. One of the inhibitory boutons is 'presynaptic' with respect to the excitatory synapse. In this context, the inhibitory axosomatic bouton shown is 'postsynaptic'. *All primary afferent fibers receive presynaptic boutons.* When the boutons are active, impulses in the primary neuron may be rendered ineffective. For example, the sensation of pain may be abolished in this way when inhibitory internuncials are excited by impulses descending from the brain.

In *dendrodendritic (DD) synapses* the soma and axon of the target neuron are bypassed. Synaptic knobs occur direct between dendrites (Fig. 1-11). In *non-reciprocal* DD synapses one dendrite contains synaptic vesicles and the other does not. In *reciprocal* synapses both contain vesicles; the 'recurrent' half of the double synapse may contain either excitatory or inhibitory synaptic vesicles. The passage of negative electrotonus along the dendrites appears to be sufficient to cause transmitter release at DD synapses, which modifies the electrotonus of the adjacent dendrite. DD synapses are quite common throughout the gray matter of the CNS.

Somato-somatic, somato-dendritic, and somato-axonic synapses have also been described, but they are relatively rare.

Electrical synapses

Electrical synapses consist of gap junctions (nexuses) between dendrites or somas of contiguous neurons. They permit electrotonus to spread from one neuron to

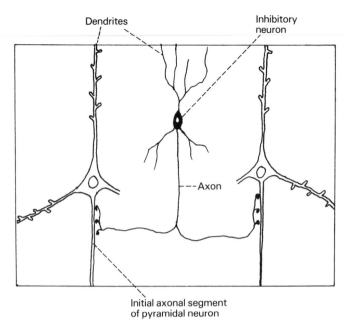

Fig. 1-9 Axo-axonic synapses in the cerebral cortex.

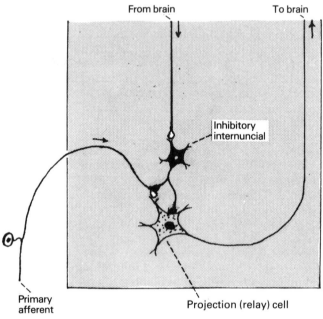

Fig. 1-10 Presynaptic and postsynaptic inhibition by an inhibitory internuncial.

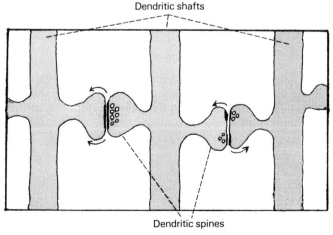

Fig. 1-11 Dendrodendritic excitation. The dendrites belong to three separate neurons. On the left is a reciprocal synapse.

another. They are structurally and functionally identical to the gap junctions occurring between cardiac muscle cells and between smooth muscle cells. The true incidence of electrical synapses in the CNS is uncertain because they easily escape detection in electron micrographs. Their role seems to be to ensure synchronous activity of neuron groups having a common action. For example, the neurons of the inspiratory center in the medulla oblongata are linked electrotonically and exhibit synchronous discharge during inspiration.

APPLIED ANATOMY

Wounds contaminated by agricultural soil or street dust may harbor *Clostridium tetani*. The tetanus toxin binds to the axolemma of any nerve endings in the vicinity of the wound. It is taken up by pinocytosis and ferried to the spinal cord, where other neurons pick it up by pinocytosis. The toxin blocks an inhibitory transmitter substance (glycine) normally acting on motoneurons, with the result that the motoneurons go out of control, especially the short motoneurons supplying the facial and mandibular muscles and the erector spinae. These muscles show *rigidity*, with agonizing *spasms* superimposed. About half of the patients who show the classical signs die of exhaustion within a few days. Tetanus is entirely preventable by appropriate immunization.

Readings

Baudet, A. and Rambourg, A. (1983) The tri-dimensional structure of Nissl bodies. *Anat. Rec., 207:* 539–546.

Bray, D. and Gilbert, D. (1981) Cytoskeletal elements in neurons. *Annu. Rev. Neurosci., 4:* 505–523.

Cotman, C.W. and Kelly, P. (1980) Macromolecular architecture of CNS synapses. In *The Cell Surface and Neuronal Function* (Cotman, C.W., Poste, C. and Nicolson, G.L., eds.), pp. 505–533. Amsterdam: Elsevier/North-Holland Biomedical Press.

Crick, F. (1982) Do dendritic spines twitch? *Trends Neurosci., 5:* 44–46.

Dustin, P. (1980) Microtubules. *Sci. Am., 243:* 67–76.

Ellisman, M.H. (1981) Beyond neurofilaments and microtubules. *Neurosci. Res. Prog. Bull., 19:* 43–58.

Forman, D.S. (1984) New approaches to the study of the mechanism of fast axonal transport. *Trends Neurosci., 6:* 112–116.

Ghabriel, M.N. and Allt, G. (1982) The node of Ranvier. In *Progress in Anatomy*, Vol. 2 (Harrison R.J. and Navaratnam, V., eds.), pp. 137–160. Cambridge: Cambridge University Press.

Gonatas, N.K. (1982) The role of the Golgi apparatus in a centripetal membrane vesicular traffic. *J. Neuropathol. Exp. Neurol., 41:* 6–17.

Gozes, I. (1982) Tubulin in the nervous system. *Neurochem. Int., 4:* 101–120.

Grafstein, B. and Forman, D.S. (1980). Intracellular transport in neurons. *Physiol. Rev., 60:* 1167–1283.

Gray, E.G. (1983) Neurotransmitter release and microtubules. *Proc. R. Soc. Lond., B218:* 253–258.

Jones, D.G. (1981) Ultrastructural approaches to the organization of central synapses. *Am. Sci., 69:* 200–210.

Jones, D.G. (1983) Development, maturation, and aging of synapses. *Adv. Cell. Neurobiol., 4:* 163–221.

Lasek, R.J. (1980) Axonal transport: a dynamic view of neuronal structures. *Trends Neurosci., 3:* 87–91.

Lasek, R.J. and Brady, S.T. (1982) The axon: a prototype for studying expressional cytoplasm. *Cold Spring Harbor Symp. Quant. Biol., 46:* 113–123.

Metuzals, J., Montpetit, V. and Clapin, D.F. (1981) Organization of the neurofilamentous network. *Cell Tissue Res., 214:* 455–482.

Peters, A., Palay, S.L. and Webster, H. de F. (1976) Synapses. In *The Fine Structure of the Nervous System: the Neurons and Supporting Cells*, pp. 118–180. Philadelphia: Saunders.

Rambourg, A. and Droz, B. (1981) Smooth endoplasmic reticulum and axonal transport. *J. Neurochem., 35:* 16–25.

Schwartz, J.H. (1980) The transport of substances in nerve cells. *Sci. Am., 42:* 122–135.

Spacek, J. and Lieberman, A.R. (1980) Relationships between mitochondrial outer membrane and agranular reticulum in nervous tissue: ultrastructural observations and a new interpretation. *J. Cell Biol., 46:* 129–148.

Stromska, D.P. and Ochs, S. (1981) Patterns of slow transport in sensory nerves. *J. Neurobiol., 12:* 441–453.

Trubatch, J.R. and Van Harraveld, A. (1981) Anatomical correlates of synaptic transmission. In *Chemical Neurotransmission 75* (Stjarne, L., Hedquist, P., Lagercrantz, H. and Wennmalm, A., eds.), pp. 139–151. London: Academic Press.

2
Neuroglia

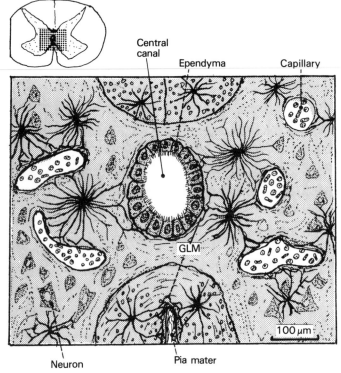

Neuroglial cells (*gliocytes*) outnumber neurons by ten to one; they are supporting cells. *Central gliocytes* comprise astrocytes, oligodendrocytes, microglia and ependymal cells. *Peripheral gliocytes* are the Schwann cells. All except microglia are of ectodermal origin.

ASTROCYTES (Fig. 2-1)

Astrocytes (Gr. star-cells) resemble small neurons. They have dozens of radiating processes. They contain filaments, which are more numerous in the *fibrous astrocytes* of white matter than in the *protoplasmic astrocytes* of gray matter. At the outer and inner surfaces of the CNS, astrocyte processes are loosely interwoven to create outer and inner *glial limiting membranes*. The outer surface of the brain is covered with pia mater, hence the term 'pia–glial membrane' for the composite external covering of the brain. The ventricular system is lined by ependymal cells (see later), hence the term 'ependyma–glial membrane' for the composite lining of the ventricles and central canal of the cord.

Fig. 2-1 Enlargement of rectangle in upper figure, to show astrocytes in spinal cord. GLM, glial limiting membranes.

Functions of astrocytes

1 A notable feature of the astrocytes is a *vascular process*, or vascular 'end foot', applied to the surface of a blood vessel. The brain capillaries are completely invested with vascular processes, which appear to maintain the unique structure of these capillaries (see Chapter 24).

2 Astrocytes invest most of the synaptic contacts between neurons (Fig. 2-2). Astrocytes are involved in the metabolism of some neurotransmitters: in particular, they retrieve the two commonest CNS transmitters, γ-aminobutyric acid and glutamate, after their release from nerve endings. The perisynaptic sheath also has a phagocytic function: any degenerating synaptic boutons are taken up by endocytosis, to be digested in lysosomes.

3 Potassium extruded during neuronal activity is taken up by astrocytes, as well as being pumped into the blood by capillary endothelium. A low extracellular K^+ concentration is essential for normal neuronal function.

4 Astrocytes are the primary glycogen store in the CNS. All astrocytes are in contact with varicosities of norepinephrine-releasing (noradrenaline-releasing) neurons. Norepinephrine released into the extracellular fluid acts upon β receptor molecules in astroglial plasma membranes. Through the cAMP 'second messenger' system, β receptor activation causes glycogen breakdown and the release of glucose for general consumption by neurons. (For α and β receptors in general, see Chapter 6.)

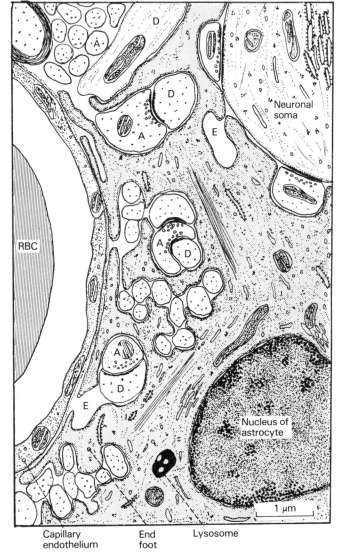

Fig. 2-2 Astrocyte in gray matter. A, axon; D, dendrite; E, extracellular space; RBC, erythrocyte.

5 In embryonic life precursors of astrocytes known as radial glial cells extend from the ventricular surface to the pial surface of the brain. They provide a scaffolding for the migration of young neurons from the ventricular zone of the neural tube to the outer surface, where the neurons form the cerebral and cerebellar cortex (see embryology texts for details).

6 In postnatal life astrocytes retain their capacity to multiply, whereas neurons do not. From a clinical standpoint, this is the most important fact about astrocytes (see 'Applied Anatomy').

OLIGODENDROCYTES (Figs. 2-3, 2-4)

Oligodendrocytes (Gr. few branches) are responsible for the myelination of axons within the CNS (see later). They come to lie in rows between the fibers they have myelinated. In the gray matter, oligodendrocytes form plump *satellite cells* along the somas of nerve cells. Their function here is unknown.

MICROGLIA (Fig. 2-3)

These rod-like cells are of mesodermal origin. They are macrophages, and they invade the embryonic CNS together with the blood vessels. Most are perivascular in the adult, and they are probably replenished from the circulation. When the CNS is injured, many phagocytes leave the blood and share with microglia the task of ingesting myelin droplets and axonal debris. Both types of cell become large and foamy ('Gitterzellen') before discharging debris into the capillary bed.

EPENDYMAL CELLS (Fig. 2-1)

These cuboidal, ciliated cells line the ventricular system of the brain and the central canal of the cord. They assist circulation of the cerebrospinal fluid (CSF). *Tanycytes* are specialized ependymal cells capable of selecting molecules from the CSF of the third ventricle (Chapter 16).

PERIPHERAL GLIOCYTES

Schwann cells ensheath the axons of peripheral nerves and are responsible for peripheral nerve myelination. They also form the *satellite cells* surrounding the somas of spinal and autonomic ganglia, and they contribute *terminal gliocytes* to encapsulated nerve endings in the skin and elsewhere. Terminal gliocytes participate in mechanoelectrical coupling during stimulation of sensory nerve endings.

Following nerve injury, Schwann cells are of particular importance in sustaining and guiding regenerating nerve sprouts.

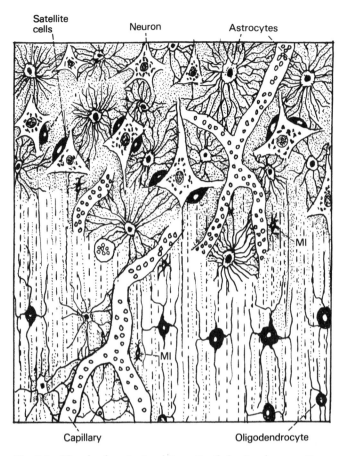

Fig. 2-3 Oligodendrocytes in white matter (below) and gray matter (satellite cells, above). MI, microglia.

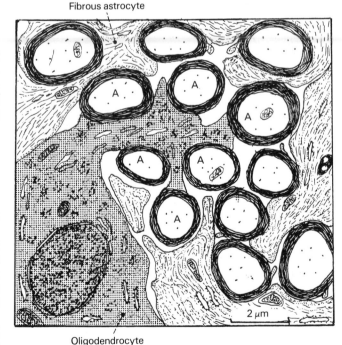

Fig. 2-4 Oligodendrocyte process with six axons (A) attached.

MYELINATION

Myelination commences during weeks 16–20 of pre-natal life, on CNS axons of 0.3 μm diameter and on peripheral nervous system (PNS) axons of 1 μm diameter. Diameter alone is not a sufficient signal for myelination since some PNS axons remain unmyelinated despite reaching a diameter greater than 1 μm.

Central myelin

In the CNS, myelination commences in the phylogenetically oldest pathways (vestibular and spinocerebellar), whereas the youngest (pyramidal and large posterior column fibers) are incompletely myelinated at birth. Fresh myelin lamellae are added to pathways in the CNS and PNS well into the second decade of life, and a few further lamellae are added during adult life.

In the CNS a single oligodendrocyte confers myelin on up to three dozen axons. A flange passes along each axon and encloses it. One lip of the flange passes inside the other and spirals around the axon (Fig. 2-5). Cytoplasm recedes from the spirals and the cytoplasmic surfaces of the cell membrane come into apposition as the continuous *major dense lines* seen in transverse sections (Fig. 2-6). The external surfaces also meet, forming continuous *minor dense lines*.

At the ends of each flange the cytoplasmic faces remain separate, enclosing pockets of cytoplasm. The pockets are applied to the surface of the axolemma (Fig. 2-5). The interval between two successive glial wrappings is a *node*.

The minor dense line ('intraperiod line') contains a minute *intraperiod gap* through which the extracellular space is continuous with the periaxonal space (Fig. 2-6). An important function of the intraperiod gap during the growth period is to allow the lamellae to slip on one another, in order to accommodate the increasing girth of the axon. Such slippage should tend to reduce the total number of lamellae, but it is more than compensated for by the progress of the inner tongue of glia around the axon. Fresh myelin is added to the outermost lamella during growth (Fig. 2-7).

A second function of the intraperiod gap is to permit metabolic exchange. In particular, the component

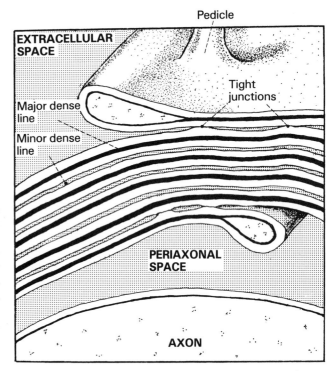

Fig. 2-6 Diagram to show continuity of extracellular space with periaxonal space. The myelin lamellae are held together by 'leaky' tight junctions at the outer and inner ends of the intraperiod gap.

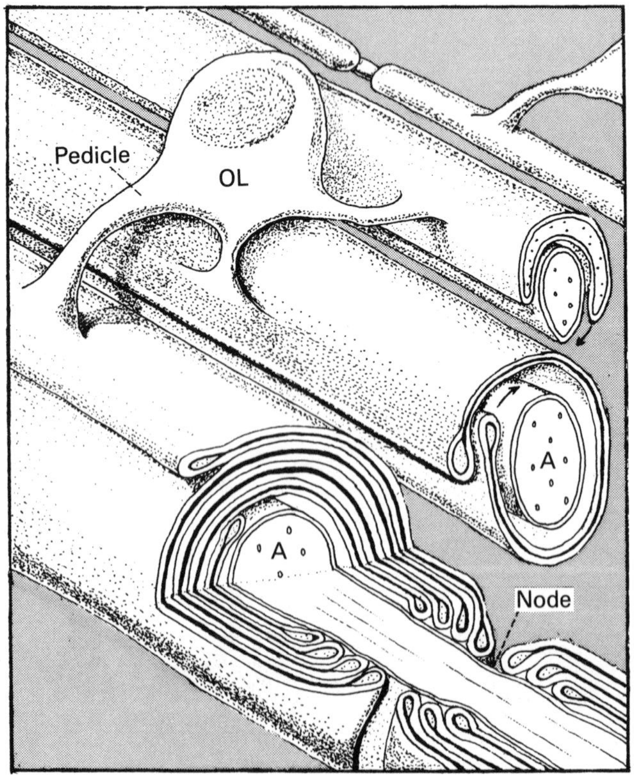

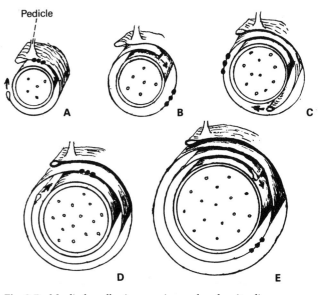

Fig. 2-7 Myelin lamellae increase in number despite slippage caused by axonal expansion. The three dots indicate newly formed external mesaxon membrane in A. This piece of membrane is followed in B through E. The arrow indicates progressive spiraling of inner mesaxon.

Fig. 2-5 Myelination in the CNS. A, axon; OL, oligodendrocyte.

molecules of myelin undergo continuous slow turnover throughout life. The individual proteolipid and glycolipid molecules have half-lives of weeks or months, and they are replaced from the blood plasma. The blood capillaries occupy the extracellular space, and access to the deeper lamellae is provided by the intraperiod gap. This route is obviously required for the largest fibers, which are wrapped by 150–200 lamellae.

Unmyelinated axons

Unmyelinated axons, particularly those of short-axon internuncial neurons, abound in the gray matter. No special provision is made for their accommodation by neuroglial cells. Such naked axons often run in small groups (Fig. 2-2).

Peripheral myelin

In the PNS, a single Schwann cell confers a length of myelin on one axon only. In the embryo, Schwann cells initially enclose many axons. Later, the axons come to lie in individual gutters near the cell surface. This is the permanent arrangement for axons that are not to be myelinated (Fig. 2-8C).

If an axon is to be myelinated, it receives the attention of a chain of individual Schwann cells along its length. Each Schwann cell encloses the axon completely, creating a 'mesentery' of plasma membrane known as a *mesaxon* (Fig. 2-8D). The mesaxon is

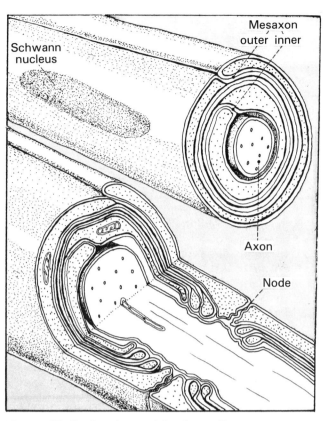

Fig. 2-9 Myelination of two peripheral nerve fibers.

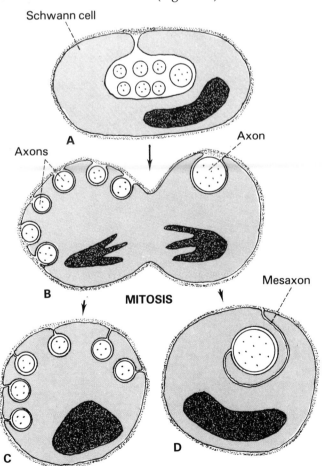

Fig. 2-8 Schwann cell–axon relationships in development. The axon on the right in B is to be myelinated (D).

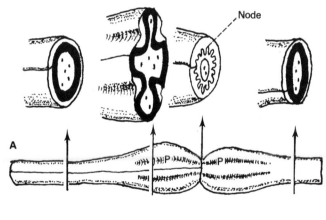

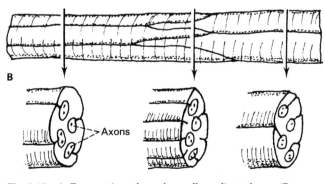

Fig. 2-10 A, Four sections through a well-myelinated axon (P, paranodal bulbs). B, Three sections through unmyelinated axons. Successive Schwann cells interdigitate deeply and there is no node of Ranvier.

11

displaced progressively, being rotated around the axon. Schwann cytoplasm is withdrawn from the interval between the layers of plasma membrane and major and minor dense lines are formed. For a time a sleeve of Schwann cytoplasm surrounds the periaxonal space, and an internal (or inner) mesaxon can be seen as well as an external (outer) one (Fig. 2-9).

Successive Schwann cells interdigitate at *nodes of Ranvier*. The nodal gap is only 0.5 µm wide because of apposition of Schwann cell protoplasm. In large peripheral fibers the axon expands on each side of the nodes, forming *paranodal bulbs*, and here the myelin lamellae have wavy instead of circular profiles. The axon is pinched at these nodes (Fig. 2-10).

Between successive nodes (that is, along the internodes) the major dense lines open at intervals to accommodate glial cytoplasm (Fig. 2-11). The function of these *incisures* is obscure. In the CNS they are found only in the largest fibers. Fig. 2-12 indicates the continuity of cytoplasm in the incisures and paranodal (terminal) pockets.

Internodal segments

Myelin is an insulator with high electrical resistance. During impulse conduction the underlying axolemma is not depolarized: instead, the current spreads electrotonically from node to node (saltatory conduction). In the PNS, there is a linear relationship between the diameter (including myelin) of the larger myelinated fibers and conduction velocity. A factor of six applies to fibers in excess of 5 µm diameter: thus, a 10 µm fiber conducts at 60 meters per second. The underlying explanation is that thicker fibers have longer internodal segments: the finest (2 µm) have segments 0.15 mm long, and the thickest (20 µm) have segments 1.5 mm long. There is a high correlation between myelin thickness and the surface area of the underlying axon.

Strictly speaking, internodal length is determined by the degree of growth of a nerve fiber after the onset of myelination. This principle is well exemplified by comparison of two sets of nerves which undergo unusual elongation during prenatal life:

1 The recurrent laryngeal nerves (especially the left) are displaced in a caudal direction by the descent of the fourth aortic arterial arches, around which they are obliged to loop to reach the larynx. This event occurs during weeks 6–10 of development. In neither of these nerves are length/diameter ratios exceptional after myelination.

2 The lower spinal nerve roots elongate during ascent of the spinal cord within the vertebral canal from the 13th week until birth. Their internodal segments become greatly elongated, without a proportionate increase in diameter.

The difference between the two cases lies in the fact that myelination of peripheral nerves commences during weeks 16–20, *after* the recurrent nerves have attained their final position, but *during* the period of ascent of the spinal cord. (Before myelination commences, Schwann cells continue to divide; hence the equal internodal lengths in the two recurrent laryngeal

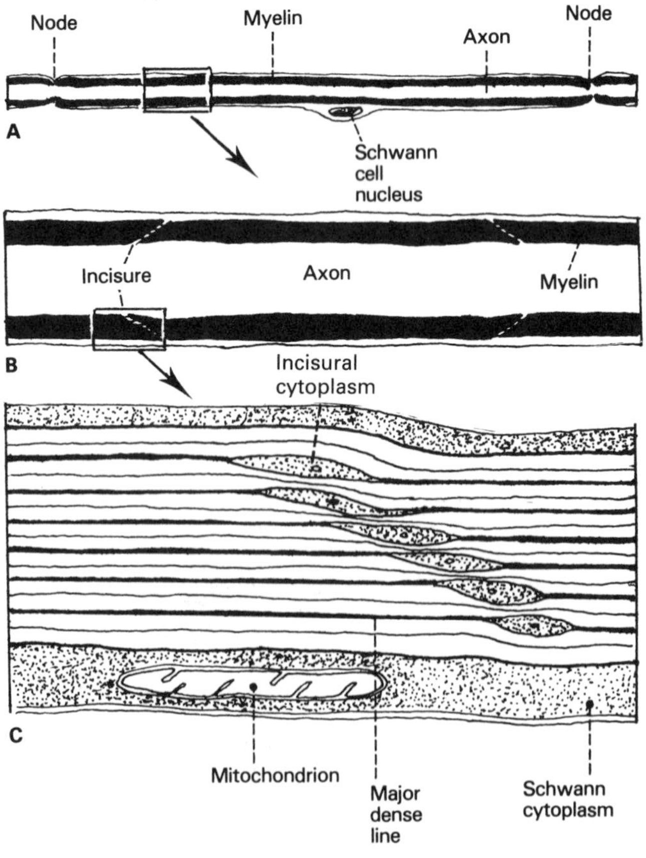

Fig. 2-11 A, An internodal segment. B, Enlargement from A, showing incisures. C, Enlargement from B, showing incisural cytoplasm.

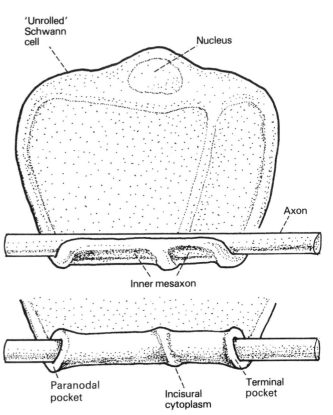

Fig. 2-12 Schematic 'unrolling' of a Schwann cell from a myelinated fiber.

nerves, even though the left is twice as long as the right.)

In fetal life, myelination of peripheral motor nerves is not a prerequisite for impulse conduction. Limb movements are detectable at 10 weeks, more than a month before myelination gets under way (Fig. 2-13). However, demyelination of adult nerve fibers seriously impairs impulse conduction.

APPLIED ANATOMY

Gliomas

Glial cells are the commonest source of *brain tumors*. The majority are *astrocytomas*, which grow to the size of a golf ball over a period of about a year. The edges of astrocytomas are difficult to define during surgery because they infiltrate the surrounding brain tissue; postoperative recurrence is therefore frequent.

Symptoms of brain tumors are both general and local. *General* symptoms are those of *raised intracranial pressure*, produced by the tumor itself and by surrounding cerebral edema. They include headache, drowsiness and vomiting. Midline structures (third ventricle, anterior cerebral arteries and pineal gland) are displaced to the opposite side if the tumor lies above the tentorium cerebelli. Tumors below the tentorium (usually cerebellar) are likely to block the exit of cerebrospinal fluid from the fourth ventricle, in which case ballooning of the lateral ventricles (hydrocephalus) adds to the intracranial pressure.

Unchecked supratentorial tumors may give rise to *uncal herniation* – protrusion of the ipsilateral temporal lobe through the tentorial notch (Fig. 2-14). As a result, (a) the midbrain may be compressed on one or both sides, (b) the brain stem as a whole may be displaced toward the foramen magnum and (c) the oculomotor and abducens nerves may be compressed or stretched (Chapter 31).

A *tonsillar hernia (coning)* is produced by displacement of the hindbrain toward the foramen magnum. It occurs earlier and more often with cerebellar tumors. The tonsils are the lowest elements of the cerebellum (Fig. 2-15), and they may

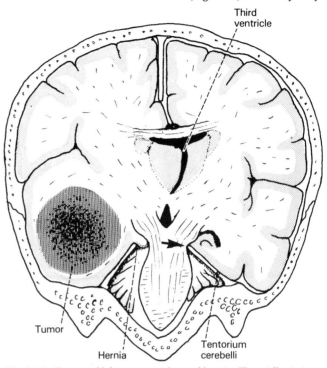

Fig. 2-14 Temporal lobe tumor with uncal hernia. The midbrain is compressed ipsilaterally by the hernia, contralaterally (arrow) by the edge of the tentorium cerebelli.

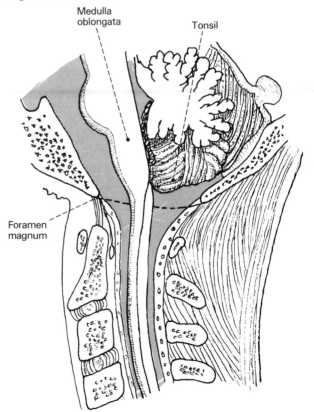

Fig. 2-15 Sagittal section of posterior cranial fossa.

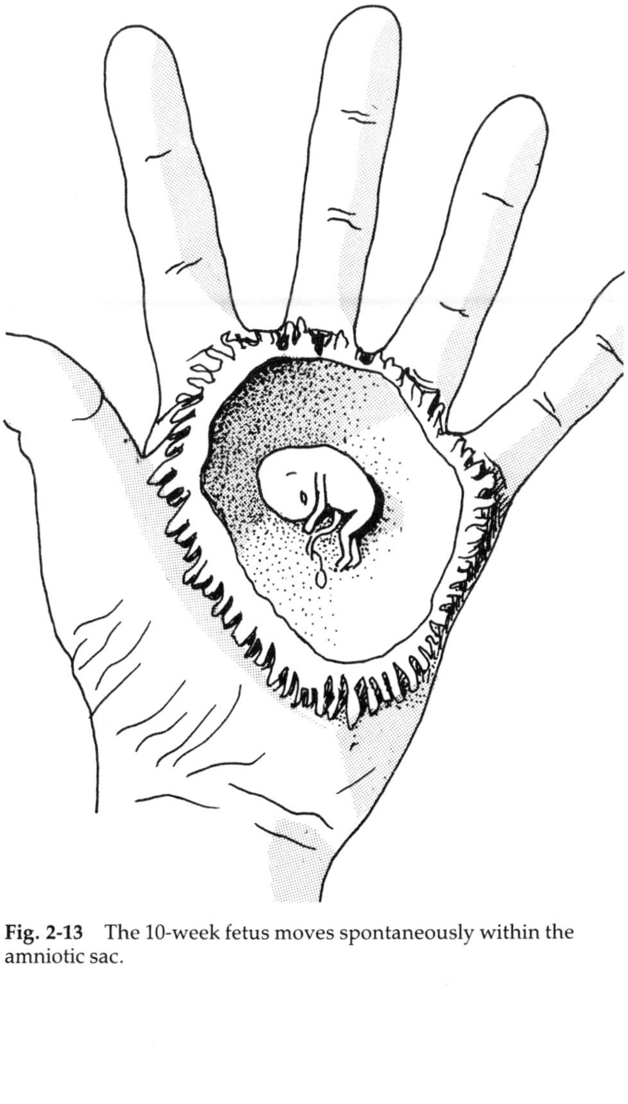

Fig. 2-13 The 10-week fetus moves spontaneously within the amniotic sac.

sink into the foramen magnum. Being a tight fit, they squeeze the medulla oblongata and compress the vital centers (cardiovascular and respiratory), so that coma quickly supervenes. A notoriously dangerous procedure in the presence of raised intracranial pressure from *any* cause (tumor, hematoma, abscess, cyst) is the performance of a spinal tap (lumbar puncture). During a spinal tap several milliliters of CSF are taken from the lumbar subarachnoid space, and this permits descent of the hindbrain. The optic fundi are always examined before a spinal tap is undertaken (see papilledema, Chapter 29).

Local symptoms and signs depend upon the location of the tumor (for example, incoordination of movement with cerebellar tumors, and motor weakness and/or visual pathway involvement with cerebral tumors).

Gliosis

Wherever neurons are injured by trauma, vascular lesions or infections, they are replaced by a proliferation of astrocyte processes (gliosis). The end result is a dense, *glial scar*.

Multiple sclerosis

The most important and commonest cause of *demyelination* is multiple sclerosis (MS). MS is characterized by the appearance of plaques (patches) of demyelination, notably in the spinal cord, cerebellum and optic nerve (Fig. 2-16). Symptoms include motor weakness (pyramidal tract), incoordination (cerebellum), bladder dysfunction (autonomic fibers descending through spinal cord) and blind patches in the visual fields (optic nerve). If the oligodendrocytes are destroyed they are not replaced, because white matter oligodendrocytes do not multiply in response to injury. However, intact oligodendrocytes can remyelinate injured myelin sheaths; this may account for *remissions* of symptoms in this disease.

Malnutrition

Myelin deposition is most active in the perinatal period. Severe *malnutrition* in infancy is accompanied by deficient myelination throughout the nervous system. In the adult, myelin turnover is slow and adult sheaths are virtually unaffected by dietary energy deprivation. The brain does not waste. Ultimately, however, both central and peripheral nerves are severely affected in the absence of B-complex vitamins.

NORMAL WHITE MATTER

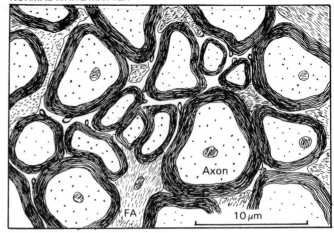

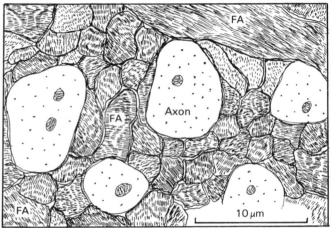

MULTIPLE SCLEROSIS

Fig. 2-16 In multiple sclerosis demyelination is followed by proliferation of fibrous astroglia (FA).

Readings

Bunge, R.P. (1981) The development of myelin and myelin-related cells. *Trends Neurosci., 4:* 175–177.

Fraher, J.P. (1978) Quantitative studies on the maturation of central and peripheral parts of individual ventral motoneurons in animals. *J. Anat., 127:* 1–11.

Friede, R.L., Benda, M., Dewitz, A. and Stoll, P. (1984) Relations between axon length and axon caliber. *J. Neurol. Sci., 63:* 369–380.

Friede, R.L., Meier, T. and Diem, M. (1981) How is the exact length of an internode determined? *J. Neurol. Sci., 50:* 217–228.

Henn, F.A. and Henn, S.W. (1983) The psychopharmacology of astroglial cells. *Prog. Neurobiol., 15:* 1–17.

Hertz, L. (1981) Functional interactions between astrocytes and neurons. In *Glial and Neuronal Cell Biology*, pp. 45–68. New York: Alan R. Liss.

Imamoto, U. (1981) Origin of microglia: cell transformation from blood monocytes into macrophagic ameboid cells and microglia. In *Glial and Neuronal Cell Biology*, pp. 125–139. New York: Alan R. Liss.

Landon, D.N. and Hall, S. (1976) The myelinated nerve fibre. In *The Peripheral Nerve* (Landon, D.N., ed.), pp. 1–105. London: Chapman and Hall.

MacKenzie, M.L., Shorer, Z., Ghabriel, M.N. and Allt, G. (1984) Myelinated nerve fibres and the fate of lanthanum tracer: an *in vivo* study. *J. Anat., 138:* 1–14.

Ochoa, J. (1976) The unmyelinated nerve fibre. In *The Peripheral Nerve* (Landon, D.N., ed.), pp. 106–158. London: Chapman and Hall.

O'Reilly, P.M.R. and FitzGerald, M.J.T. (1985) Internodal lengths in human laryngeal nerves. *J. Anat., 140* (in press).

Peters, A., Palay, S.L. and Webster, H. de F. (1976) The sheaths of myelinated nerve fibers. In *The Fine Structure of the Nervous System*, pp. 190–225. Philadelphia: Saunders.

Robertson, M. (1981) Nerves, myelin and multiple sclerosis. *Nature, 290:* 357–358.

Smith, K.J., Blakemore, W.F., Murray, J.A. and Patterson, R.C. (1982) Internodal myelin volume and axon surface area. *J. Neurol. Sci., 55:* 231–246.

Turzinski, H.-J. and Friede, R.L. (1984) Internodal length in ventral roots of bovine spinal nerves varies independently of fibre calibre. *J. Anat., 138:* 423–433.

Degeneration and Regeneration

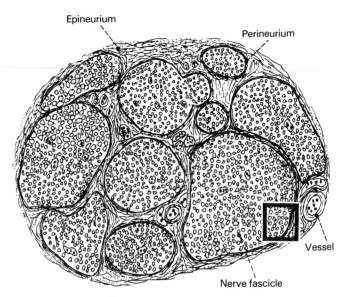

Fig. 3-1 Nerve trunk in transverse section.

STRUCTURE OF PERIPHERAL NERVES

Peripheral nerves are invested with *epineurium*, a loose, vascular connective tissue sheath which passes inward between the nerve fascicles (bundles) (Fig. 3-1). Each fascicle is invested with *perineurium*, which is composed of several layers of pavement epithelium linked by tight junctions (Fig. 3-2). Internal to this is the *endoneurium*, composed of reticular connective tissue and surrounding individual Schwann cells (Fig. 3-2). The endoneurium contains capillaries similar to those within the CNS, and they provide a *blood–nerve barrier* which is comparable to the blood–brain barrier (Chapter 24).

The term 'nerve fiber' denotes an axon with its related Schwann cell and endoneurium. (The cytoplasm of Schwann cells is sometimes called the neurolemmal sheath.)

The perineurium provides a protective barrier for peripheral nerves in local tissue inflammations. However, the perineurial sleeve is open-ended at neuromuscular junctions and at free nerve endings in the skin. The *leprosy bacillus* attacks nerves by entering the skin and travelling proximally within the endoneurium, damaging Schwann cells in its path. In the larger nerves the fascicles form plexuses (Fig. 3-3), and motor as well as sensory fibers degenerate when the bacilli invade neighboring endoneurial tubes.

When nerve fibers are cut or crushed, their axons degenerate distal to the lesion. This is because axons are pseudopodial processes which depend upon their parent cells for survival. In the PNS, the severed proximal stumps of motor and sensory neurons regenerate more or less completely. In the CNS, on the other hand, regeneration of the great motor and sensory pathways does not progress for more than a few millimeters, not because of inherent inability of central neurons to regenerate, but because of an unfavorable microenvironment around the regenerating nerve tips.

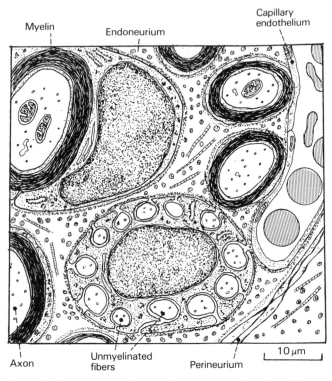

Fig. 3-2 The right edge of a nerve fascicle (rectangle in Fig. 3-1).

WALLERIAN DEGENERATION OF PERIPHERAL NERVES (WALLER, 1816–1870)

Events in degeneration

When a nerve is cut, the distal segment degenerates simultaneously along its entire length. In experimental animals, myelin begins to retract within two minutes from nodes and incisures.

A single normal myelinated fiber is depicted in Fig. 3-4A, together with an endoneurial macrophage. In

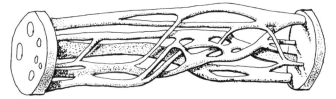

Fig. 3-3 Nerve trunk teased to show fascicular plexuses. (Adapted from Sunderland.)

Fig. 3-4B the myelin has retracted to form a series of *ellipsoids*. The axon has broken down and is contained within the ellipsoids. Fig. 3-4C shows *droplets* formed by the action of hydrolytic enzymes secreted by lysosomes which multiply in the Schwann cells and even appear in the degenerating axons; the axons also secrete a protease enzyme. Schwann cells multiply during the first week, while the macrophages are ingesting debris. By day 6 the Schwann cells form a chain within the endoneurium (Fig. 3-4D). After two weeks the macrophages have departed, and there remain endoneurial tubes filled with Schwann cells.

With a clean cut the proximal stump of nerve does not die back significantly, but in the commoner crush or tear injuries seen clinically it may degenerate for a centimeter or more.

REGENERATION OF PERIPHERAL NERVES (Fig. 3-5)

Following a clean cut, axons begin to sprout after six hours, but after crush or tear injuries sprouting may be delayed for up to a week. Each axon emits several sprouts, but successful regeneration requires that contact be made with Schwann cells of the peripheral stump. Having made contact, the sprouts grow distally within the endoneurial tubes. At the tip of each is a *growth cone* surmounted by fine *filopodia*, which sample the environment. In man, regeneration proceeds at about 5 mm per day in the larger nerve trunks and slows down to 2 mm per day in the finer branches.

If the appropriate endoneurial tubes have been entered, complete functional recovery is likely. Good recovery depends on accurate coaptation of proximal and distal stumps, because peripheral nerve trunks are mixed. Sensory sprouts are quite capable of growing along former motor tubes, and motor sprouts along sensory ones, but neither will establish functional connections. For this reason the outlook is better following a crush injury (endoneurium preserved) than after a cut injury. After a cut the ends need to be accurately aligned by microsurgical apposition of the severed perineurial sheaths.

A delay of several months between nerve section and microsurgical reunion is immaterial to the functional outcome.

RETROGRADE CHANGES FOLLOWING PERIPHERAL NERVE INJURY

1 Within three days of peripheral nerve section the Nissl bodies of parent cells (motoneurons in the spinal cord, unipolar neurons in posterior root ganglia) can no longer be identified by staining with basic dyes (Fig. 3-6). This reaction is called *chromatolysis* (from Gr. *chroma*, color, and *lysis*, dissolution). However, electron microscopy has shown that the total amount of granular endoplasmic reticulum is in fact increased; it is dispersed in the perikaryon, with local accumulation deep to the plasma membrane.

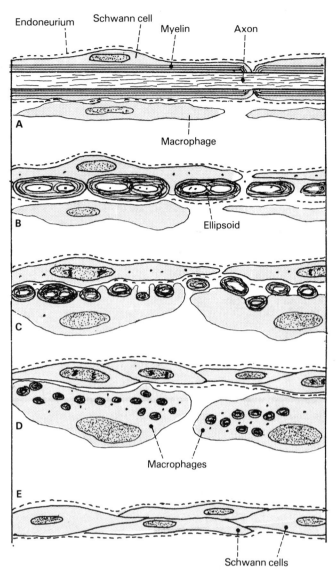

Fig. 3-4 Single nerve fiber. A, normal; B–D, degenerating; E, end stage.

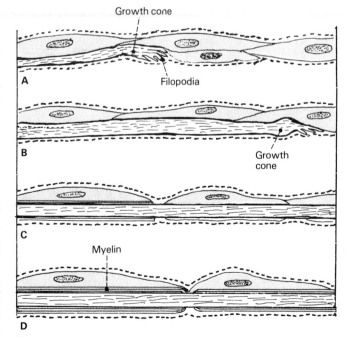

Fig. 3-5 Regenerating nerve fiber.

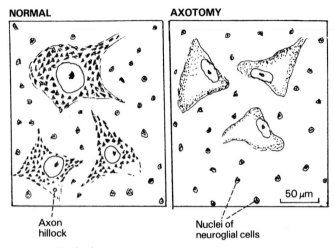

Fig. 3-6 Nissl substance in motoneurons.

2 The nucleus becomes eccentric because of osmotic changes in the perikaryon.

3 The synaptic contacts on affected motor neurons withdraw a little, and astrocyte processes penetrate the synaptic clefts. It seems that the motor neurons are no longer recognized by neighboring internuncial neurons. The inference is that the motor neurons are no longer 'labeled' by molecules taken up from muscle fibers and taken to the soma and dendrites by retrograde transport. Stripping of synapses persists until regeneration has been completed.

The above changes are sometimes called the 'axon reaction'.

DEGENERATION IN THE CNS

Following injury to the white matter, distal degeneration occurs in a manner comparable with Wallerian degeneration of peripheral nerves. Myelin and axonal debris are digested by phagocytes and terminal knobs by astrocytes. Clearance is much slower in the CNS: debris can still be identified after six months, whereas in the PNS it is virtually cleared in six days.

Chromatolysis is unusual in the CNS. Instead, large-scale necrosis (death) of injured neurons is the rule. Those that survive may appear wasted, with permanent stripping of synaptic contacts.

Transneuronal atrophy

CNS neurons have a trophic (sustaining) effect upon one another. If the main input to a particular group of cells is destroyed, the group is likely to waste away and die. This is known as *orthograde transneuronal (trans-synaptic) atrophy*, and it is comparable to the atrophy of muscle that occurs when its motor supply is cut. In some situations *retrograde transneuronal degeneration* takes place – in neurons 'upstream' to those destroyed by the lesion.

End result

If the lesion has been small, the neuronal debris is ultimately replaced by a glial scar composed of astrocyte processes. A large lesion may result in cystic cavities walled by glial scar tissue and containing cerebrospinal fluid and hemolyzed blood.

REGENERATION IN THE CNS

Remarkable degrees of functional recovery are often observed after CNS lesions. However, the major motor and sensory pathways do not re-establish their original connections. They regenerate for a few millimeters at most, and such synapses as develop are upon other neurons close to the site of injury. A variety of recovery mechanisms come into operation, as outlined in Chapter 26.

The general failure of anatomical regeneration of CNS neurons has been variously ascribed: to the absence of endoneurial sheaths in the CNS, to the obstructive effects of hemorrhagic exudates and glial scar tissue, and to possible inhibitory effects of the products of degeneration. Such explanations are insufficient, because regeneration is vigorous and complete in the amphibian CNS, whose structure closely resembles that of mammals. Even in mammals certain fine, *aminergic neurons* (Chapter 15) regenerate well.

The mammalian CNS in general appears to be lacking in growth factors required for successful regeneration. Such factors are evidently present in embryonic neurons because transplanted embryonic neurons grow well when inserted into the adult brain. In rats, parts of the adult gray matter can be replaced by equivalent pieces from embryos. The implants extend axons into the host tissue and they establish functional connections. The blood–brain barrier (Chapter 24) protects these grafts from destruction by the immune system. This approach has some prospect of being applied to patients with restricted areas of brain pathology.

In adult laboratory mammals, central neurons which usually regenerate for only a few millimeters will grow for several centimeters along a peripheral nerve graft inserted into the CNS. Such a graft contains living Schwann cells, which provide a suitable microenvironment for growth cones. However, when the cones reach the end of the graft and make contact with CNS glial cells, further growth ceases. The same effect is seen when a posterior nerve root is crushed; regeneration ceases when the growth cones come into contact with central glial cells.

APPLIED ANATOMY

In *skin grafts* the donor skin is denervated by being removed, but it contains the Schwann-cell and endoneurial skeleton of the cutaneous nerve plexus. The endoneurial tubes are invaded by sprouts entering the donor skin from the host site. Regeneration is usually incomplete because of scarring in the wound bed, but the pattern of reinnervation resembles that of the donor skin.

An *amputation neuroma* is a common sequel of limb amputations, especially at mid-thigh. Regenerating nerve sprouts form a tumor-like ball embedded in scar tissue where a main limb nerve has been transected. Patients may experience a distressing 'phantom limb' sensation. The sympathetic nervous system has some unknown function here; the 'phantom' can be abolished by blocking the sympathetic supply to the limb. 'Phantoms' are less likely to appear if the freshly cut nerve is capped with some inert material.

Readings

Abrahams, Y.H., Day, A. and Alt, G. (1981) The node of Ranvier in early Wallerian degeneration: a freeze-fracture study. *Acta Neuropathol. (Berl.), 54:* 95–100.

Aguayo, A.J., Benfey, M. and David, S. (1983) A potential for axonal regeneration in neurons of the adult mammalian nervous system. In *Birth Defects: Original Article Series*, Vol. 19, No. 4, pp. 327–340.

Barron, K.D. (1983) Axon reaction and central nervous system regeneration. In *Nerve, Organ, and Tissue Regeneration: Research Perspectives*, pp. 3–35. New York: Academic Press.

Baxter, C.F. (1983) Some thoughts concerning the study of intrinsic and extrinsic factors that promote neuronal injury and recovery. In *Nervous System Regeneration*, Vol. 19 (Haber, B., Perez-Polo, J.R., Hashim, G.A. and Guiffrida Stella, A.M., eds.), pp. 241–245. New York: Raven Press.

Bernstein, J.J. and Bernstein, E.M. (1971) Axonal regeneration and formation of synapses proximal to the site of lesion following hemisection of the rat spinal cord. *Exp. Neurol., 30:* 336–351.

Berry, M. (1983) Regeneration of axons in the central nervous system. In *Progress in Anatomy*, Vol. 3 (Navaratnam, V. and Harrison, R.J., eds.), pp. 213–234. Cambridge: Cambridge University Press.

Björklund, A., Wiklund, L. and Descarries, L. (1981) Regeneration and plasticity of central serotonergic neurons: a review. *J. Physiol. (Paris), 77:* 247–255.

Foerster, A.P. (1982) Spontaneous regeneration of cut axons in adult rat brain. *J. Comp. Neurol., 210:* 335–356.

Gibson, J.D. (1979) The origin of the neuronal macrophage. A quantitative ultrastructural study of cell population changes during Wallerian degeneration. *J. Anat., 129:* 1–20.

Guth, L., Reier, P.J., Barrett, C.P. and Donati, E.J. (1983) Repair of the mammalian spinal cord. *Trends Neurosci., 5:* 20–23.

Kiernan, J.A. (1979) Hypotheses concerned with axonal regeneration in the mammalian nervous system. *Biol. Rev., 54:* 155–197.

Low, F.N. (1976) The perineurium and connective tissue of peripheral nerve. In *The Peripheral Nerve* (Landon, D.N., ed.), pp. 159–187. London: Chapman and Hall.

Mackel, R., Kunesch, E., Waldör, F. and Struppler, A. (1983) Reinnervation of mechanoreceptors in the human glabrous skin following peripheral nerve repair. *Brain Res., 268:* 49–65.

Marx, J. (1980) Regeneration in the central nervous system. *Science, 209:* 378–380.

McQuarrie, I.G. (1983) Role of the axonal cytoskeleton in the regenerating nervous system. In *Nerve, Organ, and Tissue Regeneration: Research Perspectives*, pp. 51–88. New York: Academic Press.

Messenger, K.K. and Kingsley, R.E. (1983) Reinnervation in the spinal cord: another look. In *Developing and Regenerating Vertebrate Nervous System*, pp. 231–238. New York: Alan R. Liss, Inc.

Perlow, M.J. (1983) Functional recovery after transplantation of fetal nervous and neuroendocrine tissue into adult brain. In *Nerve, Organ, and Tissue Regeneration: Research Perspectives*, pp. 359–374. New York: Academic Press.

Pollock, M. and Harris, A.J. (1981) Accuracy in peripheral nerve regeneration. *Trends Neurosci., 2:* 18–21.

Richardson, P.M., Issa, V.M.K. and Aguayo, A.J. (1984) Regeneration of long spinal axons in the rat. *J. Neurocytol., 13:* 165–182.

Sunderland, S. (1968) *Nerves and Nerve Injuries*. London and Edinburgh: Livingstone.

Veraa, R.P. and Grafstein, B. (1981) Cellular mechanisms for recovery from nervous system injury. *Exp. Neurol., 71:* 6–75.

Wall, P.D. and Devor, M. (1978). Physiology of sensation after peripheral nerve injury, regeneration, and neuroma formation. In *Physiology and Pathology of Axons* (Wasman, S.G., ed.), pp. 377–388. New York: Raven Press.

II

PERIPHERAL NERVOUS SYSTEM

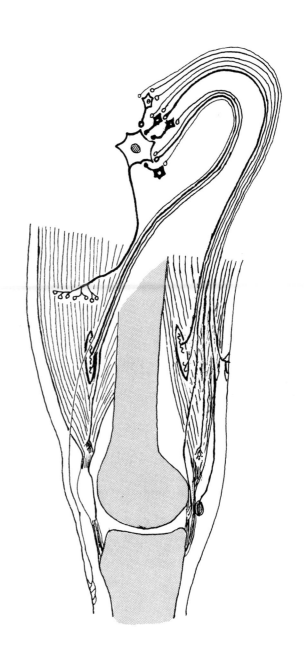

4
Innervation of Muscles and Joints

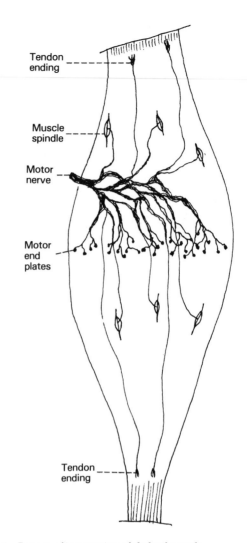

Fig. 4-1 Pattern of innervation of skeletal muscle.

About 60% of myelinated fibers in the motor nerves to skeletal muscles terminate in motor end plates. The rest are sensory fibers to neuromuscular spindles, tendons and joints.

The nerve of supply enters at the junction of the proximal and middle thirds of a muscle (Fig. 4-1). The fibers branch within an intramuscular nerve plexus before proceeding to their destinations. The motor end plates are disposed in bands, each plate being at the middle of its muscle fiber, with one plate per fiber (Fig. 4-2).

A *motor unit* comprises an anterior horn cell together with its family or squad of muscle fibers. In large muscles (for example, the tibialis anterior) a unit contains 1000 muscle fibers or more; in small ones (such as the lumbricals), about ten. Muscle contraction is produced by activation of motor units, and smaller units give finer gradations of contraction.

Muscle fiber types

There are three principal types of skeletal muscle fiber. *Slow*, oxidative (SO) fibers are small, rich in mitochondria and blood capillaries (hence, they are red), exert small forces and are fatigue-resistant. They are deeply placed and suited to postural activities, including antigravity posture. *Fast*, glycolytic (FG) fibers are large, mitochondria-poor, capillary-poor (and hence are white) and produce brief, powerful contractions. They predominate in superficial muscles. *Intermediate* (fast, oxidative–glycolytic, FOG) fibers have properties intermediate between the other two.

Each motor unit contains muscle fibers of only one of the three types. However, the fibres are widely scattered amd interdigitate with those of other units. The type of muscle fiber in a motor unit is determined by the nature of the impulse traffic in the neuron. For example, high-frequency, low-amplitude action potentials impose slow–oxidative properties on a squad.

MOTOR END PLATES

At the *myoneural junction* the axon forms a handful of branchlets which sink into *synaptic gutters* on the surface of the muscle fiber (Figs. 4-2, 4-3). The underlying sarcolemma is thrown into *junctional folds*. The basement membrane of the muscle fiber traverses the synaptic cleft and lines the folds. The sarcoplasm shows a local accumulation of nuclei, mitochondria and ribosomes known as the *sole plate*.

Each axonal branchlet forms an elongated terminal bouton, with thousands of synaptic vesicles containing

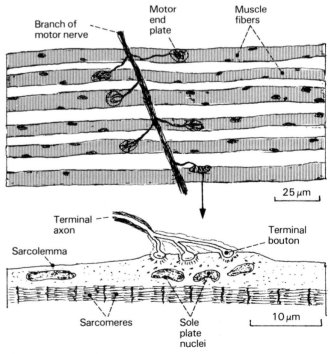

Fig. 4-2 Motor end plates.

22

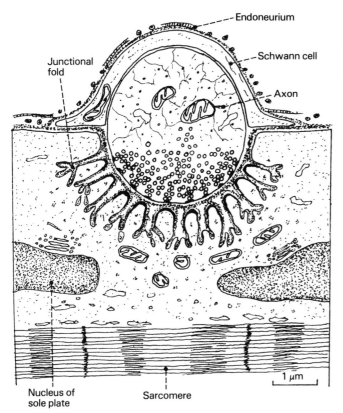

Fig. 4-3 Cross section of one axon terminal at a motor end plate.

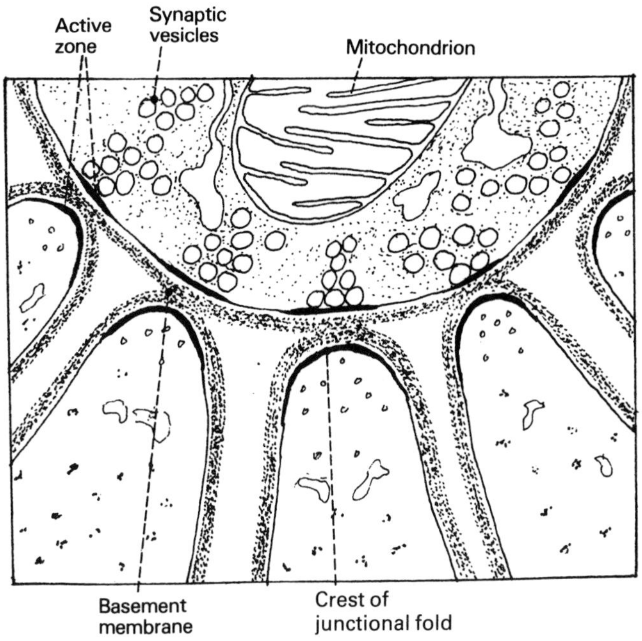

Fig. 4-4 Five active zones at a myoneural junction.

acetylcholine (ACh). Synaptic transmission takes place at *active zones* which show pre- and postsynaptic densities related to the crests of the junctional folds (Fig. 4-4). ACh is extruded by exocytosis into the synaptic cleft. It diffuses through the basement membrane to reach the receptors in the sarcolemma (Fig. 4-5). Activation of the receptors is followed by spreading depolarization of the sarcolemma; the depolarization is continued into the interior of the muscle fiber by T-tubules, leading to the release of Ca^{2+} ions by the sarcoplasmic reticulum and activation of the sarcomeres.

Cholinesterase enzyme is concentrated in the basement membrane. About 30% of released ACh is hydrolyzed without reaching the postsynaptic membrane. After hydrolysis, choline is returned to the axoplasm by active transport.

The enzymes required for synthesis of several other transmitter substances have been discovered in motoneurons, but their significance is unknown.

NEUROMUSCULAR SPINDLES

Muscle spindles are up to one centimeter in length and range in number from about a dozen to several hundred in different muscles. They are numerous in the antigravity muscles close to the vertebral column (especially in the neck) and close to the long bones of the thigh and leg. They are also numerous in the intrinsic muscles of the hand. The muscles mentioned are rich in slow, oxidative muscle fibers. Spindles are scarce where FG or FOG muscle fibers predominate.

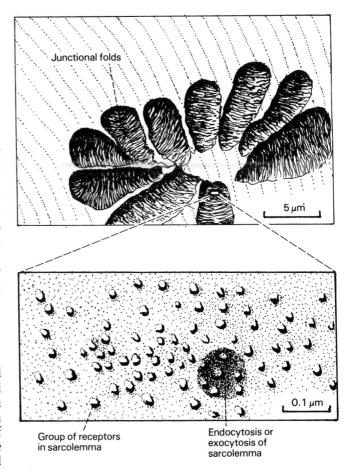

Fig. 4-5 Surface view of motor end plate after removal of axon and basement membrane. (Adapted from Desaki and Uehara, 1981.)

Structure of spindles (Fig. 4-6)

Muscle spindles contain up to a dozen *intrafusal* muscle fibers. (In this context, ordinary muscle fibers are *extrafusal*.) The larger intrafusal fibers emerge at the ends (poles) of the spindle and are attached to connective tissue (perimysium) or to a tendon. The smaller ones are anchored to the collagenous capsule of the spindle. At the spindle centers (equators) the sarcomeres are replaced almost entirely by nuclei, in the form of 'bags' (in large fibers) or 'chains' (in small fibers).

Muscle spindles have a motor and a sensory nerve supply. The motor fibers, called *fusimotor*, are in the Aγ size range, in contrast to the Aα axons supplying extrafusal muscle fibers (Table 4-1). Each fusimotor

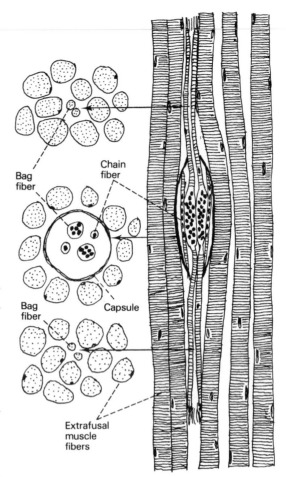

Table 4-1 Peripheral nerve fibers classified by the A,B,C system

Group	Diameter (μm)	Source/function
Aα	12–22	Motor to skeletal muscle
Aβ	5–13	Meissner's and Pacinian corpuscles
Aγ	3–8	Fusimotor
Aδ	1–5	Pain, temperature
B	1–3	Preganglionic autonomic
C (unmyelinated)	0.3–1.5	Postganglionic sympathetic Pain, temperature

Table 4-2 Peripheral sensory nerve fibers classified by the type I–IV system

Type	Diameter (μm)	Source/function
Ia	12–22	Muscle spindle primaries
Ib	10–15	Golgi tendon organs, Ruffini corpuscles
II	5–15	Meissner's and Pacinian corpuscles Large hair receptors, muscle spindle secondaries, paciniform corpuscles
III	2–7	Small hair receptors, pain, temperature
IV (unmyelinated)	0.3–1.5	Pain, temperature

Fig. 4-6 Structure of a muscle spindle.

axon forms either a discrete 'plate' ending on each end of an intrafusal fiber, or an elongated 'trail' ending (Fig. 4-7). In humans, 'plates' and 'trails' are found on all fibers.

The sensory supply is also often double. A single *primary* sensory axon supplies all of the equators in a given spindle. The axon is of Ia caliber (Table 4-2). Its equatorial endings are called *annulospiral* from their appearance in the cat, but in humans they are more often claw-like. *Secondary* sensory endings (if present) are juxta-equatorial, on one or both sides of the primary one. They are type II (Table 4-2).

Activation

Muscle spindles are stretch receptors. The sensory endings are activated by stretching of the equator. The receptor potential travels by electrotonic spread as far as the final heminode, where nerve impulses are

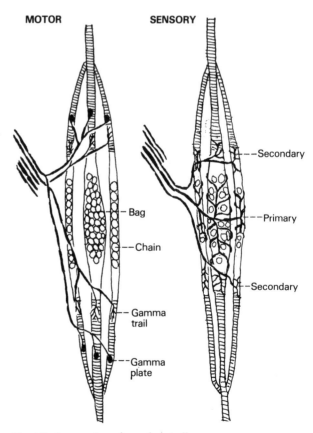

Fig. 4-7 Innervation of muscle spindles.

generated. Equatorial stretching may be passive or active (Fig. 4-8).

Passive stretch

In passive stretch the entire muscle belly is passively lengthened. Such momentary lengthening is produced when tendon reflexes (tendon jerks) are elicited by striking tendons with a patellar hammer. The reflexes arise within the muscle belly, and are equally brisk if the tendon has first been infiltrated with local anesthetic.

The *knee jerk* or *patellar reflex* is a typical example of a tendon reflex (Fig. 4-9). When the patellar tendon is struck, the muscle spindles in quadriceps are stretched and discharge synchronously to the spinal cord. Here the types Ia and II afferents synapse direct upon α motoneurons (which are so called because they give rise to Aα axons). The α motoneurons respond by causing the extrafusal muscle fibers to contract. This is a *monosynaptic reflex*, with a latency (stimulus–response interval) of 10 milliseconds.

In addition to exciting homonymous motoneurons (that is, motoneurons supplying the same muscle), the spindle afferents inhibit the α motoneurons supplying antagonist muscles: some collateral branches synapse upon inhibitory internuncials which synapse in turn on the α motoneurons to the antagonists. This effect is called *reciprocal inhibition*.

Phasic and tonic responses Spindle primary endings are most active *during* the stretching process. The more rapid the stretch, the more impulses they fire off. They therefore signal the *rate* of stretch, by a *phasic* (movement-related) response.

Spindle secondary endings do not show the same peak discharge during the stretching process. However, they are more active than the primaries when a given position is held, and their impulse frequency is related to the degree of maintained stretch. This is called the *tonic response*.

Active stretch

In active stretch the striated segments of the intrafusal muscle fibers are made to contract by γ motoneurons (the parents of the Aγ axons). Because of the dearth of sarcomeres at their equators, the intrafusal muscle fibers stretch their own equators (like pulling a Christmas cracker). During voluntary movements α and γ motoneurons are activated together by the pyramidal tract. Active contraction greatly increases the sensitivity of the spindle to passive stretching, if this is encountered during movement (Chapter 10).

Dynamic and static fusimotor neurons The phasic response of primary spindle afferents is greatly increased when 'plate' γ motoneurons are active. The 'plate' neurons are called *dynamic* because they augment the phasic response. *Static* fusimotor neurons supply the 'trail' endings and they augment the tonic response of spindle secondaries.

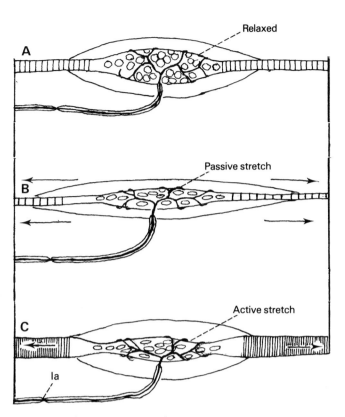

Fig. 4-8 Activation of muscle spindles. In B the whole muscle is stretched. In C the intrafusal muscle contracts.

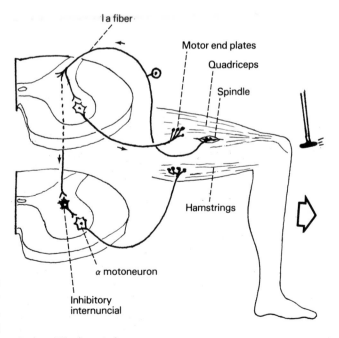

Fig. 4-9 The knee jerk.

TENDON ENDINGS

Golgi tendon organs (neurotendinous spindles) are found at muscle–tendon junctions (Fig. 4-10) at each end of muscles. Their distribution in relation to muscle fiber types resembles that of muscle spindles. A single Ib diameter nerve fiber forms elaborate sprays which become lodged between bundles of collagen within the encapsulated organ. The nerve endings are activated by being squeezed when tension develops during muscle contraction. Up to 25 muscle fibers, each from a different motor unit, insert into one end of the organ, which is therefore *in series* with the muscle fibers. Muscle spindles are *in parallel* because they lie between the muscle fibers. Muscular contraction excites tendon endings but it relaxes muscle spindles (unless the intrafusal muscles are also contracting).

Tendon endings sample the *force* of muscle contraction. They are exquisitely sensitive and respond to contraction of even one muscle fiber inserted into them. However, sampling seldom includes that of fast (FG) muscle fibers, which rarely insert into them. Tendon endings may therefore be inactivated by fast movements.

Autogenetic inhibition

The Ib afferents exert *negative feedback* on homonymous motoneurons, in contrast to the positive feedback exerted by Ia fibers from muscle spindles. The effect is called autogenetic inhibition, and the reflex is disynaptic (Fig. 4-11). There is an accompanying reciprocal excitation of motoneurons supplying antagonist muscles.

FREE NERVE ENDINGS

Muscle is rich in freely ending nerve fibers, distributed to the intramuscular connective tissue and to the walls of blood vessels. They are responsible for the sensation of pain from muscle.

JOINTS

Freely ending nerve fibers are found in joint ligaments, capsules, and intra-articular menisci. They mediate pain when a joint is strained, and they operate a protective, disynaptic reflex which causes contraction of muscles that will relax the capsule. For example, the anterior wrist capsule is supplied by the median and ulnar nerves; if it is stretched, the wrist flexors contract reflexly.

Encapsulated nerve endings found around synovial joints include Pacinian corpuscles (in periarticular connective tissue), Ruffini endings (in ligaments) and paciniform endings (in capsules). Ruffini endings (see Chapter 5) respond to tension; Pacinian and paciniform endings (see Chapter 5) respond to vibration.

At intervertebral discs, the outermost eight to ten lamellae of the annulus fibrosus are supplied with free nerve endings. The anterior and posterior longitudinal ligaments are rich in Ruffini endings, which contain

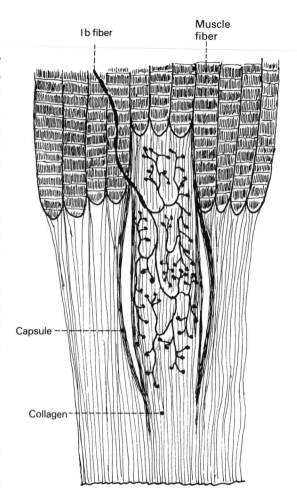

Fig. 4-10 Golgi tendon organ.

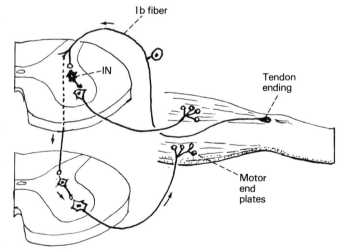

Fig. 4-11 Autogenetic inhibition of quadriceps with reciprocal excitation of hamstrings. IN, inhibitory internuncial.

collagen bundles and respond to stretching of the ligaments.

The spinal cord connections of muscle and joint afferents are described in Chapter 9.

APPLIED ANATOMY

When skeletal muscle is denervated it undergoes *wasting*. The wasting is not merely a disuse atrophy but follows the loss of a neurotrophic (nourishing) factor normally conveyed to the muscle by axoplasmic transport. The muscle fibers take about a year to waste completely.

Denervation supersensitivity to acetylcholine appears within a few days of denervation. ACh receptors appear in sites along the sarcolemma remote from the synaptic junction. Sensitivity to circulating ACh leads to *fibrillation* – minute contractions detectable by electromyography.

Fasciculation is the contraction of motor units for 0.5–2 s. It is caused by generation of action potentials in terminal branches of motoneurons before they degenerate. Fasciculations are visible through the skin: although they are a characteristic feature of motoneuron disease, they occur also in healthy muscle after vigorous exercise.

Mysathenia gravis is an autoimmune disease affecting 1 in 20 000 of the population. It is characterized by weakness and easy fatigue of skeletal muscles, especially those of the eyes, face and shoulders. In severe cases, weakness of the muscles of swallowing and respiration may be life-threatening. The motoneurons and muscles are normal, but the junctional folds at motor end plates are greatly reduced in depth and number, as is the number of ACh receptors. ACh receptors normally undergo turnover, being synthesized in Golgi complexes in muscle and inserted into the junctional sarcolemma. They have a half-life of ten days, before undergoing endocytosis and degradation in lysosomes. In myasthenics, a circulating antibody combines with the receptors. The antibody-bound receptors are removed by endocytosis one to two days after insertion into the sarcolemma, but the rate of production is not increased to balance the loss.

Readings

Barker, D. (1974) The morphology of muscle receptors. In *Handbook of Physiology, Vol. 111/2, Muscle Receptors* (Hunt, C.D., ed.), pp. 1–191. Berlin: Springer-Verlag.

Binder, M.D. and Stuart, D.G. (1980) Motor unit–muscle receptor interactions: design features of the neuromuscular control system. *Prog. Clin. Neurophysiol.*, 8: 72–98.

Bowden, R.E.M. and Duchen, L.W. (1976) The anatomy and pathology of the neuromuscular junction. In *Neuromuscular Junction* (Zaimis, E., ed.), pp. 23–43. Berlin: Springer-Verlag.

Boyd, I.A. and Davey, M.R. (1968) *Composition of Peripheral Nerves.* Edinburgh and London: Livingstone.

Buchthal, F. and Schmalbruch, H. (1980) Motor units of mammalian muscle. *Physiol. Rev.*, 60: 90–125.

Burke, D., McKeon, B. and Skuse, N.F. (1982) The muscle spindle, muscle tone and proprioceptive reflexes in normal man. In *Proprioception, Posture, and Emotion* (Ganick, D., ed.), pp. 121–134. New South Wales: Committee on Postgraduate Education.

Cargo, P.E., Houk, J.C. and Rymer, W.Z. (1982) Sampling of total muscle force by tendon organs. *J. Neurophysiol.*, 47: 1069–1083.

Chan-Palay, V., Engel, E.G., Wu, J.-Y. and Palay, S.L. (1982) Coexistence in human and primate neuromuscular junctions of enzymes synthesizing acetylcholine, catecholamine, taurine, and γ-aminobutyric acid. *Proc. Natl. Acad. Sci. USA*, 79: 7027–7030.

Desaki, J. and Uehara, Y. (1981) The overall morphology of neuromuscular junctions as revealed by scanning electron microscopy. *J. Neurocytol.*, 10: 101–110.

Drachman, D.B. (1981) The biology of myasthenia gravis. *Annu. Rev. Neurosci.*, 4: 195–225.

Drachman, D.B. (1983) Myasthenia gravis: immunobiology of a receptor disorder. *Trends Neurosci.*, 6: 446–450.

Gandenevia, S.C. and McCloskey, D.I. (1976) Joint sense, muscle sense, and their combination as position sense, measured at the distal interphalangeal joint of the middle finger. *J. Physiol.*, 260: 387–407.

Gauthier, G.F. (1976) The motor end-plate: structure. In *The Peripheral Nerve* (Landon, D.N., ed.), pp. 464–494. London: Chapman and Hall.

Hohlfield, R. (1983) Fasciculations in lower motor neuron disease. *Ann. Neurol.*, 14: 491–492.

Houk, J.C. (1981) Afferent mechanisms mediating autogenetic reflexes. In *Brain Mechanisms and Perceptual Awareness* (Pompeiano, O. and Marsan, C.A., eds.), pp. 167–181. New York: Raven Press.

Houk, J.C., Crago, P.E. and Rymer, P.Z. (1980) Functional properties of the Golgi tendon organs. *Prog. Clin. Neurophysiol.*, 8: 33–43.

Karen Pan, K.-S. and Chao, L.-P. (1981) Localization of choline acetyltransferase at neuromuscular junctions. *Muscle and Nerve*, 4: 91–93.

Kennedy, W.R. (1970) Innervation of normal human muscle spindles. *Neurology*, 20: 463–475.

Marsden, C.D., Merton, P.A., Morton, H.B., Adam, J.E.R. and Hallett, M. (1978) Automatic and voluntary responses to muscle stretch in man. *Prog. Clin. Neurophysiol.*, 4: 167–177.

Matell, G. (1982) Myasthenia gravis – an autoimmune disease. *Acta Neurol. Scand.*, 65: Suppl. 90, 112–121.

Matthews, P.B.C. (1981) Evolving views on the internal operation and functional role of the muscle spindle. *J. Physiol.*, 320: 1–30.

Morin, C., Pierrot-Descilligny, E. and Bussel, B. (1976) Role of muscular afferents in the inhibition of the antagonist motor nucleus during a voluntary contraction in man. *Brain Res.*, 103: 373–376.

Redman, S. and Walmsley, B. (1981) The synaptic basis of the monosynaptic stretch reflex. *Trends Neurosci.*, 4: 248–250.

Roll, J.P. and Vedel, J.P. (1982) Kinaesthetic role of muscle afferents in man, studied by tendon vibration and microneurography. *Exp. Brain Res.*, 47: 177–190.

Roth, G. (1982) The origin of fasciculations. *Ann. Neurol.*, 12: 542–547.

Standaert, F.G. and Dretchen, K.L. (1979) Cyclic nucleotides and neuromuscular transmission. *Fed. Proc.*, 38: 2183–2192.

Swash, M. and Fox, K.P. (1972) Muscle spindle innervation in man. *J. Anat.*, 112: 61–80.

Thibault, M.C., Havaranis, A.S. and Heywood, S.M. (1981) Trophic effect of a sciatic nerve extract on fast and slow myosin heavy chain synthesis. *Am. J. Physiol.*, 241: C269–272.

Tracey, D.J. (1980) Joint receptors and the control of movement. *Trends Neurosci.*, 2: 253–255.

Uehara, Y., Campbell, G.R. and Burnstock, G. (1976) *Muscle and its Innervation. An Atlas of Fine Structure.* London: Arnold.

5

Innervation of Skin

Having given off their muscular branches, the peripheral nerves pierce the deep fascia and form the cutaneous nerves seen in gross anatomical dissections. The cutaneous nerves occupy the tela subcutanea (subcutaneous fat). Their branches disappear from view at their points of entry into the dermis, where they join the dermal nerve plexus.

Dermal plexus (Fig. 5-1)

The *dermal nerve plexus* occupies the base of the dermis. It is a polygonal grid within which cutaneous nerve branches divide and overlap extensively. It contains sympathetic fibers (see Chapter 6) as well as somatic sensory fibers. The sensory fibers emerge from the plexus and course toward the epidermis and hair follicles.

Sensory units

A given parent fiber forms the same kind of nerve ending at all of its terminals. In physiological recordings the fiber and its family of endings are called a *sensory unit*. Together with its parent unipolar nerve cell, the sensory unit is analogous to the motor unit described in Chapter 4.

Receptive fields

The territory served by a sensory unit is its *receptive field*. The size of receptor fields diminishes as sensory acuity increases; for instance, they are $2\,cm^2$ on the arm, $1\,cm^2$ at the wrist and $25\,mm^2$ on the finger pad. Sensory units overlap so that different modalities of sensation can be perceived from a given area of skin.

Fiber diameters of several sensory units are included in Tables 4-1 and 4-2 (Chapter 4).

HAIRY SKIN AND GLABROUS SKIN

More than 90% of the body surface is covered with hairy skin (Fig. 5-2). Glabrous skin (L., *glaber*, smooth) (Fig. 5-3) covers the palmar surfaces of the hands, the plantar surfaces of the feet, the nipples and areolae, the vermilion border of the lips and the lower half of the anal canal.

NERVE ENDINGS

The morphological types are listed in Table 5-1.

Free endings

Free nerve endings emerge from a *subepidermal plexus* (SEP) of Aδ and C fibers. The SEP is better developed

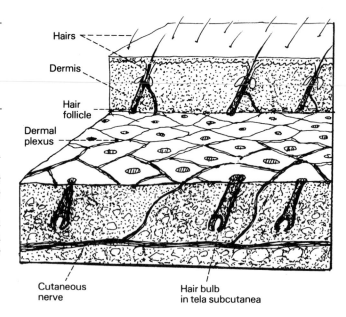

Fig. 5-1 Position of the dermal plexus.

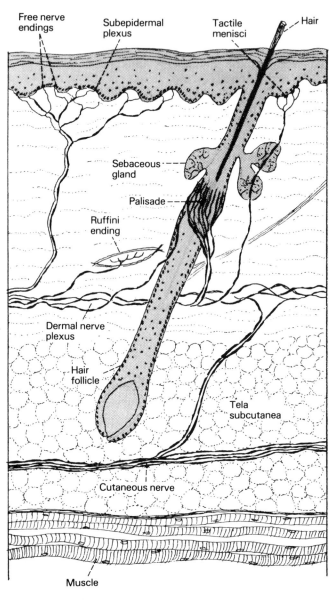

Fig. 5-2 Innervation of hairy skin.

28

Table 5-1 Morphological types of cutaneous nerve endings, related to function

Morphological type	Hairy skin	Glabrous skin	Sensory modality
Free	+	+	Pain Touch Heat Cold
Applied			
follicular	+	−	Touch
Merkel's discs	+	+	Touch
Encapsulated			
Meissner	−	+	Touch
Ruffini	+	+	Stretch
Pacinian	−	+	Vibration

in hairy skin. The perineurium is already shed within the dermal plexus, and the myelin sheath (if any) is shed prior to emergence of fibers from the SEP. The Schwann sheath and basement membrane open to permit the naked axon to contact collagen bundles (dermal nerve endings) or to pass between basal keratocytes (intraepidermal nerve endings, Fig. 5-4). Intraepidermal nerve endings are scarce. In hairy skin they occasionally penetrate to the stratum granulosum.

Plasticity

The spatial pattern of free nerve endings is not immutable. There is a slow turnover, degenerating nerve tips being regenerated by sprouting from the SEP. If the epidermis undergoes hyperplasia (thickening), as in psoriasis or in response to friction or sunburn, many fibers extend to the stratum granulosum.

Functions

Free endings must be able to serve several modalities because in hairy skin they are virtually the only endings present apart from the follicular ones (see later). Each modality is served by a separate sensory unit, although morphological distinctions are not obvious.

1, 2 *Thermosensitive units* supply 'cold spots' and 'warm spots' which are separate and lie several millimeters apart. Warm thermoreceptor units are most active between 35°C and 45°C, cold units between 33°C and 25°C.

3 Purely painful sensation (*nociception*) is served by units that respond only to noxious stimuli such as pinprick.

4 *Mechanical nociceptors* respond to mechanical stimuli of an innocuous kind, and increase their firing rate when the stimulus becomes noxious.

5, 6 *Thermal nociceptors* become active with major temperature change. *Heat nociceptors* are very active above 50°C and even more so when the stimulus is painfully hot; *cold nociceptors* are very active below 20°C and even more so when the stimulus is painfully cold.

The six kinds of sensory unit outlined above are found in both hairy and glabrous skin. Structural distinctions

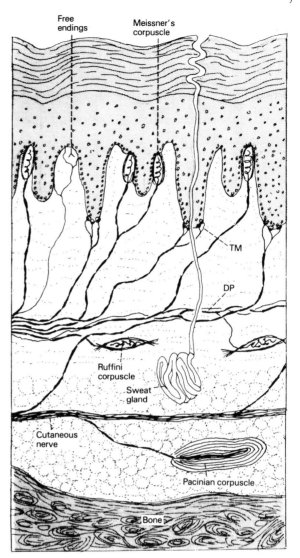

Fig. 5-3 Innervation of glabrous skin (finger pad). DP, dermal plexus; TM, tactile meniscus.

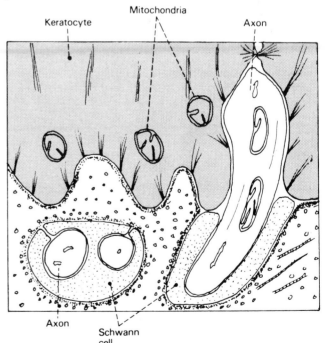

Fig. 5-4 Dermal (left) and intraepidermal (right) nerve fibers. (Adapted from Cauna, 1973.)

between them are likely to be found at a chemical rather than a morphological level. One addition should be made: the *C-fiber mechanoreceptor*, which is responsive only to mechanical stimuli. It seems to be confined to hairy skin, which has a dearth of encapsulated mechanoreceptors.

Applied endings

Follicular endings

From the dermal plexus, several myelinated fibers ascend to form a palisade of endings applied to the outer root sheath epithelium of the hair follicle immediately below the sebaceous glands. The follicular endings rapidly adapt: they give a brief burst of impulses when the hair is bent, then remain silent until the hair is released, whereupon they give a second burst. This rapid adaptation accounts for our being largely unaware of our clothing except when putting it on or taking it off.

Merkel's disks (tactile menisci)

Single fibers from the dermal plexus divide to form a cluster of endings applied to Merkel cells in the base of the epidermis (Fig. 5-5). In hairy skin the overlying epidermis is thickened to form a *tactile dome*. Tactile domes are 0.2 mm wide 'pimples' just visible beside the largest hair follicles. In glabrous skin Merkel cell–neurite complexes are found beneath epidermal ridges, such as the primary ridges in the finger pads (Fig. 5-6). Merkel disk units are slowly adapting touch receptors: they discharge continuously during sustained vertical pressure (for example, when holding a pen or wearing a belt).

Merkel cells are highly modified basal keratocytes. They contain dense-cored vesicles of uncertain content. Synapse-like contacts with apposed nerve endings (tactile menisci, Fig. 5-5) have been observed. The majority view is that the tactile menisci are depolarized by deformation of regular basal keratocytes (mechano-electrical coupling) and that the receptor potential of the menisci may be modified by discharge of vesicles from Merkel cells.

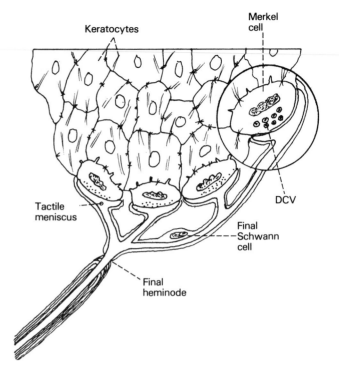

Fig. 5-5 Four Merkel cells and their tactile menisci. DCV, dense-cored vesicles.

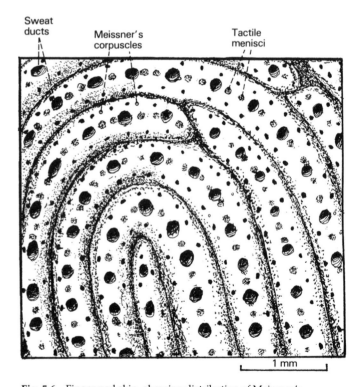

Fig. 5-6 Finger pad skin, showing distribution of Meissner's corpuscles and tactile menisci.

Encapsulated endings

The capsules of Meissner's, Ruffini's and Pacinian corpuscles are composed of connective tissue on the outside, perineurial epithelium in the middle and Schwann cells on the inside. The axons lose their myelin sheaths at their points of entry. Functionally, all encapsulated endings are mechanoreceptors: they respond to mechanical deformation.

Meissner's corpuscles are most numerous in the finger pads, where they lie beside the intermediate ridges of the epidermis (Fig. 5-3). The bulk of the capsule is composed of modified Schwann cells, and the core is occupied by up to nine axons. The corpuscles are rapidly adapting and respond best to movement of the skin across textured surfaces (as when feeling cloth or reading Braille). The slight drag on the stratum corneum is transmitted to the corpuscles by tonofilaments in the epidermis and by collagen in the dermis (Fig. 5-7).

Ruffini's corpuscles are *stretch* receptors. They contain collagen bundles which emerge at each end of the thin perineurial capsule. They are slowly adapting and give a sustained response when the skin is stretched in their long axes. They occupy the deep dermis and respond when heavy objects are gripped, for example when carrying a case. Ruffini endings beside the fingernails respond when the nails are used in scratching.

Pacinian corpuscles are visible to the naked eye (during skilled dissection), being 1–2 mm long. The capsule is mainly composed of onion-like lamellae derived from perineurial epithelium. The corpuscles are subcutaneous and are most numerous along the sides of the fingers (Fig. 5-8). They are supplied direct by the cutaneous nerves (Fig. 5-3). They are even more rapidly adapting than Meissner's corpuscles and can handle up to 600 stimuli per second, a feature rendering them optimal for signaling *vibration*, whether from the overlying skin or from the underlying bone.

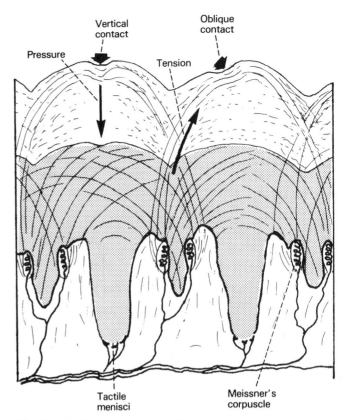

Fig. 5-7 Tactile menisci are excited by pressure through the epidermal ridges. Meissner's corpuscles are excited by tension. (Adapted from Andres, 1974.)

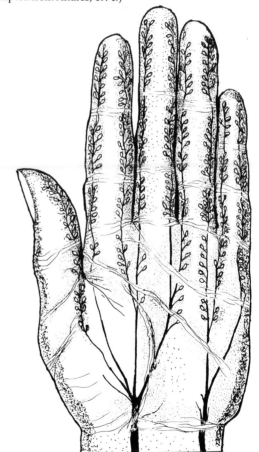

Fig. 5-8 Distribution of Pacinian corpuscles in the hand. (Adapted from Wood Jones, 1941.)

Summary

Cutaneous nerves enter the dermal plexus, from which individual fibers emerge to form nerve endings. In hairy skin, follicular endings take the form of palisades applied to the outer root sheath epithelium. They are rapidly adapting. The interfollicular epidermis is supplied by fine fibers serving different individual functions. Encapsulated (Ruffini) nerve endings are rare.

In glabrous skin separate units supply Meissner's corpuscles, tactile menisci, Ruffini's corpuscles and free nerve endings. Pacinian corpuscles occupy the subcutaneous tissue of the hands and feet.

Functionally, the encapsulated nerve endings and tactile menisci are all mechanoreceptors. Meissner's and Pacinian corpuscles are rapidly adapting, tactile menisci and Ruffini's corpuscles are slowly adapting. Six different kinds of free nerve ending are found in hairy and glabrous skin: warm thermoreceptors, cold thermoreceptors, heat nociceptors, cold nociceptors, mechanical nociceptors and pure nociceptors. In addition, hairy skin is supplied with C-fiber mechanoreceptors.

Readings

Andres, K.H. (1974) Morphological criteria for the differentiation of mechanoreceptors in vertebrates. *Rheinisch-Westfälische Akademie der Wissenschaften Abhandlung 53* (Symposium on Mechanoreception), pp. 135–152.

Andres, K.H. and v. Düring, M. (1973) Morphology of cutaneous receptors. In *Handbook of Physiology, Vol. 2, Somatosensory System* (Iggo, A., ed.), pp. 3–28. Berlin, Heidelberg and New York: Springer-Verlag.

Breathnach, A.S. (1977) Electron microscopy of cutaneous nerves and receptors. *J. Invest. Dermatol., 69:* 8–26.

Cauna, N. (1973) The free penicillate nerve endings of the human hairy skin. *J. Anat., 115:* 277–288.

Cunningham, F.O. and FitzGerald, M.J.T. (1972) Encapsulated nerve endings in hairy skin. *J. Anat., 112:* 93–97.

FitzGerald, M.J.T., Folan, J.C. and O'Brien, T.M. (1975) The innervation of hyperplastic epidermis in the mouse: a light microscopic study. *J. Invest. Dermatol., 64:* 169–174.

Halata, Z. and Munger, B.L. (1981) Identification of the Ruffini corpuscle in human hairy skin. *Cell Tissue Res., 219:* 437–440.

Hallin, R.G., Torebjork, H.E. and Wiesenfeld, Z. (1982) Nociceptors and warm receptors innervated by C fibres in human skin. *J. Neurol. Neurosurg. Psychiatry, 45:* 313–319.

Hammond, D.L. and Yaksh, T.L. (1981) Peripheral and central pathways in pain. *Pharmacol. Ther., 14:* 459–475.

Horsch, K.W., Tuckett, R.P. and Burgess, P.R. (1977) A key to the classification of cutaneous mechanoreceptors. *J. Invest. Dermatol., 69:* 75–82.

Hoyes, A.D. (1983) The primary afferent nociceptive neuron. In *Progress in Anatomy*, Vol. 3 (Navaratnam, V. and Harrison, R.J., eds.), pp. 143–164. Cambridge: Cambridge University Press.

Iggo, A. (1982) Morphology of cutaneous receptors. *Annu. Rev. Neurosci., 5:* 1–31.

Johansson, R.S. and Vallbo, A.B. (1983) Tactile sensory coding in the glabrous skin of the human hand. *Trends Neurosci., 5:* 27–29.

LaMotte, R.H. (1984) Cutaneous nociceptors and pain sensation in normal and hyperalgesic skin. In *Advances in Pain Research and Therapy*, Vol. 6 (Kruger, L. and Liebeskind, J.C., eds.), pp. 69–82. New York: Raven Press.

Montagna, W. (1977) Morphology of cutaneous sensory receptors. *J. Invest. Dermatol., 69:* 4–7.

Perl, E.R. (1980) Afferent basis of nociception and pain: evidence from the characteristics of sensory receptors and their projections to the spinal dorsal horn. In *Pain*, Vol. 58 (Bonica, J.J., ed.), pp. 19–46. New York: Raven Press.

Poulos, D.A. (1981) Central processing of cutaneous temperature information. *Fed. Proc., 40:* 2825–2829.

Wood Jones, F. (1941) *Principles of Anatomy as Seen in the Hand*, 2nd ed. London: Baillière, Tindall and Cox.

6
Autonomic Nervous System

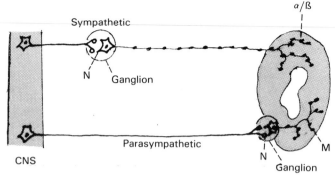

Fig. 6-1 Traditional concept of the peripheral autonomic system. M, muscarinic receptor; N, nicotinic receptor; α/β, alpha or beta receptor.

The autonomic nervous system (ANS) is partly contained within the central nervous system and partly within the peripheral nerves. The main control center is the hypothalamus, from which axons descend to the reticular formation of the brain stem and to the spinal cord.

Peripheral autonomic effects

The ANS is largely outside voluntary control (hence the name). The *sympathetic* system prepares the body for 'fight or flight'. It speeds up the heart and makes the ventricles contract more forcefully. It constricts the arterioles of the skin and intestine but dilates those of skeletal muscle. It dilates the pupils and 'pops' the eyes. It inhibits the smooth muscle of the bronchi, intestine and bladder (except for the sphincters, which it stimulates). It causes the hairs to stand on end and the skin to sweat, and it liberates epinephrine (adrenaline) from the adrenal medulla.

The *parasympathetic* system is more active at rest, especially after meals. It produces gastric secretion and aids intestinal peristalsis. It slows the heart, constricts the pupils and empties the bladder.

During sexual intercourse, both ANS components are active: the parasympathetic relaxes the arteries to the cavernous tissue, initiating tumescence. The sympathetic causes ejaculation of semen into the urethra by contracting smooth muscle in the vas deferens, seminal vesicles and prostate.

DESIGN FEATURES

The peripheral ANS is immensely complex at the biochemical–functional level. For a basis of understanding, it is helpful first to review its design features from the classical viewpoint, which still contains fundamental truths, and then to consider some of the new insights.

The classical view

The classical view of autonomic function regarded the sympathetic and parasympathetic systems as anatomically and chemically independent, exerting their opposing effects directly upon the target tissues. The only known transmitters were acetylcholine, for all preganglionic fibers and for postganglionic parasympathetic fibers, and norepinephrine (noradrenaline), for sympathetic postganglionic fibers (Fig. 6-1).

Receptors for acetylcholine in the ANS are of two kinds: nicotinic (so-called because they can be activated by nicotine) in the autonomic ganglia, and muscarinic (which can be activated by the alkaloid muscarine) in target tissues.

Adrenoceptors – *receptors* activated by adrenergic (norepinephrine-secreting) nerve endings – were classed as α receptors or β receptors. Activation of α receptors, located on smooth muscle, initiates biochemical events leading to contraction (of the pupillary dilator or the vas deferens, for example). Activation of β receptors, located in the heart, leads to increased rate and strength of cardiac contractions. Although the situation is now known to be more complex, the unqualified terms 'α receptor' and 'β receptor' retain their original significance.

Modern revisions

Although useful as a starting point, the classical view has been modified by the research findings of the 1970s and early 1980s. Major modifications are as follows:

1 The sympathetic and parasympathetic systems are not independent at target tissue level. Adrenergic and cholinergic nerve endings are often found side by side in the heart, bronchi and alimentary tract. Release of acetylcholine from the cholinergic nerve endings inhibits the release of norepinephrine from the adrenergic nerve endings, and vice versa.

2 In addition to the two classical transmitters, autonomic ganglia contain a variety of other 'transmitter candidates'. This is especially true of ganglia in the wall of the intestine designated as parasympathetic. The terms 'transmitter candidates' and 'putative transmitters' are no longer satisfactory since some fulfill all the necessary criteria for transmitters in some locations but are only modulators in others. Most are peptides, and many coexist with a classical transmitter.

3 *Modulation* has emerged as a very important feature of autonomic activity, particularly at the level of target tissues. Modulators are not transmitters (at least in the particular location being considered) but they influence neurotransmission by affecting either transmitter release or transmitter effectiveness. Modulators may be 'transmitter candidates', blood-borne hormones or tissue metabolites.

4 In the sympathetic system the original concept of an α receptor initiating contraction of smooth muscle and a β receptor initiating increased cardiac output has been complicated by the existence of other adrenoceptors.

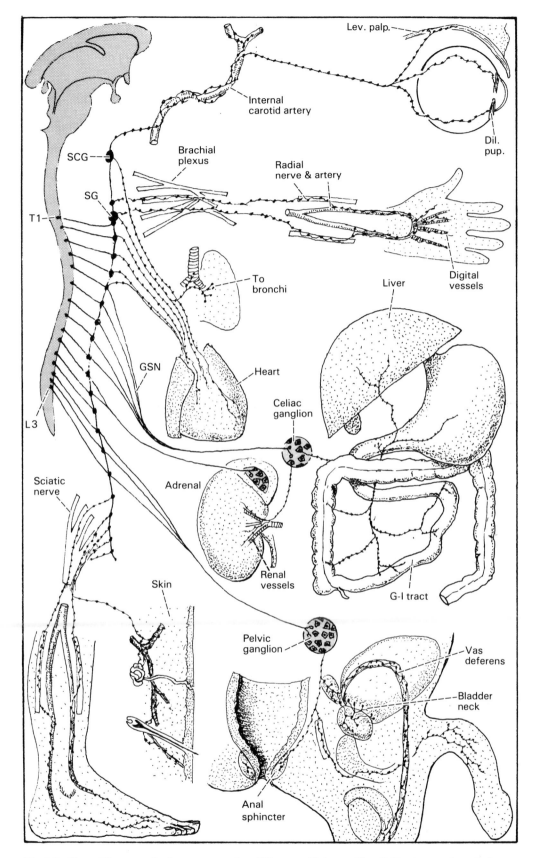

Fig. 6-2 Plan of the sympathetic nervous system. Dil. pup., dilator pupillae; G-I tract, gastrointestinal tract; GSN, greater splanchnic nerve; Lev. palp., levator palpebrae superioris; SCG, superior cervical ganglion; SG, stellate ganglion.

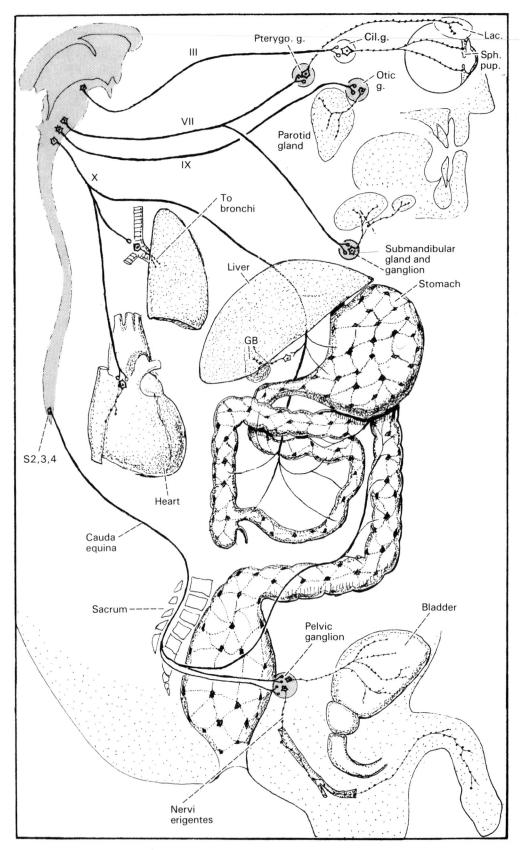

Fig. 6-3 Plan of the parasympathetic nervous system. III, oculomotor nerve; VII, facial nerve; IX, glossopharyngeal nerve; X, vagus nerve; Cil. g., ciliary ganglion; Otic g., otic ganglion; Lac., lacrimal gland; Pterygo. g., pterygopalatine ganglion; Sph. pup., sphincter pupillae.

LAYOUT OF THE SYMPATHETIC AND PARASYMPATHETIC SYSTEMS

The general layout of the two systems can be compared in Figs. 6-2 and 6-3.

Preganglionic fibers

The sympathetic outflow from the CNS is *thoracolumbar*, emerging only from spinal cord segments T1–L3. About half of the fibers are myelinated. The parasympathetic outflow is *craniosacral*, emerging in the oculomotor, facial, glossopharyngeal and vagus nerves (cranial nerves III, VII, IX and X), and from cord segments S2, S3 and S4. All fibers are myelinated.

Ganglia

Sympathetic ganglia comprise (a) those of the sympathetic chain and (b) the splanchnic ganglia of the abdomen and pelvis.

Parasympathetic ganglia comprise (a) four autonomic ganglia contained within the head and (b) thousands of small ganglia lying beside or within target tissues. The intramural ganglia (in the wall) of the alimentary tract contain as many neurons as the spinal cord. Its relative independence from the CNS has led this part of the ANS to be called the *enteric nervous system* (Chapter 39).

The interposition of ganglia in the peripheral ANS permits *diffusion* of preganglionic impulses, because each entering fiber makes synapses (of classical type) upon several ganglion cells. The output of impulses may also be modified by inhibitory internuncial neurons contained within the ganglia, and by collateral branches of postganglionic fibers and of visceral afferents (Fig. 6-4). The visceral afferents traverse autonomic ganglia on their way to entering the cord by posterior nerve roots. Most sympathetic ganglia contain small, intensely fluorescent (SIF) cells which contain *dopamine* (a precursor of epinephrine). The SIF cells exert an inhibitory action on the main relay neurons.

Postganglionic fibers

These are all unmyelinated, and have innumerable varicosities (swellings) in their course within the target tissues. The larger varicosities are local transmitter storage sites; the smaller are *en passant* boutons from which transmitters are released.

Neuroeffector junctions

The smaller varicosities are separated from tissue cells by a *junctional cleft*. Unlike a synaptic cleft, which has a

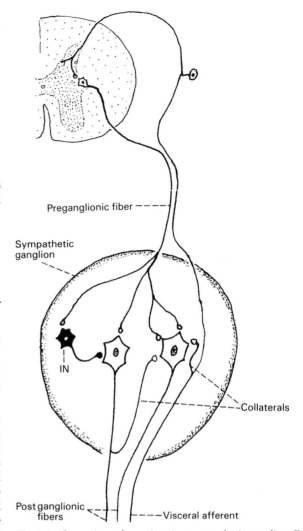

Preganglionic fiber

Sympathetic ganglion

IN

Collaterals

Postganglionic fibers

Visceral afferent

Fig. 6-4 Synaptic configurations in a sympathetic ganglion. IN, inhibitory internuncial.

fixed diameter of about 20 nm, the junctional cleft may be as narrow as 20 nm or as wide as 2000 nm (2 μm). Apart from occasional prejunctional densities, the clefts show no membrane specializations. Narrow clefts characterize the rapidly responding smooth muscle of the iris and vas deferens. Wide clefts characterize cardiovascular and alimentary muscle. The wider the cleft, the more space is provided for modulation of transmitter effects by hormones and metabolites.

THE SYMPATHETIC SYSTEM

The chief sympathetic pathways are summarized in Table 6-1.

Table 6-1 Segmental origins and peripheral distribution of the sympathetic system

Cord levels of outflow	Ganglionic relays	Distribution*
T1–T2	Superior cervical	Eye (31), brain, head and neck
T1–T5	3 cervical, upper 5 thoracic	Heart (37)
T2–T7	Middle cervical, stellate	Upper limb
T2–T3	Upper thoracic chain	Lungs, wall of trunk
T5–T12	Preaortic	G-I tract (39), adrenal medulla
T12–L3	Lumbosacral chain	Wall of trunk, lower limb, perineum
T12–L3	Pelvic	Bladder sphincter, ductus deferens, rectum (40, 41)

*Numbers in parentheses refer to the chapters giving details

Sympathetic chain

The sympathetic chain extends along the entire length of the vertebral column on each side. At T1–L3 levels many preganglionic fibers synapse at their own segmental level and the postganglionic fibers accompany the spinal nerves into the wall of the trunk, for distribution to blood vessels and skin. The preganglionic fibers give rise to a *white ramus communicans* from spinal nerve to ganglion. The postganglionic fibers give rise to a *gray ramus communicans* from ganglion to spinal nerve (Fig. 6-5).

The cervical sympathetic chain receives its preganglionic supply entirely from below, from fibers emerging at T1–T6 segmental levels of the cord and ascending the chain. The postganglionic fibers are widely distributed:

1 to the cerebral arteries and the eye, by fibers surrounding the internal carotid artery;
2 to the face and neck, along the external carotid branches and via the cervical plexus;
3 to the heart, by fibers descending along the trachea.

Stellate ganglion

The inferior cervical and first thoracic ganglia are usually fused, as the stellate ganglion (Fig. 6-6). The entire sympathetic supply to the head, neck, and upper limb enters the stellate, although not all fibers relay there.

Sympathetic supply to the hand

The preganglionic fibers relay in the stellate and middle cervical ganglia (Fig. 6-6). The postganglionic fibers enter the brachial plexus, most of them passing over the first rib in the lower trunk of the plexus. The hand fibers leave the radial, ulnar and median nerves and run along the accompanying arteries.

The lower lumbar and sacral sympathetic chain receives its preganglionic supply entirely from above, by fibers descending the chain from T10–L3 segmental levels. Postganglionic fibers enter the lumbosacral plexus for distribution to the vessels and skin of the lower limb (Fig. 6-2).

Splanchnic ganglia and splanchnic nerves (Fig. 6-7)

The splanchnic ganglia are the (preaortic) celiac and mesenteric ganglia in the abdomen, and the pelvic ganglia on each side of the rectum. To reach the abdominal ganglia, preganglionic fibers from spinal segments T5–T12 pass through the chain without relay, emerge as the (preganglionic) *thoracic splanchnic nerves*, and pierce the diaphragm. From the preaortic ganglia, postganglionic fibers accompany the arteries to the foregut (celiac), midgut (superior mesenteric), hindgut (inferior mesenteric) and kidney (renal). The medulla of the adrenal is supplied *direct* by preganglionic fibers (see later).

To reach the pelvic ganglia, preganglionic fibers from cord segments T10–L3 pass through the chain without relay, emerge as the (preganglionic) *lumbar splanchnic nerves*, and descend in front of the aortic

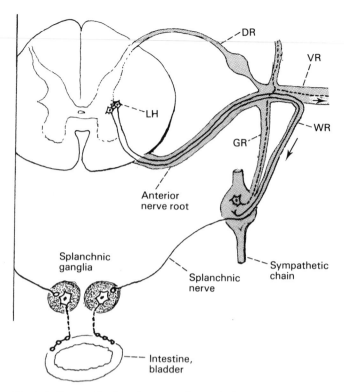

Fig. 6-5 Preganglionic and postganglionic (dashed lines) sympathetic fibers. DR, VR, dorsal and ventral nerve roots; GR, WR, gray and white rami communicantes; LH, lateral gray horn.

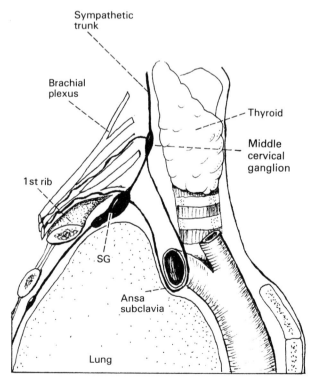

Fig. 6-6 Stellate ganglion (SG) seen from the right. The ansa subclavia is a sympathetic loop around the subclavian artery.

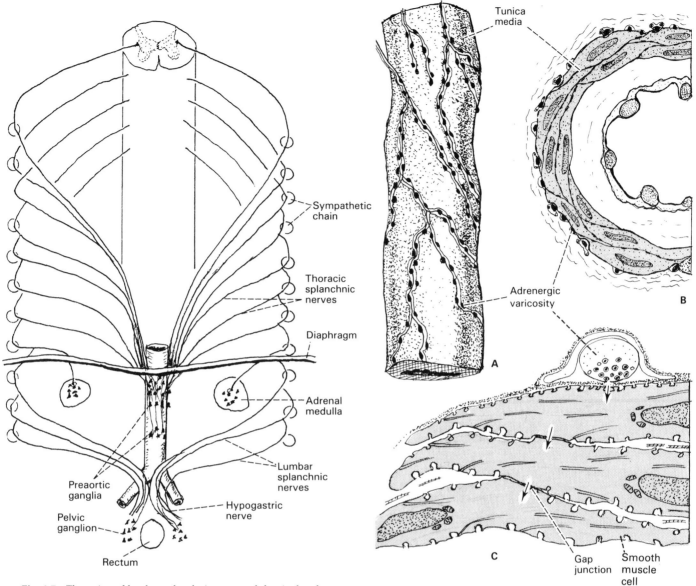

Fig. 6-7 Thoracic and lumbar splanchnic nerves; abdominal and pelvic splanchnic ganglia.

Fig. 6-8 Adrenergic innervation of an arteriole.

bifurcation to enter the pelvic ganglia. Postganglionic fibers emerge from the pelvic ganglia and supply the male genital tract in particular, but also the rectum and bladder.

Neuroeffector junctions

The primary transmitter released from postganglionic sympathetic fibers is norepinephrine. Notable exceptions are the fibers to eccrine sweat glands of the general hairy skin and to the arteries supplying the limb muscles: these are cholinergic. The norepinephrine is contained in 50 nm dense-cored vesicles where it is bound to a carrier protein.

In the fast-responding dilator pupillae and vas deferens the musculature is pervaded by sympathetic fibers, and virtually every muscle cell is in contact with a varicosity. In the blood vessels, varicosities are deployed along the surface of the tunica media, and depolarization is propagated inward from cell to cell by gap junctions (Fig. 6-8).

Excitatory and inhibitory effects of norepinephrine

As already mentioned, target-cell adrenoceptors were initially thought to be of only two kinds, designated α and β. The α receptor initiates contraction of smooth muscle (and secretion in some glands). The β receptor improves the performance of the heart. Both are postjunctional receptors, occupying the plasma membrane of target cells. α and β receptors are now subdivided, as follows:

1 A prejunctional receptor – called α_2 – is found on adrenergic and cholinergic nerve endings (and elsewhere). On adrenergic endings it is called an *autoreceptor* and it inhibits the further release of noradrenaline. In this context the original α receptor is called α_1 (Fig. 6-9).

Although still 'official', the existence of autoreceptors has been questioned.

2 A postjunctional receptor initiating *relaxation* of some smooth muscle (notably in the bronchi) is designated β_2. The β receptor in the heart is designated β_1 in this context.

The unqualified terms α *and* β *adrenoceptors signify* α_1 *and* β_1.

Although α_1 and α_2 receptors had an anatomical connotation at first (post- and prejunctional, respectively), they are now categorized in accordance with their pharmacological properties. Thus, α_2 receptors are found on blood vessels (in addition to α_1) and on postsynaptic membranes in the brain.

Innervation of the skin

The skin is supplied by adrenergic and cholinergic fibers of the sympathetic system. Adrenergic fibers act upon α receptors to cause contraction of arterioles and secretion of the odoriferous apocrine sweat glands of the axillae, pubic region and areolae. Cholinergic fibers act upon muscarinic receptors (see later) to cause secretion of the eccrine sweat glands covering the body surface. Vasoactive intestinal polypeptide (VIP) (discovered first in the intestine) is liberated together with acetylcholine, and (together with locally released bradykinin) it provides the required local vasodilatation around the glands (Fig. 6-10).

Innervation of the adrenal medulla (Fig. 6-11)

Preganglionic fibers of the lowest thoracic splanchnic nerves synapse directly upon chromaffin cells, which are the secretory cells. This is because these are modified ganglion cells (a few even have short processes). The cells abut on a rich, fenestrated capillary bed typical of endocrine tissue. The cytoplasm next to the capillaries is packed with dense-cored vesicles (DCV). The larger DCVs (about 80%) contain epinephrine; the smaller contain norepinephrine.

Synthesis of catecholamines

Epinephrine is one of three catecholamines, the others being dopamine and norepinephrine. All are synthesized from the amino acid tyrosine, the sequence (a–d) being tyrosine → dopa (dihydroxyphenylalanine) → dopamine → norepinephrine → epinephrine. Dopaminergic neurons contain the requisite enzymes for steps a and b. Adrenergic neurons also contain enzyme c. Chromaffin cells have enzyme d as well, to complete the sequence.

The primary action of epinephrine is on β_2 receptors, which have been called hormonal receptors for this reason. When abundant epinephrine is liberated during the defense reaction to sudden threat, β_2 receptors are activated:

1 in the heart, to relax the coronary vessels,
2 in the lungs, to relax the bronchi,
3 in skeletal muscle, to relax arterioles,
4 in the eye, to relax the ciliary and sphincter pupillae muscles,
5 at sympathetic nerve endings, to assist release of norepinephrine.

Dopamine and the sympathoadrenal system

Sympathetic nerve endings and chromaffin cells normally release small amounts of dopamine into the

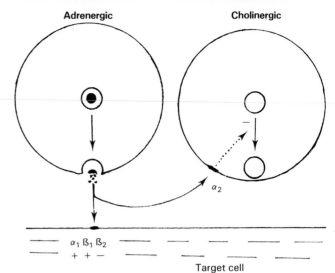

Fig. 6-9 Released norepinephrine binds with α_1 or β_2 receptors on smooth muscle and with β_1 receptors on heart muscle. Release of acetylcholine is inhibited by prejunctional α_2 receptors on cholinergic varicosities.

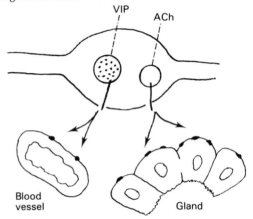

Fig. 6-10 Cotransmission of acetylcholine (ACh) and vasoactive intestinal polypeptide (VIP), causing glandular secretion and vascular dilatation.

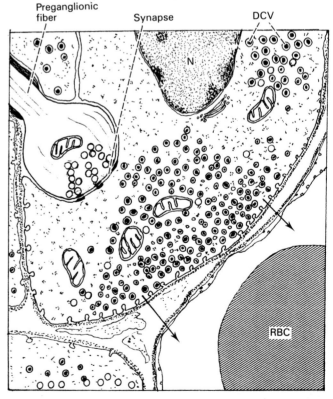

Fig. 6-11 Suprarenal medulla. The synapse is cholinergic. DCV, dense-cored vesicle; N, nucleus of chromaffin cell; RBC, erythrocyte.

Table 6-2 Components of the peripheral parasympathetic nervous system

Nucleus of origin	Peripheral nerve (preganglionic)	Ganglionic relays	Target organs (postganglionic)*
Edinger–Westphal	Oculomotor (III)	Ciliary	Sphincter pupillae, ciliary muscle (31)
Salivatory	Facial (VII) (greater petrosal)	Pterygopalatine	Lacrimal and nasal glands (35)
Salivatory	Facial (VII) (chorda tympani)	Submandibular	Submandibular, sublingual, intralingual glands (35)
Salivatory	Glossopharyngeal (IX) (tympanic branch)	Otic	Parotid gland (36)
Vagus and nucleus ambiguus	Vagus (X)	Cardiac and intramural	Heart (37), lower respiratory system (36), foregut and midgut (39)
S2,3,4	Pelvic splanchnic	Pelvic	Bladder (40), erectile tissue (41)
		Intramural	Hindgut (40)

*Numbers in parentheses refer to the chapters giving details.

circulation, where it is degraded by the blood. In conditions of stress, including vigorous exercise, dopamine release is greatly increased: chromaffin cells may release dopamine and norepinephrine in equal amounts. Dopamine in these high concentrations has a supportive action on α and β receptors (as well as on specific dopamine receptors), helping to raise the blood pressure by accelerating the heart and by constricting appropriate arterioles.

THE PARASYMPATHETIC SYSTEM

The chief parasympathetic pathways are listed in Table 6-2. Details for each are to be found in the corresponding chapters.

Neuroeffector junctions (Fig. 6-12)

Released acetylcholine acts upon the local muscarinic receptors on heart, smooth muscle and exocrine glands. Accumulation of transmitter in the junctional cleft is prevented (a) by cholinesterase enzyme in the cleft (the choline moiety is actively taken up by the nerve ending) and perhaps (b) by muscarinic autoreceptors on the nerve ending (compare the α_2 autoreceptors on sympathetic nerve endings). At the same time, release of norepinephrine from nearby sympathetic fibers is inhibited by muscarinic receptors on the sympathetic fibers (compare the α_2 receptors on cholinergic fibers).

In the exocrine glands (lacrimal, salivary, gastric and pancreatic) VIP is liberated together with acetylcholine, to dilate the local blood vessels and stimulate secretion.

Non-adrenergic, non-cholinergic neurons

So-called 'NANC' neurons are abundant in the intramural ganglia of the gut and in the pelvic ganglia (the latter are shared by preganglionic sympathetic and parasympathetic fibers). Some of these contain excitatory transmitters or modulators (notably serotonin or substance P). Others contain inhibitory transmitters or modulators (notably ATP, VIP or enkephalin). The role of the many 'transmitter candidates' in controlling smooth muscle is largely unknown.

APPLIED ANATOMY

Stellate block
The stellate ganglion lies in front of the neck of the first rib. *Stellate block* (injection of an anesthetic or destructive solution into the ganglion) is often performed for relief of vascular spasm in the hands (Reynaud phenomenon), for hyperhidrosis (excessive sweating) and for pain relief (see 'Applied anatomy', Chapter 7). After injection, the hand becomes warm and dry, and Horner's syndrome appears in the eye (constriction of the pupil by the unopposed parasympathetic supply to the iris, and drooping of the upper eyelid; details in Chapter 31).

Sympathectomy
Surgical sympathetic denervation of the upper limb may be performed in two ways. *Anatomical* denervation follows removal of the stellate ganglion because the postganglionic fibers degenerate. *Physiological* denervation is done by merely cutting the sympathetic trunk below the stellate; the ganglion cells are rendered inactive by interruption of nerve impulses from the spinal cord. (A variant is to cut the trunk just below the entry of the T1 contribution; T1 supplies the eye and cerebral vessels, whereas T2–6 supply the upper limb, so this variant prevents Horner's syndrome.)

Any procedure on the stellate interrupts the sympathetic supply to the cerebral arteries. This is not important because the cerebral vessels are largely controlled by autoregulation (Chapter 24).

For the lower limb, the ischemic effects of vascular disease may be alleviated by removing lumbar ganglia 2 and 3, thus

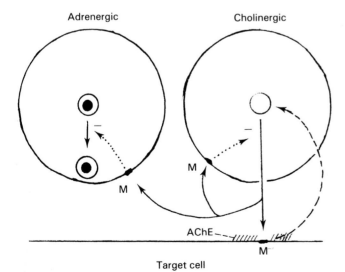

Adrenergic   Cholinergic

AChE

Target cell

Fig. 6-12 Three muscarinic (M) receptors related to a cholinergic nerve ending. Also shown is acetylcholinesterase (AChE); choline is actively taken up for recycling (dashed line at right).

interrupting the descending preganglionic fibers (Fig. 6-2). The procedure may be only partly successful because scattered ganglion cells often occupy the lumbar rami communicantes.

Vagotomy is considered in Chapter 39.

AUTONOMIC PHARMACOLOGY

Drugs and the sympathetic system

Considerable scope is offered for pharmacological interference at sympathetic nerve endings. It must be borne in mind that adrenergic nerve endings, and α and β receptors, are numerous in the brain as well. Drugs which cross the blood–brain barrier may exert their most significant effects centrally rather than peripherally.

Potential sites of drug action (Fig. 6-13)
1 A satisfactory drug for blocking the norepinephrine-synthesizing enzyme has not been found. This enzyme is found only within the dense-cored vesicles (DCV).

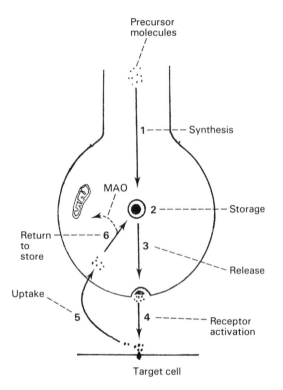

Fig. 6-13 Some potential sites of drug action at adrenergic nerve endings. MAO, monoamine oxidase.

2 Norepinephrine is loosely bound to a protein in the DCV. It can be unbound by specific drugs, whereupon it diffuses into the axoplasm and is degraded by a mitochondrial enzyme known as monoamine oxidase (MAO). This method can be used to deplete norepinephrine reserves when the sympathetic is overactive (such as in hypertension).
3 Norepinephrine release can be accelerated. Amphetamine, for example, exerts its central stimulant effect by flooding the extracellular space with norepinephrine expelled from DCVs.
4 The α and β receptors can be selectively either stimulated or blocked by suitable drugs (see below).
5 An 'amine pump' returns norepinephrine to the cytoplasm. The tricyclic antidepressant drugs and cocaine cause norepinephrine to accumulate in the brain extracellular fluid by interfering with the uptake pump.

6 Some norepinephrine is normally degraded by monoamine oxidase. MAO inhibitors are used for their central effects in the treatment of depression (Chapter 21).

Drug action at adrenoceptors
The chief targets are the α_1 and β_1 receptors. Alpha or beta *agonists* are drugs which *activate* the receptor (they are sympathomimetic). *Antagonists* occupy the receptor but do not activate it. They *block* it.
1 α agonists contract arteriolar and sphincteric smooth muscle. In practise, central effects of such drugs predominate.
2 α antagonists are used in hypertension and peripheral vascular disease (to prevent access of epinephrine and norepinephrine to arteriolar smooth muscle).
3 β_1 agonists are used in acute heart failure to stimulate nodal and ventricular muscle.
4 β_1 antagonists (commonly known as beta blockers) reduce heart rate and myocardial contractility. They are widely used in the treatment of angina pectoris and hypertension.
5 β_2 agonists are especially useful in the treatment of asthma; they relax the bronchial smooth muscle.
6 β_2 antagonists are not required.

Peripheral actions of dopamine
Dopamine as such does not cross the blood–brain barrier; otherwise, it would have major effects on CNS function. It is the drug of choice for treating the cardiovascular collapse associated with shock. It acts upon α and β receptors to restore blood pressure by constricting peripheral arterioles and accelerating the heart.

Cholinergic and anticholinergic drugs

Acetylcholine is a transmitter at all autonomic ganglia, as well as at postganglionic parasympathetic nerve endings. It is also a transmitter at some synapses in the CNS.

Stimulation or blockade of ACh at autonomic ganglia is no longer used in general practice (for example, in hypertension, where the sympathetic is overactive), because of the inevitably widespread effects produced. Fortunately, the ACh receptor in the ganglia is different from that at postganglionic parasympathetic nerve endings. At the ganglia it is nicotinic, but at the postganglionic endings it is muscarinic. The CNS contains both kinds of receptor.

Cholinergic drugs in common use bind with muscarinic receptors in tissues innervated by postganglionic cholinergic neurons, including sympathetic fibers to eccrine sweat glands and to some arterioles. In addition they bind with 'free' receptors on arterioles having no detectable cholinergic innervation. The reason for nerve-free arteriolar receptors is not clear.

The regional effects of peripherally active cholinomimetic (ACh-imitating) drugs are listed in Fig. 6-14. Drugs have been developed to affect particular organs; for example, pilocarpine eye drops constrict the pupil and carbachol stimulates the bladder and bowel.

Anticholinergic drugs are mainly used to prevent access of ACh to muscarinic receptors. In the musculoskeletal system, anticholinergic drugs are used to produce relaxation during surgery. The regional effects are listed in Fig. 6-14. Atropine is the prototype.

Anticholinergic drugs are used (a) to dilate the pupil (using eye drops) by allowing dilator pupillae unrestricted action, (b) as premedication for surgery, by drying the bronchi, (c) in cardiac arrest, by blocking vagal action on nodal tissue, (d) as antiemetics (vomiting cannot occur if the stomach is relaxed), (e) for diarrhea, (f) when morphine is administered for any purpose, to counter its spastic effect on the intestine, (g) to relax the bladder in patients suffering from cystitis and (h) to

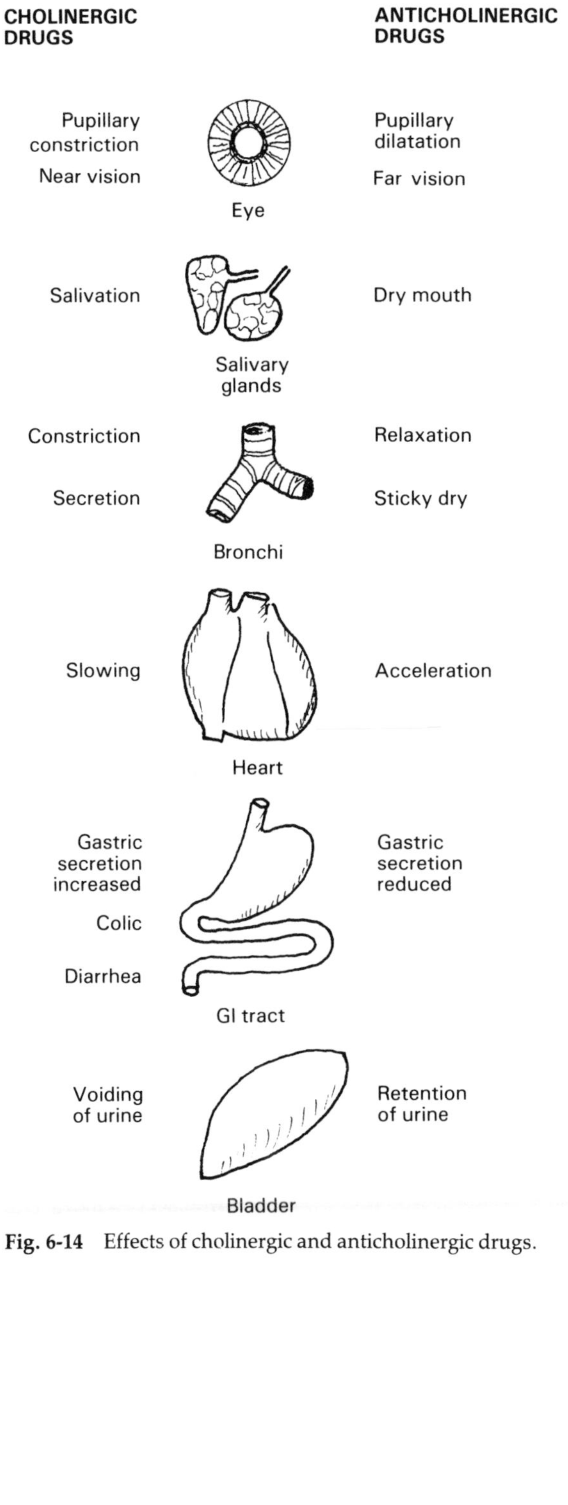

CHOLINERGIC DRUGS		ANTICHOLINERGIC DRUGS
Pupillary constriction		Pupillary dilatation
Near vision		Far vision
	Eye	
Salivation		Dry mouth
	Salivary glands	
Constriction		Relaxation
Secretion		Sticky dry
	Bronchi	
Slowing		Acceleration
	Heart	
Gastric secretion increased		Gastric secretion reduced
Colic		
Diarrhea		
	GI tract	
Voiding of urine		Retention of urine
	Bladder	

Fig. 6-14 Effects of cholinergic and anticholinergic drugs.

treat poisoning by overdose of cholinergic drugs or by drugs that inhibit cholinesterase.

Readings

Ahlquist, R.P. (1980) Historical perspective: classification of adrenoceptors. *J. Auton. Pharmacol.*, 1: 101–106.

Appenzeller, D. (1982) *The Autonomic Nervous System. An Introduction to Basic and Clinical Concepts*, 3rd ed. Amsterdam: Elsevier Biomedical Press.

Bulygin, I.A. (1983) A consideration of the general principles of organization of sympathetic ganglia. *J. Auton. Nerv. Syst.*, 8: 303–330.

Burnstock, G. (1983) Recent concepts of communication between excitable cells. In *Dale's Principle and Communication between Neurones* (Osborne, N.N., ed.), pp. 7–35. Oxford and New York: Pergamon Press.

FitzGerald, G.A. (1984) Peripheral presynaptic adrenoreceptor regulation of norepinephrine release in humans. *Fed. Proc.*, 43: 1379–1381.

Gabella, G. (1976) *Structure of the Autonomic System.* London: Chapman and Hall; New York: Wiley.

Gibbins, I.L. (1982) Lack of correlation between ultrastructural and pharmacological types of non-adrenergic autonomic nerves. *Cell Tissue Res.*, 221: 551–581.

Helén, P. and Hervonen, A. (1981) Nerve endings in human sympathetic ganglia. *Am. J. Anat.*, 162: 119–130.

Kalsner, S. (1984) Limitations of presynaptic theory: no support for feedback control of autonomic effects. *Fed. Proc.*, 43: 1358–1364.

Kilbinger, H. (1984) Presynaptic muscarinic receptors modulating acetylcholine release. *Trends Pharmacol. Sci.*, 5: 103–105.

Lees, G.M. (1981) A hitch-hiker's guide to the galaxy of adrenoceptors. *Br. Med. J.*, 283: 173–178.

Lefkowitz, R.J. (1982) Clinical physiology of adrenergic receptor regulation. *Am. J. Physiol.*, 243: E43–E47.

Minneman, K.P., Pittman, R.N. and Molinoff, P.B. (1981) β-adrenergic subtypes: properties, distribution, and regulation. *Annu. Rev. Neurosci.*, 4: 414–461.

Neff, N.H., Karoum, F. and Hadjiconstantinou, M. (1983) Dopamine-containing small intensely fluorescent cells and sympathetic ganglion function. *Fed. Proc.*, 42: 3009–3011.

Robie, N.W. (1984) Controversial evidence regarding the functional importance of presynaptic α receptors. *Fed. Proc.*, 43: 1371–1374.

Snider, S.R. and Kuchel, O. (1983) Dopamine: an important hormone of the sympathoadrenal system. *Endocr. Rev.*, 4: 291–309.

Starke, K. (1980) Presynaptic receptors: a numerous family. *Prog. Pharmacol.*, 3/4: 9–17.

Szurszewski, J.H. (1981) Physiology of mammalian prevertebral ganglia. *Annu. Rev. Physiol.*, 43: 53–68.

Westfall, T.C. (1980) Neuroeffector mechanisms. *Annu. Rev. Physiol.*, 42: 383–397.

Westfall, T.C. (1984) Evidence that noradrenergic transmitter release is regulated by presynaptic receptors. *Fed. Proc.*, 43: 1352–1357.

Visceral Afferents

Afferents from the viscera utilize autonomic pathways to reach the CNS. (The viscera in this context include the heart and great vessels.) The visceral afferents initiate several important reflexes as well as signaling noxious stimulation of the viscera. Because they accompany peripheral autonomic fibers they are sometimes (incorrectly) called autonomic afferents.

Fig. 7-1 shows the general plan. The major visceral reflexes are listed in Table 7-1.

Table 7-1 Visceral afferents and their associated reflexes

Nerves	Territory	Reflexes*
Glossopharyngeal	Oropharynx	Swallowing (36)
	Carotid sinus	Baroreceptor (37)
	Carotid body	Respiratory (38)
Vagus	Laryngopharynx	Swallowing (36)
	Aortic arch	Baroreceptor (37)
	Aortic bodies	Respiratory (38)
	Trachea	Coughing (38)
	Lungs	Respiratory (38)
	Alimentary tract	Motility (39)
Sympathetic-related afferents	Heart	Pressor (37)
	Great vessels	Baroreceptor (37)
	Alimentary tract	Several (39)
	Body of uterus	
	Top of bladder	
Pelvic splanchnic afferents	Rectum	Defecation (40)
	Bladder	Micturition (40)
	Uterus	Delivery

*Numbers in parentheses refer to the chapters giving details.

AFFERENT PATHWAYS

The visceral afferents are either finely myelinated (Aδ) or unmyelinated (C) fibers. They form abundant free endings in the muscle coats and mucous membranes of the viscera. Their cell bodies are unipolar and occupy (a) the sensory ganglia of the glossopharyngeal and vagus nerves close to the jugular foramen and (b) the spinal ganglia, where they mingle with somatic sensory neurons.

Central terminations

Reflex afferents in the glossopharyngeal and vagus nerves terminate in the *nucleus solitarius*, which serves as a distribution center for several major reflex arcs (Chapters 36, 37). The corresponding spinal afferents enter the posterior nerve roots and terminate in the *intermediolateral cell column* at thoracolumbar and sacral levels. For details see the chapters listed in Table 7-1.

Nociceptive afferents in the glossopharyngeal and vagus (from pharynx, larynx and trachea) terminate in the *spinal nucleus of the trigeminal nerve* (Chapter 34). In spinal afferents (from heart, abdominal and pelvic viscera) they terminate in the posterior gray horn, which they reach via anterior and posterior roots (Fig. 7-2). In the posterior horn they synapse direct upon cells of origin of the spinothalamic and spinoreticular tracts. These tracts mediate somatic pain from the body wall and limbs, as well as visceral pain. The remainder of this chapter is devoted to pain of visceral origin.

VISCERAL PAIN

There are three fundamental types of visceral pain:
1 pure visceral pain, felt in the region of the affected organ,
2 visceral referred pain, projected into the somatic territory of the corresponding spinal nerves,
3 viscerosomatic pain, caused by the spread of visceral disease to somatic structures.

Pure visceral pain

This is characteristically vague and deep-seated and often accompanied by autonomic responses (sweating or nausea). It is experienced as the initial pain in intestinal, biliary or ureteric obstruction, or when the capsule of a solid organ (liver, kidney or pancreas) is stretched by underlying disease.

Visceral referred pain

As its severity increases, visceral pain is 'referred' to somatic structures innervated from the same segmental levels of the spinal cord. For example, the pain of myocardial ischaemia is usually referred to the chest wall, biliary and intestinal colics are referred to the anterior abdominal wall, and labor pains are referred to the sacral area of the back. From the gastrointestinal tract, pain is referred to the anterior midline area: from foregut to epigastrium, from midgut to the periumbilical region, and from hindgut to hypogastrium (Fig. 7-3). This is because the visceral afferents invade the alimentary tract during the fifth week of embryonic life, at which time the primitive gut is attached to the posterior abdominal wall by a midline dorsal mesentery.

Mechanisms of visceral referred pain

According to the 'convergence–projection theory', the brain falsely interprets the source of noxious stimulation because visceral and somatic nociceptors have spinothalamic neurons in common; in previous experience, these neurons habitually signaled somatic pain.

According to the 'convergence–facilitation theory', the visceral input to spinothalamic neurons lowers their threshold to the extent that background activity in somatic afferents is sufficient to cause firing. According to this explanation, infiltration of the somatic structure should abolish the pain. This has been investigated, with conflicting results, and the question is not resolved. However, the somatic structure to which pain is referred may exhibit *hyperalgesia* – hypersensitivity to stroking with a sharp

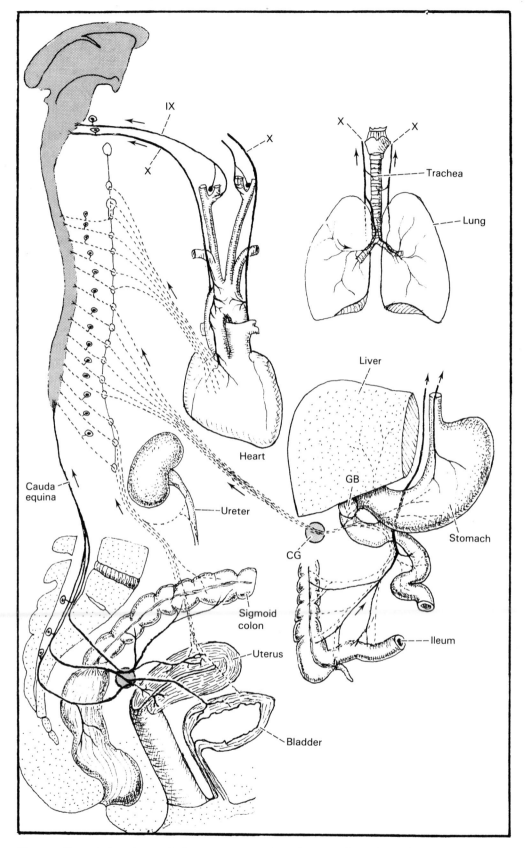

Fig. 7-1 General plan of visceral afferents. Arrows indicate direction of impulse conduction. CG, celiac ganglion; GB, gallbladder; IX, glossopharyngeal nerve; X, vagus nerve.

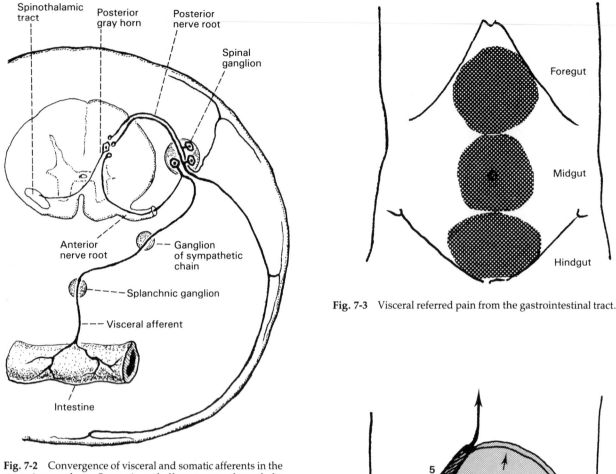

Fig. 7-2 Convergence of visceral and somatic afferents in the posterior gray horn. Some visceral afferents enter through the posterior nerve root.

Fig. 7-3 Visceral referred pain from the gastrointestinal tract.

object – an observation consistent with the 'convergence–facilitation theory'.

Viscerosomatic pain

The parietal serous membranes are supplied by the overlying somatic spinal nerves (mainly by the intercostal nerves). The membranes are exquisitely sensitive to mechanical insults of any kind and to inflammatory exudates. In the abdominal cavity the extension of inflammatory reaction to the outer surface of the intestine or gall bladder produces a severe, steady pain in the abdominal wall directly overlying the inflamed organ (Fig. 7-4).

Tenderness

Tenderness is pain elicited by palpation. In the abdomen tenderness is sought by pressure of the finger pads on the abdominal wall. The clinician is, in effect, clothing the finger pads with the patient's parietal peritoneum and using this to seek out an inflamed organ. If the organ is mobile, like the appendix, 'shifting tenderness' may be elicited if the patient is willing to roll to the right side and then to the left.

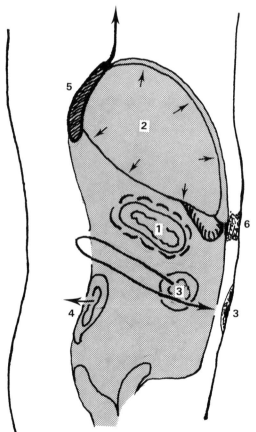

Fig. 7-4 Examples of visceral pain. 1, Contraction of stomach, gastric ulcer and, 2, stretching of liver capsule are examples of pure visceral pain. 3, Obstruction of small intestine causing visceral referred pain (periumbilical). 4, 5, 6, Viscerosomatic pain: 4, involvement of lumbar spinal nerves by disease in ascending/descending colon; 5, involvement of phrenic nerve by subphrenic abscess or hematoma (arrow indicates shoulder-top pain); 6, involvement of thoracoabdominal nerves in inflammation spreading from the gallbladder.

Rigidity

Rigidity is the board-like hardness of the abdominal wall produced by inflammation of the parietal peritoneum. It is *general* if the peritoneal cavity contains an inflammatory exudate, such as purulent material from a ruptured appendix, gastric contents from a perforated peptic ulcer, or blood from a ruptured tubal pregnancy. It may instead be *local*, over the site of acute inflammation (for example, the gallbladder or appendix).

Rigidity is a flexor reflex response mediated by internuncial neurons linking somatic afferents to somatic efferent neurons at the same segmental level. It is completely outside voluntary control and is identical in nature to the 'splinting' contraction of muscles around a fracture.

APPLIED ANATOMY

Myocardial ischemia

In acute myocardial ischemia the patient may initially experience pure visceral pain, expressed as a sense of acute epigastric discomfort. Referred pain usually supervenes or may be present from the beginning. Most commonly,

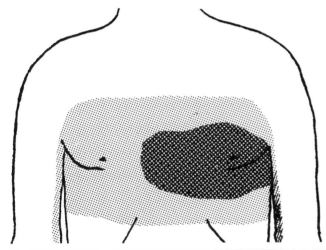

Fig. 7-5   Distribution of pain in angina pectoris.

spinothalamic neurons at T2–T5 levels are excited by cardiac C fibers traversing the sympathetic route. The stimulus is projected to the somatic territory of spinal afferents entering the cord at the same levels. The territory includes that of the intercostobrachial nerve (lateral branch of the second intercostal) which supplies the skin of the medial arm (Fig. 7-5). Reference along posterior rami may produce interscapular pain. Severe autonomic responses (sweating and pallor) are characteristic, and there may be a sense of impending death.

For no clear reason, pain of myocardial origin may be felt mainly or even entirely outside the thorax – notably in the epigastrium (where it may be interpreted as 'indigestion') or in the neck and lower jaw.

Acute appendicitis

The initial, diffuse pain of appendicular obstruction (the lumen is occluded by swollen lymphoid tissue) is periumbilical. Classically, the pain shifts to the right lower quadrant of the abdomen after 6–12 hours and becomes constant. The right lower quadrant pain signifies extension of inflammatory exudate to the outer surface of the appendix. Tenderness can be elicited at the same site.

Acute cholecystitis

The initial pain is colicky, central and epigastric. The later pain is steady, is perceived in the right upper quadrant and is caused by inflammatory exudate. Tenderness may be elicited at the costal margin if the gallbladder is pendulous. If it is not pendulous, pain may be elicited by sinking the finger pads into the abdominal wall below the costal margin, and asking the patient to take a deep breath. The inspiratory movement will be arrested if an inflamed gallbladder descends (with the liver) into contact with the parietal peritoneum infolded by the clinician.

Peptic ulcer

Although the healthy gastric and duodenal mucous membranes are insensitive to acid, they become sensitized by the inflammatory reaction around a peptic (gastric or duodenal) ulcer. Peptic ulcer pain is initially central, steady and epigastric, but it may move to the right side in established cases of duodenal ulcer (inflammatory surface exudate). Tenderness, if elicited, overlies the ulcer site.

Acute pancreatitis

In the Western world acute pancreatitis nearly always results either from a gallstone lodged in the lower end of the bile duct, with consequent obstruction of the pancreatic duct, or from excessive intake of alcohol. The pain is violent and continuous and is accompanied by clinical shock and collapse. Tenderness and rigidity, however, may be absent because the stomach intervenes between the pancreas and the anterior parietal peritoneum.

Colitis

The pain of colonic obstruction or inflammation is initially central and hypogastric. In the case of the ascending and descending parts of the colon, later pain may be felt in the corresponding lumbar region because of involvement of somatic nerve endings on the posterior abdominal wall (these sections of the colon lack mesenteries).

Ureteric colic

The passage of a stone down the ureter elicits intense peristaltic activity. The ureter is innervated by afferent fibers entering L1 and L2 segments of the spinal cord. The pain is excruciating – the patient rolls around the floor – and is referred to the territory of the iliohypogastric and ilioinguinal nerves: the loin, the groin and the scrotum or labium majus (Fig. 7-6). In males, the pain may be felt exclusively in the testis.

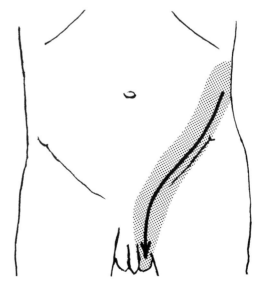

Fig. 7-6   Radiation of pain during an attack of ureteric colic.

Ruptured ectopic gestation

A tubal pregnancy exceeds the capacity of the tube during the sixth week. About four weeks after a missed menstruation, the woman is struck by violent abdominal pain, vomiting and shock. Upon lying down, free intraperitoneal blood may accumulate under the diaphragm and cause additional pain referred to the shoulder (see later).

Acute pleurisy

Acute inflammation of the pleura is accompanied by very severe pain which is exacerbated by deep inspiration. The pain is usually experienced in the chest wall overlying the affected parietal pleura (the visceral pleura is insensitive).

Diaphragmatic pleurisy excites branches of the lower six intercostal nerves, which supply a 'rind' of body wall mesoderm incorporated into the diaphragm during embryonic life. The lower six intercostals are the *thoracoabdominal nerves*, and the pain is referred to the anterior abdominal wall. On the right side, it may be referred to the lower quadrant, but diagnostic confusion with acute appendicitis should not arise, although the abdominal skin will be hyperesthetic.

Uterine pain

The uterus has a dual visceral afferent innervation (Fig. 7-1). The fundus and body are mainly supplied by sympathetic-related afferents entering the cord via the lumbar splanchnic route. These nerves respond to the contractions of *spasmodic dysmenorrhea*, a distressing condition in which menstruation is accompanied by crampy lower abdominal pain. Should drug treatment fail, the pain can be abolished by section of the lumbar splanchnic nerves at the level of the aortic bifurcation.

Hypogastric pain is also characteristic at the onset of labor.

The cervix is supplied by visceral afferents entering the sacral segments of the spinal cord. Pain over the sacrum (somatic territory of posterior roots S2, S3 and S4) may be severe during the first stage of labor, when the cervix is slowly drawn up over the fetal head. Sacral pain is also a feature of cervical disease, as well as of disease of other pelvic organs (rectum, prostate and bladder base).

Shoulder-top pain

Stimulation of sensory fibers in the phrenic nerve may cause a referred 'ache' at the shoulder top (above the acromion process). The nerve roots concerned are C3 and C4 (entering the phrenic and supraclavicular nerves). Causes of shoulder-top pain include diaphragmatic pleurisy, perforated peptic ulcer, ruptured ectopic gestation, ruptured spleen (left shoulder), acute cholecystitis (right shoulder) and acute pancreatitis (both shoulders).

Blocking visceral afferents

The injection of local anesthetics or destructive chemicals (alcohol or phenol) into visceral afferent pathways can be very helpful in treating intractable pain of visceral origin. This is especially true of advanced cancerous conditions of the stomach, pancreas, biliary tract and liver, in which the pain may not be controlled by narcotic analgesics. Infusion of a blocking solution into the retroperitoneal space surrounding the abdominal splanchnic ganglia may produce complete relief. Infusion at a lower level, to block the lumbar splanchnic nerves, may afford at least temporary relief in advanced cancers of pelvic viscera.

Stellate ganglion block (Chapter 6) is often used to relieve painful conditions in the head, neck and upper limb. In these regions, blockade of somatic nerves is often required as well.

Readings

Challenger, J.H. (1974) Sympathetic nervous system blocking and pain relief. In *Monographs in Anesthesiology*, Vol. I. (Smerdlow, M., ed.), pp. 176–194. New York: Excerpta Medica.

Coggleshall, R.E., Hancock, M.B. and Appelbaum, M.L. (1976) Categories of axons in mammalian rami communicantes. *J. Comp. Neurol., 167:* 105–124.

Coleridge, H.M. and Coleridge, J.C.G. (1980) Cardiovascular afferents involved in regulation of peripheral vessels. *Annu. Rev. Physiol., 42:* 413–427.

Crousillat, J. and Ranieri, F. (1980) Mécanorécepteurs splanchniques de la voie biliare at son péritoine. *Exp. Brain Res., 40:* 146–153.

de Dombal, F.T. (1980) *Diagnosis of Acute Abdominal Pain.* Edinburgh: Churchill Livingstone.

Ellis, H. (1980) *Clinical Anatomy*, 6th ed. Oxford and London: Blackwell Scientific.

Gelin, L.-E., Nyhus, L.M. and Condon, R.E. (1969) *Abdominal Pain. A Guide to Rapid Diagnosis.* Philadelphia and Toronto: Lippincott.

Leek, B.F. (1977) Abdominal and pelvic visceral receptors. *Br. Med. Bull., 33:* 163–168.

Mei, N. (1983) Recent studies on intestinal vagal afferent innervation. Functional implications. *J. Auton. Nerv. Syst., 9:* 199–206.

Morgan, C., Nadehaft, I. and de Groat, W.C. (1981) The distribution of visceral primary afferents from the pelvic nerve to Lissauer's tract and the spinal gray matter and its relationship to the sacral parasympathetic nucleus. *J. Comp. Neurol., 201:* 415–440.

Neil, E. (ed.) (1972) Enteroceptors. In *Handbook of Sensory Physiology*, Vol. III, Sec. I, pp. 1–233. Berlin and New York: Springer-Verlag.

Newman, P.P. (1974) *Visceral Afferent Function of the Nervous System.* London: Arnold.

Pack, A.I. (1981) Sensory inputs to the medulla. *Annu. Rev. Physiol., 43:* 73–90.

Paintal, A.S. (1975) Thoracic receptors concerned in sensation. *Br. Med. Bull., 33:* 169–174.

Procacci, P. and Zoppi, M. (1983) Pathophysiology and clinical aspects of visceral and referred pain. In *Advances in Pain Research and Therapy*, Vol. 5 (Bonica, J.J., Lindblom, D., Iggo, A., Jones, L.E. and Benedetti, C., eds.), pp. 643–660. New York: Raven Press.

8
Spinal Nerve Roots

The spinal nerve roots extend from their attachments to the spinal cord to the intervertebral foramina, where they unite to form the spinal nerves (Fig. 8-1). The anterior roots contain the motor fibers supplying the skeletal muscles of the trunk and limbs. At appropriate levels, they also contain preganglionic fibers of the autonomic system. The posterior roots contain somatic afferents from the body wall and limbs.

The nerve roots are sheathed by pia–glial membrane as they enter or leave the cord. They run in the subarachnoid space to their points of exit from the vertebral canal. At these points they invaginate the arachnoid and dura mater, carrying a sleeve of cerebrospinal fluid into the intervertebral foramina (Figs. 8-2, 8-3). The arachnoid blends with the perineurium of the spinal nerves and the dura blends with the epineurium.

External to the dura mater of the vertebral canal is the *epidural (extradural) space*, which contains a rich plexus of valveless veins. The epidural venous plexus drains the red bone marrow contained in the vertebral bodies and it discharges into the segmental veins (deep cervical, intercostal, lumbar and sacral). It is an important potential route of spread of cancer cells to the vertebral bodies, notably from the thyroid gland,

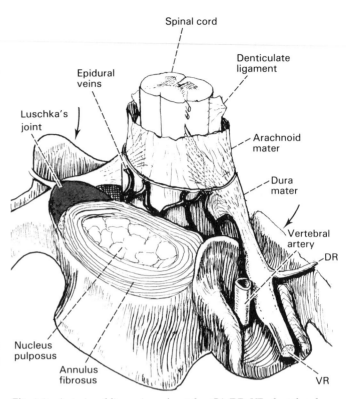

Fig. 8-2 Anterior oblique view of vertebra C6. DR, VR, dorsal and ventral rami of spinal nerve C6. Arrows indicate apophyseal joints.

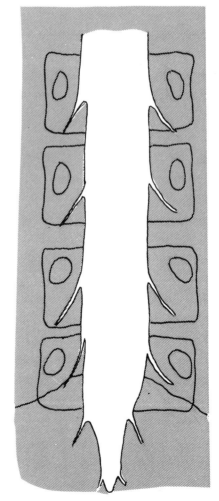

Fig. 8-3 Radiological appearance of lumbar subarachnoid cistern. Note extensions along the lumbar nerve roots.

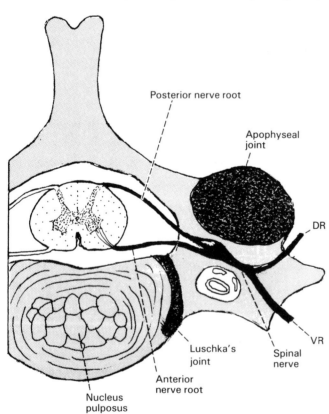

Fig. 8-1 Sixth cervical vertebra viewed from above. DR, VR, dorsal and ventral rami of spinal nerve C6.

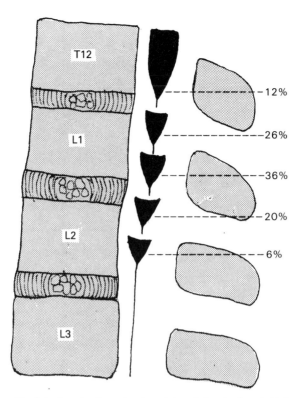

Fig. 8-4 Levels of termination of the adult spinal cord. (Adapted from Louis, 1970.)

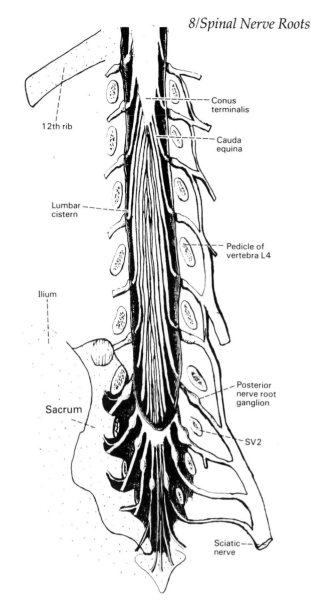

Fig. 8-5 Lumbar cistern. SV2, second sacral vertebra.

breast, lung and prostate. In fact, compression of a nerve root (due to collapse of a vertebra) may be the presenting sign of cancer in one of these organs.

Ascent of the spinal cord

The spinal cord fills the vertebral canal completely until the end of the third month of gestation. Thereafter, the vertebrae grow relatively rapidly and the cord ascends the canal (Chapter 11). The spinal nerves are anchored at the intervertebral foramina, and the nerve roots show an increasing slope from above downward. The tip of the cord reaches its adult level within two weeks after birth. In almost 90% of adults, the cord ends behind the first or second lumbar vertebra or behind the intervening disc (Fig. 8-4).

Cauda equina

The lumbar and sacral nerve roots below cord level form the cauda equina (L., horse's tail), which is suspended in the lumbar cistern. The lumbar cistern is a CSF-filled meningeal sac extending down to the level of the second sacral vertebra (Fig. 8-5). The cauda comprises nerve roots L3–S5 of both sides: in other words, 32 nerve roots at its upper end.

Filum terminale

The filum terminale (clinically unimportant) is a glial strand extending from the tip of the spinal cord all the way to the coccyx. The filum is formed in fetal life during regression of the embryonic tail: the number of coccygeal vertebrae dwindles from six to three, and the coccygeal part of the cord dies away at the same time (Fig. 8-6).

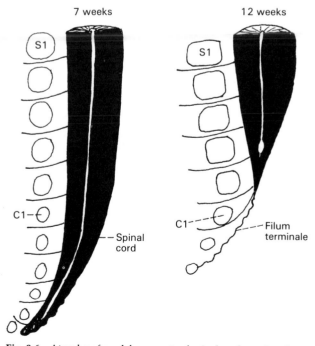

Fig. 8-6 Atrophy of caudal segments of spinal cord creating the filum terminale.

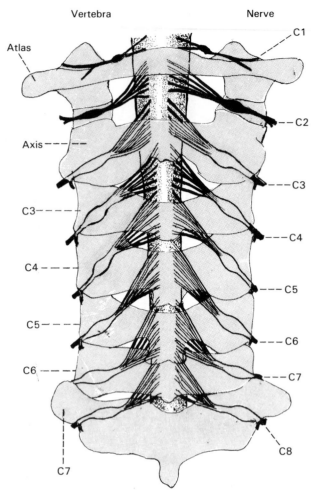

Fig. 8-7 Cervical vertebrae and spinal nerves. (Adapted from Pernkopf, 1963).

Enumeration of spinal nerves

The first seven cervical nerves emerge *above* their respective vertebrae (Fig. 8-7). The eighth emerges *below* the seventh vertebra. All of the thoracic, lumbar and sacral nerves emerge below the respective vertebrae (Fig. 8-8).

Segmental vs. vertebral levels

A spinal cord segment is the cylinder of cord to which a given spinal nerve is attached (Fig. 8-9). The upper cervical nerve roots are nearly horizontal, and the segmental and vertebral levels are similar. The levels diverge progressively at lower levels:

Cord segment	Vertebral body
C8	C7
T6	T5
T12	T10
S1	L1

Collapse of the *first lumbar* vertebra from secondary cancer or injury is likely to produce 'root pain' in the sensory territory of the *first sacral* nerve.

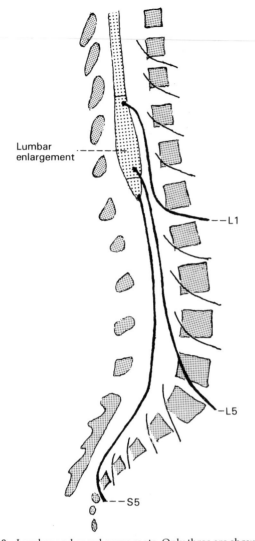

Fig. 8-8 Lumbar and sacral nerve roots. Only three are shown in continuity.

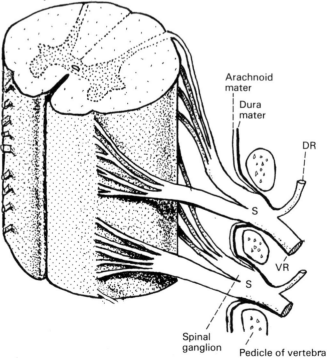

Fig. 8-9 Two thoracic spinal cord segments and spinal nerves. DR, dorsal ramus; S, spinal nerve; VR, ventral ramus.

Descent of the cord

After the age of 50, shrinkage of intervertebral discs may cause the cord to descend. In the elderly, it may reach as low as the third lumbar vertebra.

Innervation of dura mater and vertebral ligaments

Each spinal nerve gives off a recurrent branch within the intervertebral foramen. The recurrent branch supplies the dura mater, the posterior longitudinal ligament of the vertebral column, and the outermost 8–10 lamellae of the annulus fibrosus of the intervertebral disc. The dura mater is exquisitely sensitive to stretching, and clinical evidence indicates extensive overlap of innervation. Stretching of the dural sheath of a single spinal nerve gives rise to pain over five or more dermatomes on the back (see later).

The *synovial* joints are supplied by the corresponding anterior and posterior rami of the spinal nerves. The articular processes make synovial joints with one another (so-called apophyseal joints, Fig. 8-1). In most adults cervical vertebrae 3 to 7 have additional synovial joints (of Luschka) at the scalloped lateral edges of the vertebral bodies (Fig. 8-1).

Pain from disease of the vertebral ligaments, discs, and synovial joints is referred to the sensory territory of the dorsal rami of the spinal nerves (Fig. 8-10).

THE DERMATOMES

The clinical dermatome is the strip of skin supplied by a posterior nerve root. The dermatomes are orderly in the embryo (Fig. 8-11), but they become distorted by the later growth of the limbs. Fig. 8-12 shows the

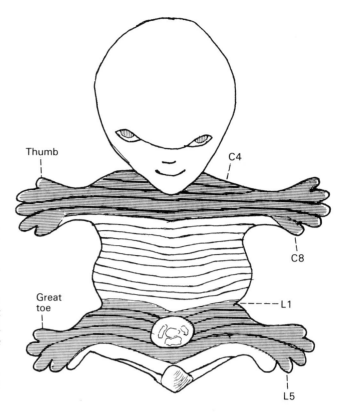

Fig. 8-11 Dermatomes of a 6-week embryo. Cervical and lumbar are shaded. (Adapted from Langman, 1975.)

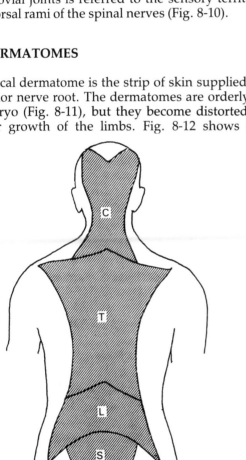

Fig. 8-10 Cutaneous distribution of dorsal rami. C, cervical; T, thoracic; L, lumbar; S, sacral.

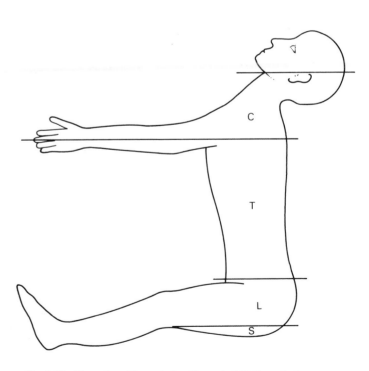

Fig. 8-12 Dermatomal boundaries. C, cervical; T, thoracic; L, lumbar; S, sacral.

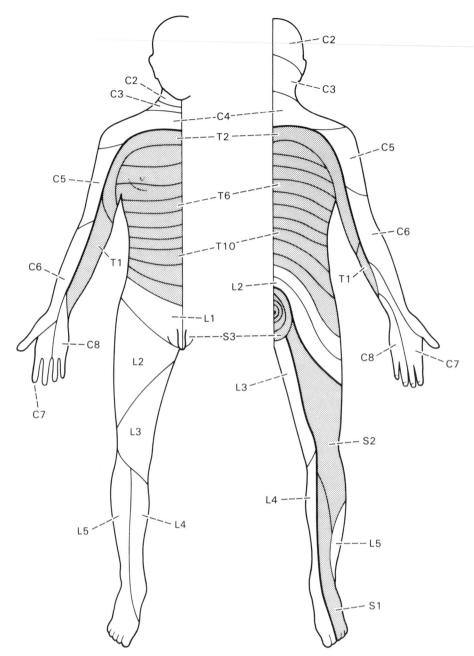

Fig. 8-13 Dermatomes: left, anterior aspect; right, posterior aspect.

boundaries between the adult cervical, thoracic, lumbar, and sacral dermatomes. Dermatomes C5 to T1 are pulled into the upper limbs during fetal life, and C4 later abuts on T2 on the upper thorax (Fig. 8-13).

Overlap

Successive dermatomes overlap extensively with one another. A given patch of skin is supplied by the cutaneous branches of three posterior roots – possibly even five (Chapter 15). However, non-contiguous roots overlap for only a few millimeters, along the *axial lines* (the heavy lines in Fig. 8-13). Overlap across the midline is also negligible.

The cutaneous territories of the *peripheral nerves* are given in the Appendix to this Chapter.

APPLIED ANATOMY

Nerve root compression
Root compression syndromes are most frequent where the spine is most mobile, at lower cervical and lower lumbar levels. Compression of posterior root fibers produces paresthesia (tingling, or 'numb' sensations) or pain in the dermatome supplied by the affected root. In accordance with Fig. 8-13, the distribution of the pain gives an immediate clue to the spinal nerve involved. On the other hand, sensory testing (with a pin, for example) may be uninformative because of sensory overlap.

Cervical roots
Vertebra C6 is the fulcrum for flexion–extension movements of the neck. The discs and synovial joints immediately above and below vertebra C6 have degenerative disease (*cervical spondylosis*) in about 50% of 50-year-olds and 70% of 70-year-olds. Spinal nerves C6 (above) and/or C7 (below)

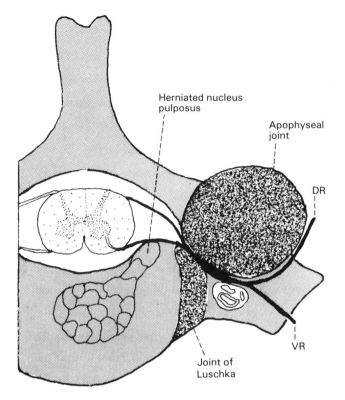

Fig. 8-14 Degenerative joint disease compressing a cervical spinal nerve. DR, VR, dorsal and ventral rami.

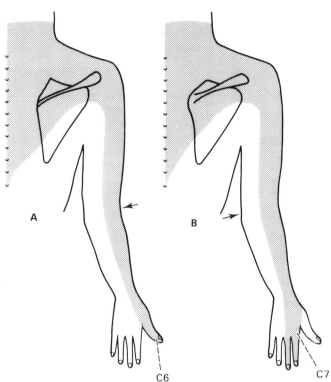

Fig. 8-15 Dermatomes most involved in cervical spondylosis. Arrow in A indicates weakness of elbow flexion ± loss of biceps tendon jerk. Arrow in B indicates weakness of elbow extension ± loss of triceps tendon jerk. (Adapted from de Palma and Rothman, 1970.)

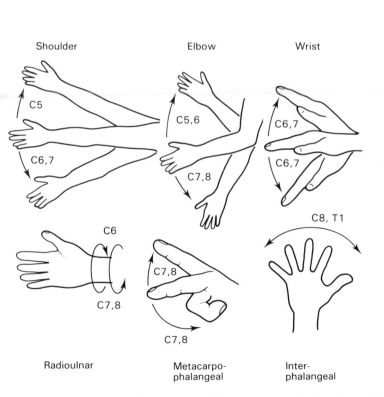

Fig. 8-16 Segmental control of upper limb movements. (Adapted from Last, 1973, and Rosse and Clawson, 1980.)

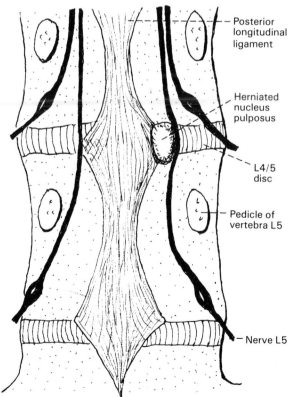

Fig. 8-17 Prolapse of L4/5 disc usually presses on L5 nerve roots. (Only posterior roots are shown.)

may be pinched either by prolapsed disc material (herniated nucleus pulposus) or by bony excrescences (osteophytes) at the margins of the synovial joints (Fig. 8-14).

The commonest dermatome distributions for nerves C6 and C7 are shown in Fig. 8-15. The index finger may be supplied by *either* C6 or C7. Pain in the arm overlies the distributing nerve trunks (radial and median). Pain in the back is attributed to tension on the dura mater.

Prolonged compression leads to motor weakness and diminished reflexes in the territory of the affected ventral ramus. The segmental supply of the upper limb is expressed in terms of the movements shown in Fig. 8-16. The arc for the biceps jerk passes through segment C6 and that for the triceps jerk through C7.

Thoracic roots

These are rarely affected, because only rotary movements are permitted between the thoracic vertebrae. However, nerve roots may be compressed by vertebral collapse from trauma or metastatic cancer.

The *T1 syndrome* is a rare condition in which the first thoracic anterior root is torn from the spinal cord by violent traction, for instance when someone is pulled along the ground by one hand. The two presenting features are (a) wasting of the intrinsic muscles of the hand, and (b) Horner's syndrome (pupillary constriction, drooping of the upper eyelid (Chapter 31).

Lumbar roots

Fully 95% of all cases of prolapsed intervertebral disc occur just above or below the fifth lumbar vertebra. The nucleus pulposus herniates posterolaterally as a rule and compresses the pair of roots traveling to the *next* foramen of exit (Fig. 8-17).

Lumbar disc protrusions are characterized by backache and sciatic pain. Backache is caused by tearing of the annulus fibrosus and by pressure on the dura mater. The sciatica is caused by pressure on posterior root fibers. It is felt in the buttock and in the back of the thigh and leg. It is increased by pressure within the lumbar cistern, for example by coughing or sneezing. It is also increased by stretching the affected root, as by having the straightened leg raised by the examiner.

An L4/5 disc prolapse produces pain over the L5 dermatome (Fig. 8-18). In accordance with the plan of motor segmental innervation (Fig. 8-19), there may be weakness of dorsiflexion of the ankle or great toe.

With an L5/S1 prolapse (the commonest), pain is felt in the back of the leg and sometimes in the sole of the foot (Fig. 8-18). Plantar flexion and eversion are weak and the ankle jerk (S1 segment) is reduced or absent.

Cauda equina syndrome

This is most often caused by a meningomyelocele (Chapter 11). In adults, the syndrome may result from vertebral collapse. The cauda is more or less completely interrupted, with motor paralysis, loss of reflexes, and anesthesia. Lesions of S3 and S4 roots (whether anterior or posterior) interrupt bladder and rectal reflexes and penile erection (Chapters 40, 41).

Lumbar puncture

To obtain a sample of cerebrospinal fluid, a needle is passed between the spines of L3 and L4 or L4 and L5. The patient lies curled up on one side during the procedure, and the skin and interspinous ligaments are anesthetized. A slight 'give' is felt when the dura and arachnoid are penetrated. There is no risk to the spinal cord, even in infancy. However, a lumbar puncture (spinal tap) is a dangerous procedure in the presence of raised intracranial pressure (Chapter 2).

Myelography

The lumbar CSF cistern may be injected with radio-opaque medium through a lumbar puncture needle. A prolapsed intervertebral disc is suspected if one of the perineural sleeves refuses to fill. An alternative to myelography is to inject medium into the epidural venous plexus by way of the great saphenous vein. A prolapsed disc will compress the local epidural veins.

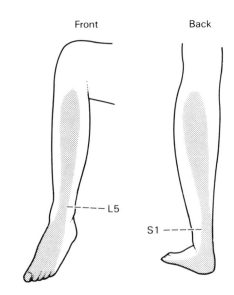

Fig. 8-18 Dermatomes most involved in lumbar disc prolapse. (Adapted from de Palma and Rothman, 1970.)

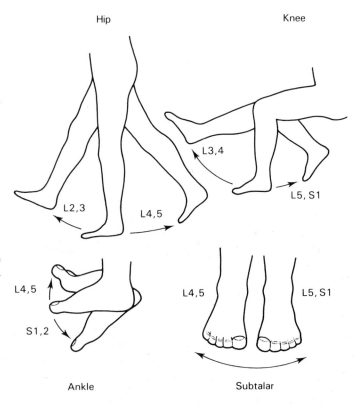

Fig. 8-19 Segmental control of lower limb movements. (Adapted from Last, 1973, and Rosse and Clawson, 1980.)

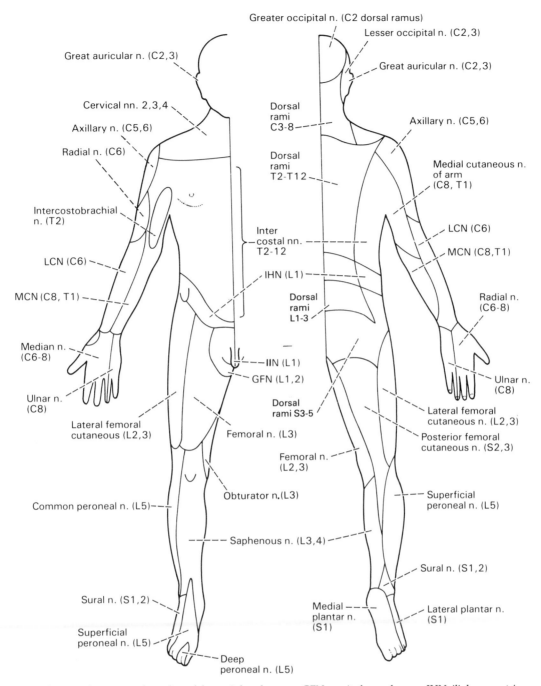

Fig. 8-20 Distribution of cutaneous branches of the peripheral nerves. GFN, genitofemoral nerve; IHN, iliohypogastric nerve; IIN, ilioinguinal nerve; LCN, MCN, lateral and medial cutaneous nerves of the forearm.

Spinal anesthesia
A 'spinal' anesthetic can be given as a prelude to surgery, by injecting anesthetic solution into the lumbar cistern to paralyze the lower thoracic, the lumbar and the sacral nerve roots. A 'spinal' is given in circumstances where general anesthesia is not available, and also for cesarean section.

Analgesia and childbirth
Pain-free labor can be assured by blocking the lumbar and sacral nerve roots extradurally. In *epidural analgesia* local anesthetic is carefully introduced into the extradural space by the lumbar route. In *caudal analgesia* the extradural space is approached by means of a catheter inserted through the sacral hiatus. In both methods the anesthetic diffuses through the dural sheath of the nerve roots as they emerge from the subarachnoid space. Labor may be prolonged

because of the interruption of reflex arcs from perineum to uterus. The use of local rather than general anesthesia is valuable, in allowing establishment of bonding between mother and child.

Chapter 9 gives details of nerve root composition.

APPENDIX

Cutaneous territories of the peripheral nerves
Except for the intercostals, all of the peripheral spinal nerves receive their cutaneous sensory fibers from more than one posterior nerve root. The mixing takes place in the cervical and lumbosacral plexuses. Cutaneous sensory maps are shown in Fig. 8-20, for comparison with the dermatomal maps in Fig. 8-13. Based on the patient's history, and on the

distribution of pain or analgesia, it is usually easy to distinguish nerve root disorders from those of the mixed peripheral nerves. The extent of analgesia caused by section of an individual nerve trunk (for example, ulnar or common peroneal) is usually less than the maps suggest because of overlap of adjacent nerves within the dermal plexus (Chapter 5).

Readings

Adams, C.B.T. and Logue, V. (1971) Studies in cervical spondylitic myelopathy. 1. Movement of the cervical roots, dura and cord, and their relation to the course of extrathecal roots. *Brain, 94:* 557–568.

Barson, A.J. (1970) The vertebral level of termination of the spinal cord during normal and abnormal development. *J. Anat., 106:* 489–497.

Bogduk, N., Tynan, W. and Wilson, A.S. (1981) The nerve supply to the human lumbar intervertebral discs. *J. Anat., 132:* 39–56.

De Palma, A.F. and Rothman, R.H. (1970) *The Intervertebral Disc.* Philadelphia: Saunders.

Gamble, H.J. (1976) The spinal and cranial nerve roots. In *The Peripheral Nerve* (Landon, D.N., ed.), pp. 330–354. London: Chapman & Hall.

Hoppenfeld, S. (1977) *Orthopaedic Neurology: A Guide to Neurologic Levels.* Philadelphia and Toronto: Lippincott.

Howe, J.F., Loeser, J.D. and Calvin, W.H. (1977) Mechanosensitivity of dorsal root ganglia and chronically injured axons: a physiological basis for the radicular pain of nerve root compression. *Pain, 3:* 25–41.

Jackson, H.C., Winkelmann, R.K. and Bickel, W.H. (1966) Nerve endings in the human lumbar spinal column and related structures. *J. Bone Joint Surg., 48A:* 1272–1281.

Langman, J. (1975) *Medical Embryology,* 3rd ed. Baltimore: Williams & Wilkins.

Last, R.J. (1973) *Anatomy: Regional and Applied,* 5th ed. Edinburgh: Churchill Livingstone.

Lieberman, A.R. (1976) Sensory ganglia. In *The Peripheral Nerve* (D.N. Landon, ed.), pp. 188–278. London: Chapman & Hall.

Louis, R. (1970) Topographie vertébro-médullaire. *Bull. Assoc. Anat. (Nancy), 54:* 272–284.

Meehan, M.P. (1969) Continuous caudal analgesia in obstetrics. *Proc. R. Soc. Med., 62:* 185–186.

Nathan, H. and Feuerstein, M. (1970) Angulated course of spinal nerve roots. *J. Neurol., 32:* 349–352.

Pernkopf, E. (1963) *Atlas of Topographical and Applied Human Anatomy, Vol. 1, Head and Neck* (Ferner, H. and Monse, H., eds.). Philadelphia: Saunders.

Renard, M., Larde, D., Masson, J.P. and Roland, J. (1980) Anatomical and radio-anatomical study of the lumbo-sacral intervertebral venous plexus. *Anatomia Clinica, 2:* 21–28.

Rosse, C. and Clawson, D.K. (1980) *The Musculoskeletal System in Health and Disease.* Hagerstown: Harper & Row.

Sunderland, S. (1974) Meningeal–dural relations in the intervertebral foramen. *J. Neurosurg., 40:* 756–763.

III
SPINAL CORD

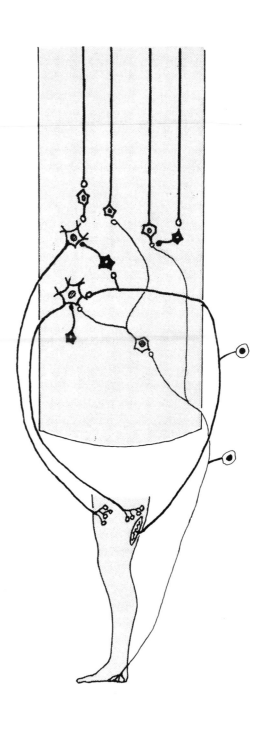

9

General Anatomy and
Ascending Pathways

The spinal cord extends from the foramen magnum to the level of the first or second lumbar vertebra. It is intimately invested with pia mater and is surrounded by cerebrospinal fluid. The cord is anchored to the dura mater by the denticulate ligament. The *cervical* and *lumbar enlargements* are produced by expansions of the gray matter serving the upper and lower limbs (Fig. 9-1). The lumbar enlargement tapers into the *conus terminalis* (conus medullaris), which contains the sacral segments of the cord. The *anterior median fissure* extends the full length of the cord; it is created during fetal life by expansion of the anterior gray horn (Chapter 11).

TRANSVERSE SECTIONS (Figs. 9-1, 9-2)

The gray matter is like a butterfly and surrounds the minute *central canal. Anterior* (ventral) and *posterior* (dorsal) *horns* of gray matter are present at all levels of the cord. A *lateral horn* (intermediolateral cell column) is present at T1–L3 segmental levels, housing preganglionic sympathetic somas. The anterior median fissure is separated from the gray matter by the *white commissure.* Anterior and posterior *gray commissures* extend across the midline around the central canal.

The white matter is incompletely divided into *anterior, lateral,* and *posterior funiculi* by the entering and emerging nerve roots (Fig. 9-2). (The term 'dorsal columns' is clinically more current than 'posterior funiculi'.) The posterior funiculi are separated by the *posterior median septum,* composed of neuroglia. The funiculi contain myelinated tracts linking the brain with the spinal cord, and vice versa. (A *tract* is a collection of fibers having common functions; a *fasciculus,* or *bundle,* contains fibers of diverse functions.)

Microscopy

Fully 90% of spinal cord neurons are *propriospinal,* lying entirely within the cord. They are small (somas 5–20 μm). Some are contained within a single segment, linking the posterior horns to one another or to the anterior horns; others are intersegmental, their axons running beside the gray matter in the *propriospinal tract* before re-entering (Fig. 9-3).

Medium-sized neurons (somas 20–50 μm) occupy the middle and base of the posterior horn and the intermediate gray matter. They include the *nucleus proprius,* the *dorsal (thoracic) nucleus* (Clarke's column), and the intermediolateral cell column (Fig. 9-4). They contain *relay cells* projecting to the brain.

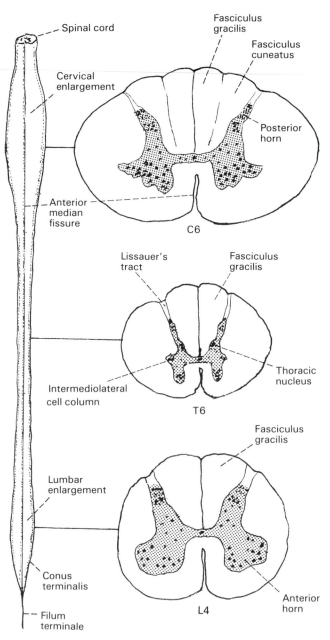

Fig. 9-1 Representative transverse sections of the spinal cord.

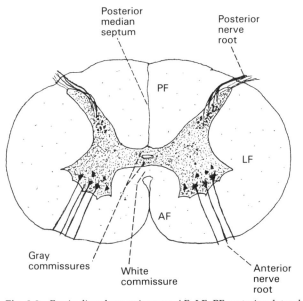

Fig. 9-2 Funiculi and commissures. AF, LF, PF, anterior, lateral, posterior funiculi.

60

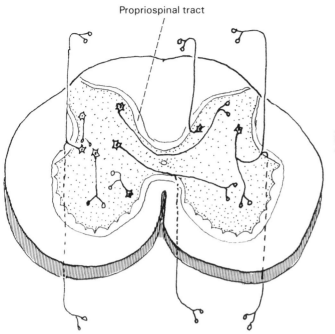

Propriospinal tract

Fig. 9-3 Propriospinal neurons.

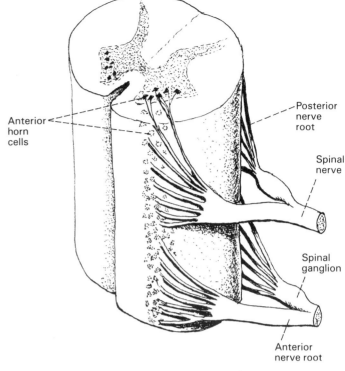

Anterior horn cells

Posterior nerve root

Spinal nerve

Spinal ganglion

Anterior nerve root

Fig. 9-5 The gray matter is not interrupted by segmentation.

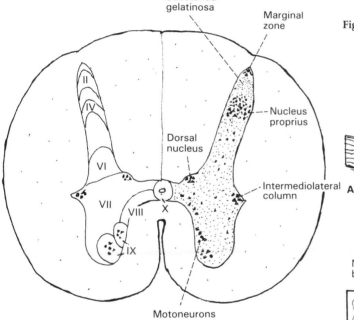

Substantia gelatinosa

Marginal zone

Nucleus proprius

Dorsal nucleus

Intermediolateral column

Motoneurons

Fig. 9-4 Mid-thoracic cord. The laminae of gray matter are shown on one side and the nuclear groups on the other.

The largest neurons in the cord are the α motoneurons (somas 50–100 μm). The γ motoneurons to muscle spindles are scattered between α cells and are about one-third their size.

Laminae (Fig. 9-4)

In thick sections, spinal cord neurons appear to have a laminar (layered) arrangement. True lamination is confined to the posterior horn (Fig. 9-4), but ten laminae have been defined in the whole of the gray matter in order to correlate research findings. There is considerable overlap among the laminae of the posterior horn; for example, dendrites of cells in laminae III–VI extend outward to lamina II.

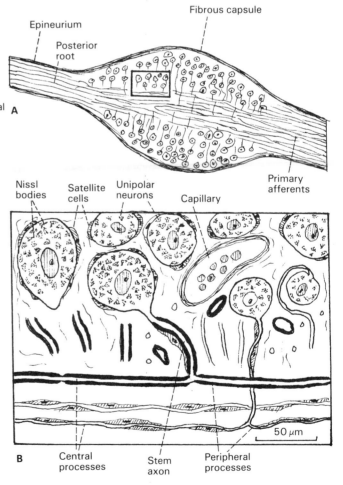

Fibrous capsule

Epineurium

Posterior root

Primary afferents

A

Nissl bodies

Satellite cells

Unipolar neurons

Capillary

50 μm

B Central processes

Stem axon

Peripheral processes

Fig. 9-6 A, spinal ganglion. B, enlarged rectangle from A.

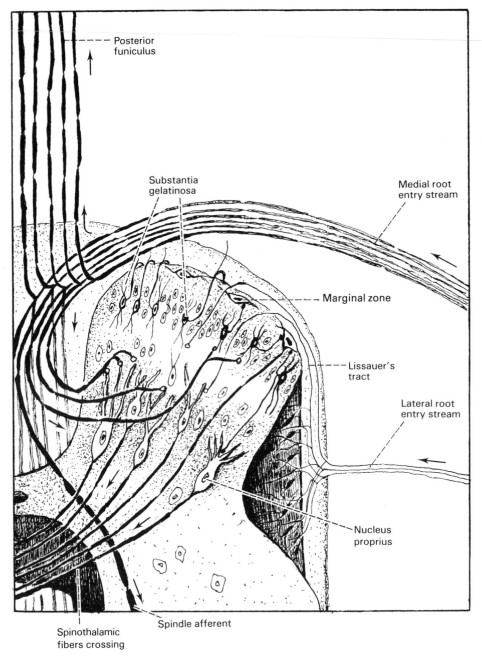

Fig. 9-7 Course of posterior nerve root axons into the spinal cord.

Segmentation (Fig. 9-5)

A spinal cord segment is defined in Chapter 8 as the block of cord to which a given pair of nerve roots is attached on each side. The internal structure of the cord is *not* segmented. The nerve roots enter and leave the gray matter in continuous streams. The surface impression of segmentation is brought about in embryonic life by convergence of the nerve roots onto the mesodermal somites.

SPINAL GANGLIA

The spinal ganglia (posterior root ganglia) (Fig. 9-6) lie in or near the intervertebral foramina. Each ganglion contains 50000–100000 unipolar neurons. The stem axon of each neuron sends a peripheral process into

the spinal nerve and a central process into the spinal cord. Upon peripheral stimulation, action potentials cross the axonal bifurcations without interruption. However, the cell bodies are also depolarized. The cell bodies do not normally initiate impulses but they may do so if the posterior nerve root is put under pressure, for example by a prolapsed intervertebral disc.

Cord trajectories (Fig. 9-7)

Just before entering the cord the posterior root fibers are segregated into small and large fiber streams. The small fibers are lateral and enter the *posterolateral tract (of Lissauer)*. They divide into ascending and descending branches, which span several segments and terminate in the marginal zone (lamina I) and substantia gelatinosa (II). Some Aδ fibers penetrate as far as lamina V. Neurons serving pain sensation may use substance P as transmitter at their central synapses.

The large-fiber stream enters the posterior funiculus. Most fibers divide immediately into ascending and descending branches. The descending ones enter the gray matter over three to six segments. Many ascending branches travel all the way to the medulla oblongata before terminating in the nucleus gracilis or cuneatus. They give collaterals to the gray matter as they commence their long run.

SENSORY PATHWAYS

Sensory functions

All sensations are divisible into two great classes: exteroceptive and proprioceptive (Table 9-1). *Exteroceptive* sensations arise from stimuli (touch, pain, heat, etc.) from the outside; *proprioceptive* sensations arise

Table 9-1   Sensory pathways in the spinal cord

Class	Modalities*	Pathway
Exteroceptive	Pain Temperature Touch	Spinothalamic tract (crossed)
Proprioceptive Conscious	Position sense Kinesthetic sense Vibration sense Touch	Dorsal column–lemniscal pathway (crossed in brainstem)
Unconscious		Posterior spinocerebellar tract (uncrossed)

*The term 'modality' refers only to conscious sensations.

within the body. Exteroceptive sensations are described as *conscious*; that is, they are perceived when the nerve impulses are decoded by the brain. Proprioceptive sensations may be conscious or unconscious. *Conscious proprioception* is produced by decoding impulses from the muscles and joints. It is perceived as the *sense of position* of the body parts at rest, and as the sense of movement, or *kinesthetic sense*. The term *'unconscious proprioception'* refers to activity in the spinocerebellar tracts; sensations are not perceived by the cerebellum, whose function is the co-ordination of movement.

Pathways serving conscious sensations are largely 'crossed'; that is, they cross the midline before reaching the cerebrum. This is true of vision, hearing, and balance as well as of the conscious sensations mediated by the spinal cord. Olfaction (smell) is the only uncrossed sensation.

The two great conscious sensory pathways in the spinal cord are the spinothalamic and the dorsal column–lemniscal pathways.

Spinothalamic tract (Fig. 9-8)

The cells of origin occupy the spinal cord at all segmental levels. Most are in the marginal zone (lamina I), nucleus proprius (laminae III and IV) and lamina V. Many of the cells (known as transmission, projection, or relay cells) respond only to peripheral painful stimuli; others respond only to thermal stimuli.

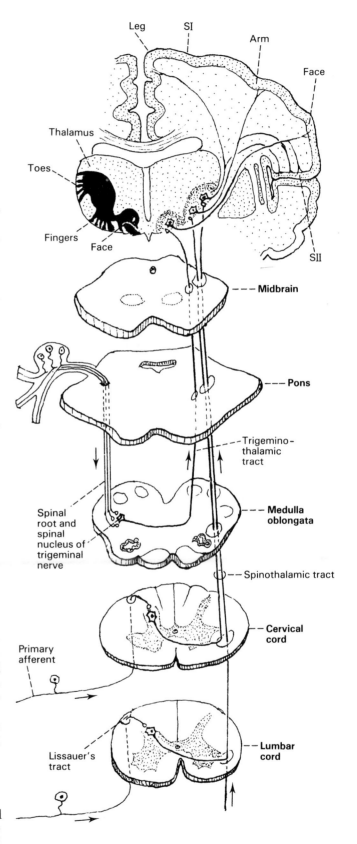

Fig. 9-8   Principal nociceptive pathways. SI, SII are subdivisions of the somatic sensory cortex. Diagrams such as this take no account of modulatory influences (cf. Chapter 15).

Some show *convergence*, a term used for two types of cell. The first type, viscerosomatic convergent cells, respond to both somatic and visceral noxious stimuli; these cells are significant in visceral referred pain (Chapter 7). The second type respond to both noxious and mechanical stimuli; these cells are involved in *diffuse noxious inhibitory control*, an important concept considered in Chapter 15.

The spinothalamic axons cross the midline in the white commissure, at all segmental levels. They ascend in the anterolateral quadrant near the cord surface and pass through the brain stem to reach the thalamus. Third-order neurons pass from the thalamus to the somatic sensory cortex (SI) and to the second somatic sensory area (SII).

Substantia gelatinosa (Fig. 9-9)

The substantia gelatinosa neurons have somas the size of erythrocytes. They are tightly packed and difficult to demonstrate by laboratory stains (hence their 'gelatinous' appearance). They receive fine primary afferents from Lissauer's tract on their external aspects. They receive coarse collaterals from medial root fibers on their deep aspects (Fig. 9-9). Their axons run outward. Some synapse immediately upon marginal cells; others run up or down for a few segments within Lissauer's tract before re-entering the gray matter, where they synapse upon transmission cells, or upon primary afferent terminals.

Some substantia gelatinosa cells (mostly medially placed) are excitatory. Others (mostly lateral) are inhibitory. Inhibitory transmitters include GABA and enkephalin.

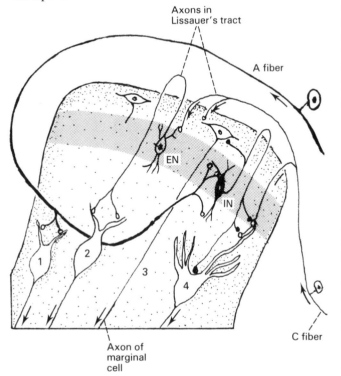

Fig. 9-9 Some connections of cutaneous fibers of the posterior root. Nociceptor activity (C fiber) excites STT relay cells 2, 3, and 4. Addition of tactile activity (A fiber) excites relay cell 1 and inhibits 3 and 4. EN, IN, excitatory, inhibitory internuncials in substantia gelatinosa. Lamina II is shaded.

Filter function The subtantia gelatinosa acts as a filter, or 'gate', controlling the admission of impulses from primary afferents to spinothalamic transmission cells. See Chapter 15 for details.

The applied anatomy of the spinothalamic tract is considered in Chapter 11.

Dorsal column–lemniscal pathway (Fig. 9-10)

The posterior funiculi contain myelinated fibers ascending uncrossed to the dorsal column nuclei located in the medulla oblongata. Up to mid-thoracic level, each posterior funiculus is made up of the *fasciculus gracilis*, which terminates in the *nucleus gracilis*. The *fasciculus cuneatus* carries information from the upper trunk and upper limb. It terminates in the *nucleus cuneatus*.

Components

1 The largest component fibers (25% of the total number) are superficial and are the axons of *primary sensory neurons*. The peripheral processes of these neurons terminate in the largest cutaneous receptors: Meissner's, Ruffini's, and Pacinian corpuscles, tactile discs, and perifollicular basketworks (Chapter 5). Implicit here is the astonishing length of some unipolar neurons, extending from the sole of the foot to the nucleus gracilis – about 150 cm (5 feet).

The fasciculus cuneatus contains, in addition, primary afferents from neuromuscular spindles and from joint capsules in the upper limb. From the lower limb, these primary afferents leave the fasciculus cuneatus to synapse in the thoracic nucleus (Clarke's column). The second-order neurons follow the posterior spinocerebellar tract as far as the medulla, then synapse in *nucleus z*, which lies immediately rostral to the nucleus gracilis.

2 The deeper fibers belong to the so-called 'indirect' dorsal column–lemniscal pathway. They are phylogenetically older than the 'direct' (superficial) fibers. They synapse upon small, peripherally placed cells in the dorsal column nuclei, from which some fibers project via the medial lemniscus to the reticular formation, where they mingle with spinoreticular fibers. They may account for the fact that electrical stimulation of the medial lemniscus in patients elicits pain.

Medial lemniscus From the dorsal column nuclei and nucleus z, axons sweep across the midline, intersecting their opposite numbers in the *sensory decussation* (Fig. 9-10). They then turn rostrally and ascend through the brain stem to reach the thalamus as a fiber tract called the *medial lemniscus*. A fresh set of neurons projects from the thalamus to the somatic sensory cortex.

Functions

Traditionally, the dorsal column–lemniscal pathway has been regarded as solely responsible for the sense of position and the sense of movement (kinesthesia). These modalities, as well as vibration sense, are lost in

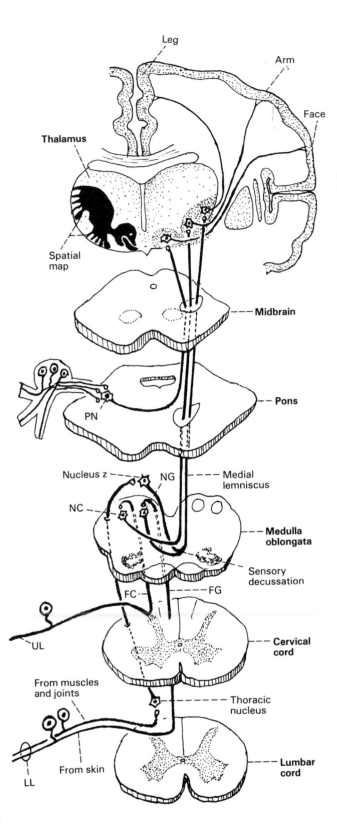

Fig. 9-10 Dorsal column–lemniscal pathway. From the upper limb (UL), afferents from skin, muscle and joints travel together in the fasciculus cuneatus (FC) to reach the nucleus cuneatus (NC). From the lower limb (LL), muscle and joint afferents leave the fasciculus gracilis (FG) and travel alongside the posterior spinocerebellar tract (not shown) to reach nucleus z. Afferents from the face synapse mainly in the pontine nucleus (PN) of the trigeminal nerve. The spatial map in the thalamus is anterior to the one shown in Fig. 9-8. NG, nucleus gracilis.

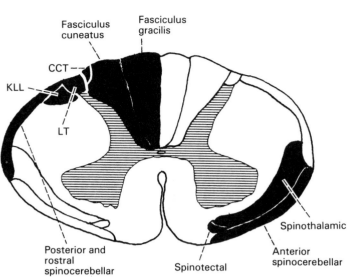

Fig. 9-11 Ascending tracts. CCT, cuneocerebellar tract; KLL, kinesthesia from lower limb; LT, Lissauer's tract.

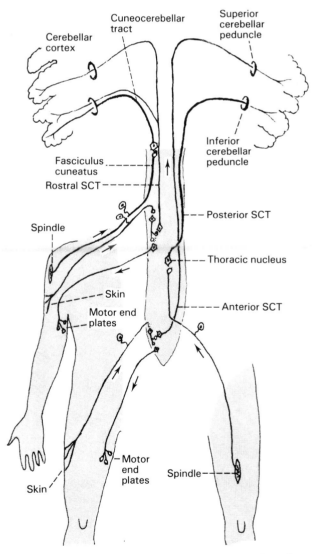

Fig. 9-12 Spinocerebellar pathways. Two cutaneomuscular reflexes are shown. SCT, spinocerebellar tract.

65

the classical dorsal column disorder known as *tabes dorsalis* (L., dorsal wasting). However, tabes dorsalis is a syphilitic disorder characterized by meningitis of posterior nerve roots, and axonal degeneration is by no means confined to fibers destined for the dorsal columns.

In a small number of patients in whom the dorsal columns have been severed either surgically or by injury, position, vibration, and kinesthetic senses were remarkably well preserved. For the lower limbs this is understandable because the main pathway from their muscles and joints runs with the posterior spinocerebellar tracts, which occupy the lateral funiculus (Fig. 9-11). Vibration sense is mediated by spinothalamic as well as by dorsal column fibers. Preservation of position and kinesthetic sense in the upper limbs may be explained by collaterals given to spinothalamic relay cells by primary afferents from muscles. Muscle afferents may be more important than joint afferents in signaling the sense of position and movement.

The only obvious deficiency after dorsal column lesions is a loss of *tactile discrimination*. The patient has difficulty in discriminating between one and two sharp points applied to the skin, in identifying numbers traced onto the skin by the examiner's finger, and in distinguishing objects of similar shape but of different textures.

In monkeys, dorsal column lesions interfere with complex motor activities. In jumping from one bar to another the animal often misses its target. For this reason the columns are seen as providing an instantaneous body image at the level of the somatic sensory cortex, to serve as a baseline for the execution of serial motor acts.

Sensory ataxia is described in Chapter 11.

Spinocerebellar pathways (Fig. 9-12)

There are two spinocerebellar systems. One transmits unconscious proprioceptive information from muscles and joints to the ipsilateral cerebellar hemisphere, and has minor inputs from cutaneous receptors. The other transmits information (mainly to the contralateral hemisphere) from reflex arcs – especially from flexor reflex arcs – and has minor inputs from muscles and joints.

Unconscious proprioception (Figs. 9-11, 9-12)

The pathways are the posterior spinocerebellar tract, from the lower trunk and lower limb, and the cuneocerebellar tract, from the upper trunk and upper limb. Both are uncrossed, in keeping with the known control by each cerebellar hemisphere of movements on its own side of the body – unlike the motor cortex, which controls contralateral movements.

Posterior spinocerebellar tract This originates in the dorsal (thoracic) nucleus (Clarke's column), which extends from segments C8 to L3. The nucleus receives first-order afferents of all kinds from the muscles of the lower limb and lower trunk, including an intense and overlapping input from spindle primaries. It also receives collaterals from cutaneous sensory fibers. To

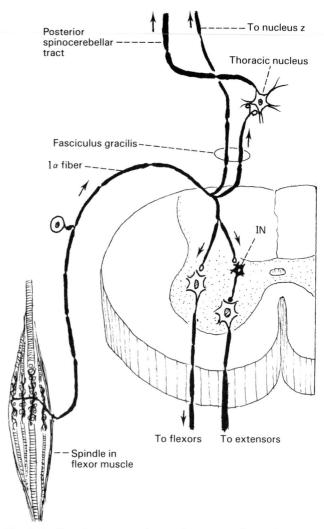

Fig. 9-13 Four destinations of a spindle primary afferent from a lower limb flexor muscle. IN, inhibitory internuncial.

reach the nucleus, lower limb fibers travel for a while in the fasciculus gracilis (Fig. 9-13).

The axons of the posterior spinocerebellar tract are about 20 µm in diameter – the largest axons in the entire CNS. They ascend close to the surface of the cord on their own side and enter the inferior cerebellar peduncle.

Cuneocerebellar tract From the upper limb and upper trunk, primary afferents from muscles and joints (and from skin) ascend within the fasciculus cuneatus to reach the *accessory cuneate nucleus*, which lies rostrolateral to the cuneate nucleus. Second-order afferents enter the ipsilateral inferior cerebellar peduncle.

Feedback from reflex arcs (Fig. 9-12)

Anterior spinocerebellar tract The transmission cells occupy the intermediate gray matter (lamina VII). They receive afferents from internuncial neurons of spinal reflex arcs – especially from flexor reflex internuncials. Their function is to provide feedback to the cerebellum about on-going spinal reflexes. However, they also receive some primary afferent collaterals from the muscles and joints of the lower limb and lower trunk.

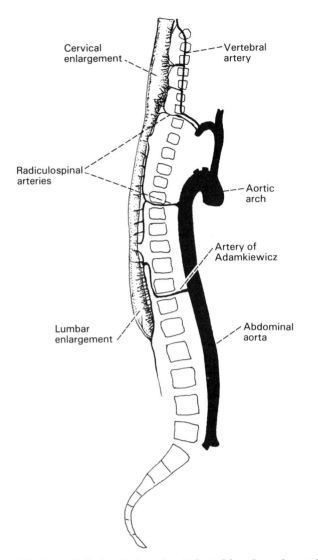

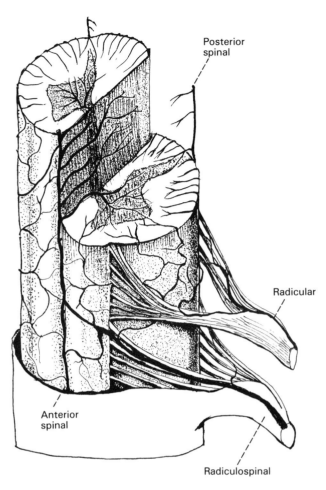

Posterior spinal

Radicular

Anterior spinal

Radiculospinal

Fig. 9-15 Arteries of spinal cord and nerve roots.

Cervical enlargement

Vertebral artery

Radiculospinal arteries

Aortic arch

Artery of Adamkiewicz

Lumbar enlargement

Abdominal aorta

Fig. 9-14 Radiculospinal arteries. (Adapted from Lazorthes et al., 1971.)

The flexor reflex is also called the *withdrawal* or *cutaneomuscular reflex* because escape does not always involve flexion of the affected part.

The anterior spinocerebellar tract crosses the midline in the white commissure and ascends as far as the midbrain before entering the contralateral superior cerebellar peduncle. Many fibers recross within the cerebellar white matter.

Rostral spinocerebellar tract This tract serves corresponding functions for the upper trunk and upper limb. However, it is uncrossed. It arises in the intermediate gray matter of the cervical and upper thoracic cord, and enters the ipsilateral superior and inferior cerebellar peduncles.

A detailed knowledge of the spinocerebellar pathways is unimportant from the clinical standpoint. Disorders of cerebellar function almost invariably arise from disease within the cerebellum itself.

Other ascending pathways

The *spinoreticular tract* arises, in company with the spinothalamic tract, from nucleus proprius and lamina V neurons along the full length of the cord. Unlike the spinothalamic tract, however, it is largely uncrossed. It terminates in the reticular formation of the brain stem. Stimulation of the spinoreticular system has an arousal (wakening) effect (Chapter 14).

The *spinotectal tract* (crossed) runs alongside the spinothalamic. The tectal fibers separate in the brain stem to terminate in the superior colliculus, an important ocular control center (Chapter 32).

The *spinocervical tract* is well developed in the cat, in which the spinothalamic tract is small. It seems to be inconstant in humans. It arises in the nucleus proprius and terminates on the same side in the *lateral cervical nucleus*, a collection of gray matter (when present) beside or within the posterior horn at C1–C2 levels. Further projection to the contralateral thalamus accompanies the spinothalamic tract.

BLOOD SUPPLY OF THE SPINAL CORD
(Figs. 9-14, 9-15)

One anterior and two posterior *spinal arteries* arise from the vertebral arteries within the foramen magnum. The gray matter is supplied by the anterior spinal and the white matter by the posterior spinals. The spinal arteries are boosted by several *radiculospinal* branches from the vertebral artery and from the aorta. These are distinguishable from *radicular* arteries, which enter every intervertebral foramen to nourish the nerve roots.

The largest radiculospinal is the *artery of Adamkiewicz*, which arises from the 10th, 11th, or 12th posterior intercostal artery of one side and descends to supply the lumbar enlargement and conus terminalis.

The *venous drainage* of the cord is by anterior and posterior spinal veins, which drain outward along the nerve roots. Any obstruction to the venous outflow is liable to produce *edema of the cord*, with progressive paralysis of function.

Readings

Albe-Fessard, D., Levante, A. and Lamour, Y. (1974) Origin of spinothalamic tract in monkeys. *Brain Res.*, 65: 503–509.

Bennett, G.J., Abdelmoumine, M., Hayashi, H. and Dubner, R. (1980) Physiology and morphology of substantia gelatinosa neurons intracellularly stained with horseradish peroxidase. *J. Comp. Neurol.*, 194: 809–827.

Campbell, J.N. (1980) Examination of possible mechanisms by which stimulation of the spinal cord in man relieves pain. *Appl. Neurophysiol.*, 44: 181–186.

Cervero, F. and Iggo, A. (1980) The substantia gelatinosa of the spinal cord. A critical review. *Brain*, 103: 717–772.

Dykes, R.W. (1983) Parallel processing of somatosensory information: a theory. *Brain Res. Rev.*, 6: 47–115.

Ekerot, C.-F., Larson, B. and Oscarsson, O. (1979) Information carried by the spinocerebellar tracts. *Prog. Brain Res.*, 50: 79–90.

Hunt, S.P. (1983) Cytochemistry of the spinal cord. In *Chemical Neuroanatomy* (Emson, P.C., ed.), pp. 53–84. New York: Raven Press.

Kerr, F.W.L. and Fukushima, T. (1980) New observations on the anatomy of the spinothalamic tract. *Pain*, 58: 47–62.

Knyihar-Csillik, B. and Rakic, P. (1982) Ultrastructure of normal and degenerating glomerular terminals of dorsal root axons in the substantia gelatinosa of the rhesus monkey. *J. Comp. Neurol.*, 210: 357–375.

Lazorthes, G., Gouaze, A., Zadeh, J.O., Santini, J.J., Lazorthes, Y. and Burdin, P. (1971) Arterial vascularization of the spinal cord. *J. Neurosurg.*, 35: 253–262.

Light, A.R., Trevino, D.L. and Perl, E.R. (1974) Morphological features of functionally defined neurons in the marginal zone and substantia gelatinosa of the spinal dorsal horn. *J. Comp. Neurol.*, 186: 151–172.

MacFadyen, D.J. (1984) Posterior column dysfunction in cervical spondylitic myelopathy. *Can. J. Neurol. Sci.*, 11: 365–370.

McCloskey, D.I. (1980) Kinaesthetic sensation and motor commands in man. *Prog. Clin. Neurophysiol.*, 8: 203–214.

Meinck, H.M., Benecke, R., Küster, S. and Conrad, B. (1983) Cutaneomuscular (flexor) reflex organization in normal man and in patients with motor disorders. In *Motor Control Mechanisms in Health and Disease* (Desmedt, J.E., ed.), pp. 787–796. New York: Raven Press.

North, R.B., Fischell, T.A. and Long, D.M. (1978) Chronic dorsal column stimulation via percutaneously inserted epidural electrodes. *Acta Neurophysiol.*, 40: 184–191.

Rethelyi, M., Light, A.R. and Perl, E.R. (1982) Synaptic complexes formed by functionally defined primary afferent units with fine myelinated fibers. *J. Comp. Neurol.*, 207: 381–393.

Ross, E.D., Kirkpatrick, J.B. and Lastimoso, A.C.B. (1979) Position and vibration sensations: function of the dorsal spinocerebellar tracts? *Ann. Neurol.*, 5: 171–176.

Smith, M.C. and Deacon, P. (1984) Topographical anatomy of the posterior columns of the spinal cord in man: the long ascending fibres. *Brain*, 107: 671–698.

Snyder, R. (1977) The organization of the dorsal root entry zone in cats and monkeys. *J. Comp. Neurol.*, 174: 47–70.

Tan, C.K. and Wong, W.C. (1982) The structure and connections of the dorsal column nuclei. In *Progress in Anatomy*, Vol. 2 (Harrison, R.J. and Navaratnam, V., eds.), pp. 161–177.

Willer, J.C., Boureau, F. and Albe-Fessard, D. (1980) Human nociceptive reactions: effects of spatial summation from relatively large diameter fibers. *Brain Res.*, 201: 465–470.

Willis, W.D. (1980) Neurophysiology of nociception and pain in the spinal cord. *Pain*, 58: 77–92.

Willis, W.D. and Coggeshall, R.E. (1978) *Sensory Mechanisms of the Spinal Cord*. New York: Plenum Press.

10

Motoneurons and Descending Pathways

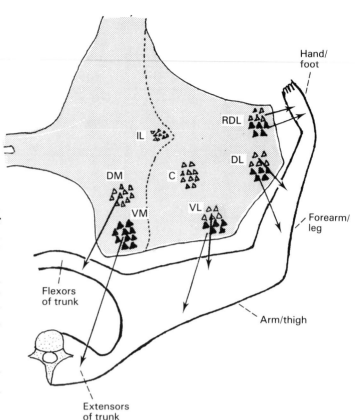

Fig. 10-1 Cell columns in the gray matter. Dotted line indicates limit of gray matter at thoracic level. C, central; DL, dorsolateral; DM, dorsomedial; IL, intermediolateral (autonomic); RDL, retrodorsolateral (for intrinsic muscles); VL, ventrolateral; VM, ventromedial nucleus.

The motoneurons of the spinal cord are arranged in *columns* which supply muscle groups having similar functions. The individual muscles are supplied from cell groups (nuclei) within the columns. Medially placed columns supply the axial (trunk) musculature. Laterally placed columns, present only in the cervical and lumbar enlargements, supply the limb musculature. Finally, motoneurons innervating extensor muscles lie in front of motoneurons innervating flexors (Fig. 10-1, Table 10-1).

Table 10-1 Motor cell columns

Cell column	Muscles
Ventromedial (all segments)	Erector spinae
Dorsomedial (T1–L2)	Intercostals, abdominals
Ventrolateral (C5–8, L2–S2)	Arm/thigh
Dorsolateral (C6–8, L3–S3)	Forearm/leg
Retrodorsolateral (C8, T1, S1, S2)	Hand/foot
Central (C3, C4, C5)	Diaphragm

ALPHA AND GAMMA MOTONEURONS

The α motoneurons (αMN) have very large dendritic trees which receive some 10 000 excitatory boutons from reflex arcs and from descending (supraspinal) pathways. Their somas receive 5000 inhibitory boutons, mainly from propriospinal neurons. Initial axonal segments are largely devoid of synaptic contacts.

'Tonic' αMNs innervate squads of slow, oxidative–glycolytic (SOG) muscle fibers. They are readily depolarized and have slowly conducting axons with small spike amplitudes. 'Phasic' αMNs are bigger and have higher thresholds and fast-conducting axons with large spikes. They supply fast, oxidative (FO) and fast, oxidative–glycolytic (FOG) muscle fibers. Before leaving the gray matter, all αMNs give recurrent branches to Renshaw cells located in the medial part of the anterior gray horn (Fig. 10-2).

Gamma motoneurons are interspersed among the αMNs. They too are subject to propriospinal and supraspinal controls.

Segmental inputs

At each segmental level, αMNs receive powerful excitation and inhibition:

1 Monosynaptic excitation from primary and secondary afferents from neuromuscular spindles. Under physiological conditions – unlike those of the clinical tendon reflex – abrupt muscle stretch adds strength to supraspinal inputs, as in running, where contact of the

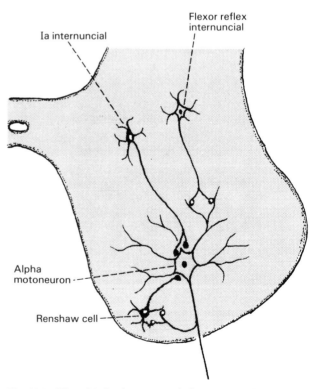

Fig. 10-2 Three kinds of internuncial playing upon alpha motoneurons.

70

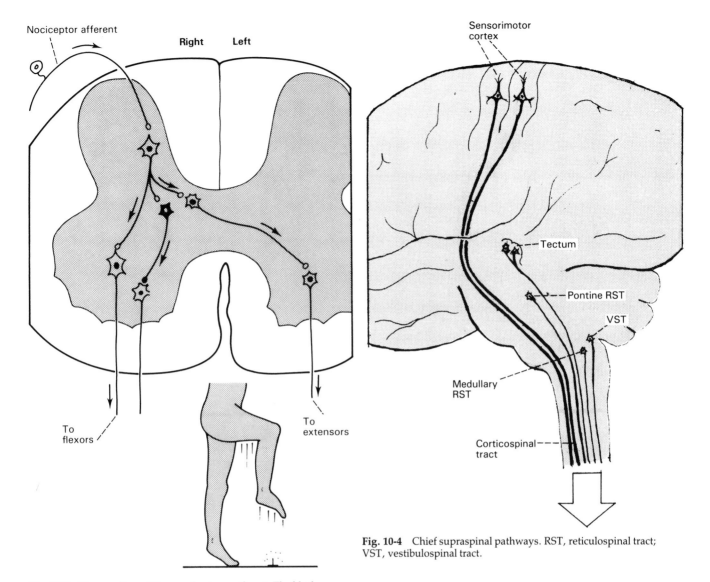

Fig. 10-3 Flexor reflex with crossed extensor thrust. The black internuncial is inhibitory.

Fig. 10-4 Chief supraspinal pathways. RST, reticulospinal tract; VST, vestibulospinal tract.

forefoot with the ground allows the heel to descend, eliciting a brisk tendon reflex in the gastrocnemius.

2 Disynaptic excitation by flexor reflex afferents. The *flexor reflex* is the withdrawal that occurs upon noxious stimulation of skin or muscle (Fig. 10-3). Large numbers of excitatory internuncials to flexor motoneurons are excited together with inhibitory motoneurons to extensors on the same side. In the lower limb, an *extensor thrust* develops on the contralateral side and sustains the body weight.

3 Disynaptic inhibition of antagonist αMNs by spindle primary (Ia) afferents (see Fig. 4-9). The internuncials concerned are called *Ia inhibitory neurons*, and they lie at the base of the anterior horn (Fig. 10-2).

4 Disynaptic, autogenetic inhibition from tendon endings (Chapter 4).

5 Disynaptic inhibition via Renshaw cells (see later).

SUPRASPINAL MOTOR PATHWAYS (Fig. 10-4)

Lateral (crossed) corticospinal tract

This descends the full length of the spinal cord, beside the base of the posterior horn (Fig. 10-5). It is the

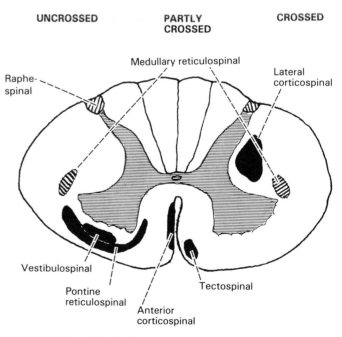

Fig. 10-5 Descending tracts.

71

principal voluntary motor pathway. It synapses (a) in the posterior horn, where it modulates sensory transmission (Chapter 20), (b) in the intermediate gray matter and base of anterior horn (lamina VII), upon excitatory and inhibitory internuncials, and (c) upon αMNs, γMNs, and Renshaw cells. Axial and proximal limb motoneurons are activated indirectly, through internuncials shared with reticulospinal pathways. Distal limb motoneurons (to extrinsic and intrinsic muscles of the hands and feet) are innervated direct by *corticomotoneuronal fibers*. Direct innervation confers on the lateral corticospinal tract the unique property of *fractionation*: the selection of individual motoneurons from a motor nucleus. This property makes it possible to move individual digits with extreme delicacy. With training (involving feedback from electromyographic recordings), even single motor units can be operated voluntarily. Fractionation is assisted by cooperation of Renshaw cells (see later).

The dependence of fractionation on corticomotoneuronal activity accounts for the permanent loss of delicate hand movements (e.g. buttoning one's coat) after a stroke (Chapter 20).

Targets

The lateral corticospinal tract synapses upon four different kinds of neurons concerned with *movement:*
1 Upon the Ia interneurons (lamina VII) serving reciprocal inhibition. These are the *first* neurons to be recruited. They cause the antagonist muscles to start relaxing before the prime movers begin to contract (Fig. 10-6).
2 Upon αMNs, directly or indirectly, as already described.
3 Upon γMNs, directly or indirectly, in company with homonymous αMNs. ('Homonymous' here refers to the same muscle or muscle group.)
4 Upon Renshaw cells.

The gamma loop

In voluntary movements αMNs and γMNs are recruited together. This is known as α-γ *coactivation* or α-γ *linkage*. The γMNs reinforce α excitation through what is known as the *gamma loop* (Fig. 10-6). Intrafusal and extrafusal muscles shorten simultaneously, and the brain is continuously informed about the state of muscle contraction, on one side of a joint (except in fast movements) and about the state of relaxation (passive stretching) on the other side.

The gamma loop provides *load compensation*. When a weight is lifted, shortening of extrafusal fibers is resisted while the intrafusal fibers continue to shorten. The additional input to αMNs through the gamma loop reinforces extrafusal contraction. This effect, through the afferent limb of the tendon reflex arc, serves for minor loads and has a latency (time lag) of 10 milliseconds. If an unexpected obstruction to movement occurs, the αMNs discharge more strongly after a 20 ms interval. This is also reflex, since voluntary effort to overcome an obstacle has a 40 ms latency (for the hand). The 20 ms response has two components: a polysynaptic reflex within the spinal cord, and a

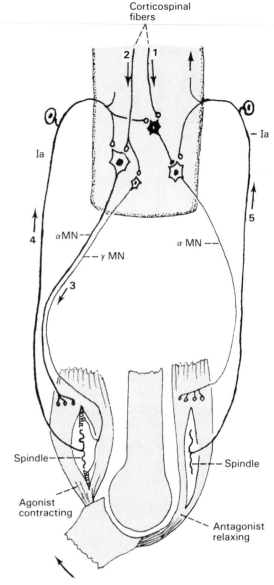

Fig. 10-6 Sequence of events in a voluntary movement (knee flexion):
1 activation of Ia internuncial inhibits antagonist αMN.
2 activation of agonist αMN and γMN.
3 contraction of extra- and intrafusal muscle.
4 feedback from contracting spindle increases αMN excitation and Ia inhibition.
5 antagonist Ia fiber finds its homonymous αMN refractory, but it transmits to higher centers (arrow).
γMN, Ia, and αMN constitute the gamma loop.

'long-loop' reflex traveling by the dorsal column–lemniscal path to the motor cortex. The long-loop reflex seems to have evolved particularly for control of the hand (see Chapter 20).

Renshaw cells

The chief characteristic of Renshaw cells is their versatility. They are in a Janus position at the gateway to the 'final common path' to the locomotor system. They receive the recurrent collaterals of αMNs. All αMNs are subject to tonic inhibition by Renshaw cells, as exemplified by the agonizing convulsions that follow poisoning with strychnine: strychnine prevents the release of glycine, the transmitter used by most Renshaw cells. Renshaw cells have several functions:

1 The order of recruitment of motor units is the same for a given movement, whether it be fast or slow. However, 'phasic' αMNs give rise to more (about six each) recurrent collaterals than do 'tonic' αMNs (about three each). The 'tonic' αMNs are silenced (via Renshaw cells) when rapid movements get under way.

2 In fractionation, Renshaw cells are used to seal off αMNs not required for a particular movement.

3 Some Renshaw cells synapse upon Ia inhibitory internuncials. This makes *co-contraction* possible. During distal limb movements, the proximal joints are *fixated* by simultaneous contraction (co-contraction) of prime movers and antagonists (for example, to keep the shoulder and elbow stable while using a screwdriver).

4 During maximal muscular effort (as in lifting a heavy weight), all of the motor units are brought to bear. This is achieved by recruitment of Renshaw cells that synapse upon one another. In effect, Renshaw activity is deleted.

Anterior corticospinal tract

This descends to cervical and upper thoracic levels. It is concerned with movements of the head (Chapter 20).

(Lateral) vestibulospinal tract

This descends in the anterior funiculus, where it is well placed for access to axial motoneurons. It stimulates appropriate antigravity muscles when the head is tilted (Chapter 33).

Reticulospinal tracts

The reticulospinal tracts (Chapter 14) arise in the reticular formation of the brain stem. The *pontine* (medial) tract descends uncrossed in the anterior funiculus. It activates extensor αMNs, mainly through the gamma loop (Fig. 10-7). The *medullary* (lateral) tract descends (partly crossed) in the lateral funiculus. It supplies αMNs serving flexor muscles.

Both reticulospinal tracts control axial and proximal limb motoneurons, and they are the principal supraspinal pathways controlling posture (such as sitting and standing) and automatic movements (such as walking and running).

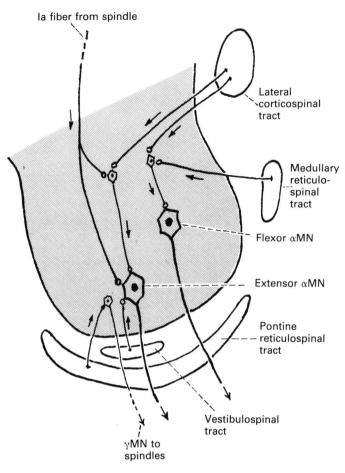

la fiber from spindle

Lateral corticospinal tract

Medullary reticulo-spinal tract

Flexor αMN

Extensor αMN

Pontine reticulospinal tract

Vestibulospinal tract

γMN to spindles

Fig. 10-7 Inputs from four motor pathways to motoneurons (MN) serving axial or proximal limb muscles.

Tectospinal tract

This is a crossed tract arising in the tectum (roof) of the midbrain. It synapses on cervical αMNs and it turns the head toward visual or auditory stimuli.

Rubrospinal tract

This is an important motor pathway in cats and dogs, where it arises in the contralateral red nucleus and descends in front of the lateral corticospinal tracts. In monkeys this tract is small and in humans it is quite negligible.

Monoaminergic fibers

Monoaminergic fibers descend from several nuclear groups in the brain stem and permeate the gray matter of the spinal cord. They are described in Chapter 15.

APPLIED ANATOMY

This is discussed in Chapter 11.

Readings

Abdel-Maguid, T.E. and Bowsher, D. (1979) Alpha- and gamma-motoneurons in the adult human spinal cord and somatic cranial nerve nuclei. *J. Comp. Neurol., 186:* 259–270.

Binder, M.D. and Stuart, D.G. (1980) Motor unit-muscle receptor interactions: design features of the neuromuscular control system. *Prog. Clin. Neurophysiol., 8:* 72–98.

Brodal, A. (1981) Pathways mediating supraspinal influences on the spinal cord. In *Neurological Anatomy in Relation to Clinical Medicine*, Chapter 4. New York & Oxford: Oxford University Press.

Burke, R.E. (1979) The role of synaptic organization in the control of motor unit activity during movement. *Prog. Brain Res., 50:* 61–67.

Commissiong, J.W. (1981) Spinal monoaminergic systems: an aspect of somatic motor function. *Fed. Proc., 40:* 2771–2777.

Commissiong, J.W., Galli, C.L., Hellstrom, S. and Karoum, F. (1984) Neurochemical aspects of spinal cord monoamines. In *Dynamics of Neurotransmitter Function* (Hanin, I., ed.), pp. 39–46. New York: Raven Press.

Coulter, J.D., Bowker, R.M., Wise, S.P., Murray, E.A., Castilioni, A.J. and Westland, K.N. (1979) Cortical, tectal and medullary descending pathways to the cervical spinal cord. *Prog. Brain Res., 50:* 263–279.

Delwaide, P.J. and Toulouse, P. (1981) Facilitation of monosynaptic reflexes by voluntary contraction of muscles in remote parts of the body. Mechanisms involved in the Jendrassik manoeuvre. *Brain, 104:* 701–719.

Freund, H.-J. (1983) Motor unit and muscle activity in voluntary motor control. *Physiol. Rev., 63:* 387–436.

Friedman, W.A., Sypert, G.W., Munson, J.B. and Flashman, J.W. (1981) Recurrent inhibition in type-identified motoneurons. *J. Neurophysiol., 46:* 1349–1359.

Ghez, C. and Shinoda, Y. (1978) Spinal mechanisms of the functional stretch reflex. *Exp. Brain Res., 32:* 369–375.

Granit, R. (1975) The functional role of the muscle spindles – facts and hypotheses. *Brain, 98:* 531–556.

Henneman, E. and Harris, D. (1976) Identification of fast and slow firing types of motoneurons in the same pool. *Prog. Brain Res., 44:* 377–382.

Jankowska, E. and Lundberg, A. (1981) Interneurones in the spinal cord. *Trends Neurosci., 4:* 230–233.

Jung, R. (1979) Two functions of reflexes in human movement: interaction with preprograms and gain of force. *Prog. Brain Res., 50:* 237–241.

Lagerbäck, P.-A. (1982) *On α Motoneuron Collateral Boutons and Renshaw Cells.* Stockholm: Karolinska Institutet.

Nathan, P.W. and Smith, M.C. (1982) The rubrospinal and central tegmental tracts in man. *Brain, 105:* 223–269.

Pierrot-Deseilligny, E. and Morin, C. (1980) Evidence for supraspinal influences on Renshaw inhibition during motor activity in man. *Prog. Clin. Neurophysiol., 8:* 142–169.

Stein, P.S.G. (1978) Motor systems, with specific reference to the control of locomotion. *Annu. Rev. Neurosci., 1:* 61–81.

Tanaka, R. (1976) Reciprocal Ia inhibition and voluntary movements in man. *Prog. Brain Res., 44:* 291–302.

White, S.R. and Nenman, R.S. (1980) Facilitation of spinal motoneurone excitability by 5-hydroxytryptamine and noradrenaline. *Brain Res., 188:* 119–127.

11
Embryology and Applied Anatomy

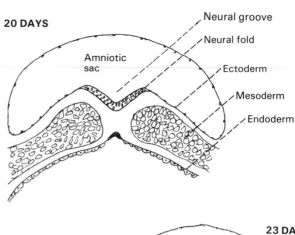

The embryology of the nervous system is not formally addressed in this book. However, a short section on spinal cord development is introduced here as an aid to understanding (a) the anatomy of the adult cord and meninges, and (b) common congenital malformations of this region.

THREE PHASES OF SPINAL CORD FORMATION

Phase of neurulation: days 18–27

The process of *neurulation* denotes the formation of the bulk of the neural tube from the neural folds. The neurectoderm can be detected in the floor of the amniotic sac on day 16 after fertilization, the neurectodermal cells being taller than the rest of the embryonic ectoderm.

On day 18 a shallow *neural groove* appears in the midline, flanked by two *neural folds* (Fig. 11-1). The underlying paraxial mesoderm commences segmentation on day 20. When six or seven mesodermal somites have been formed, the crests of the neural folds unite at cervical level to form the *neural tube*. Union of the folds proceeds both rostrally and caudally, the neurectoderm separating from the skin ectoderm (future epidermis) which unites dorsal to it. Along the line of union, the neurectodermal cells give rise to the ribbon-like *neural crest* on each side.

The open ends of the neural tube are the *neuropores*. The rostral (anterior) neuropore closes on day 24 and the caudal (posterior) neuropore closes on day 26 or 27.

Phase of secondary canalization: days 30–50

The caudal neuropore closes at the level of the first or second lumbar somite. This is the future level of the first or second lumbar segment of the spinal cord. Caudal to this the ectoderm and mesoderm mingle, forming the *caudal cell mass* (Fig. 11-2).

Ectoderm-lined vacuoles appear in the caudal cell mass. They coalesce and open into the end of the neural tube. This is known as *secondary canalization*, and it contributes the lower lumbar and sacral segments of the spinal cord. In one-third of embryos the caudal contribution to the neural tube is initially forked.

The mesoderm of the caudal cell mass gives rise to the lower lumbar and sacral somites, and to the six coccygeal somites of the embryonic tail.

Phase of regression: days 50–80

The embryonic tail regresses by a process of selective cell death (*necrobiosis*). The tip of the developing spinal

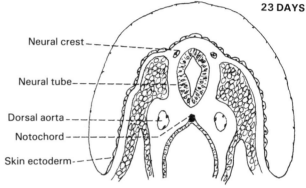

Fig. 11-1 Transverse sections of embryo showing neural folds and neural tube.

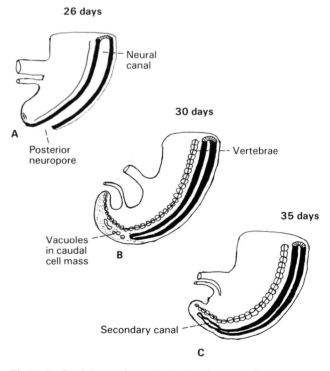

Fig. 11-2 Caudal part of neural tube showing secondary canalization.

cord becomes involved in necrobiosis, and it dwindles to form a strand of glia, the *filum terminale*, which remains attached to the tip of the definitive coccyx. The lower end of the central canal expands to form the *terminal ventricle*, which persists throughout life (Fig. 11-3).

CELLULAR DIFFERENTIATION

The early neural tube is a pseudostratified epithelium composed of *germinal cells*, which look alike and extend from the inner to the outer surface (Fig. 11-4). All of the cells synthesize DNA.

During the fourth week after fertilization, germinal cells retract in succession to the innermost or *ventricular zone*, where they divide. The daughter cells become reconnected to the outer surface of the tube. Their nuclei move out, synthesize fresh DNA, then retract and divide again. After repeated cycles of this kind the cells move to the *intermediate zone*. They include young neurons and glial cell precursors (glioblasts). The young neurons do not divide further, and the term 'neuroblast' is not appropriate.

The neural canal becomes coffin-shaped in profile. The *sulcus limitans* lies between the *alar plate*, containing connector neurons, and the *basal plate*, containing motoneurons (Fig. 11-5). The alar and basal plates give rise to the posterior and anterior gray horns. Enlargement of the posterior horns causes the ventricular zones of both sides to come together, forming the posterior median septum. Bulging of the ventral horns creates the anterior median fissure.

The nerve cells emit axons and dendrites. The initial outgrowths are independent, but full development of dendritic trees requires synaptic contacts. This interaction is mutual, because the continued growth of dendrites promotes the further development of axo-dendritic synapses.

Segmentation

Some cells of the neural crest become bipolar neurons, which quickly become unipolar. (The term 'pseudounipolar' is sometimes used to denote the initially bipolar nature of spinal ganglion cells. The bipolar state persists in the special senses, except taste.) The central processes enter the alar lamina, and the peripheral processes enter the myotomes and dermatomes as these differentiate from the somites. Other neural crest cells give rise to the ganglia of the sympathetic system and to chromaffin cells. The parasympathetic ganglia come from neural crest (and possibly other) cells that migrate along cranial nerves III, VII, IX, and X. Still other crest cells travel to the skin where they form melanocytes.

Anterior horn motoneurons innervate the myotomes, which migrate into the trunk wall and into the roots of the limbs. In the limbs, the myotomes form the girdle muscles, but the more distal musculature develops in situ from somatic mesoderm in the core of the limb buds.

From the third month onward, the outermost, *marginal zone* of the neural tube is invaded by

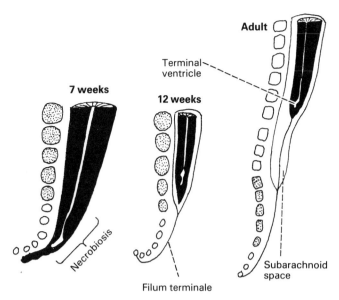

Fig. 11-3 Phase of regression. Sacral vertebrae are stippled.

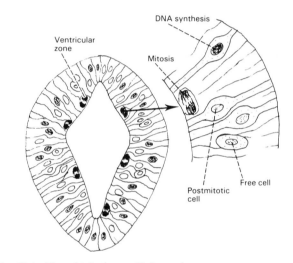

Fig. 11-4 Neural tube from a 23-day embryo.

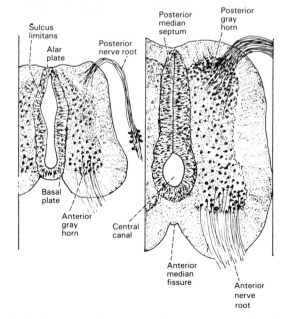

Fig. 11-5 Formation of posterior median septum, central canal, and anterior median fissure during the seventh embronic week.

77

ascending, descending, and propriospinal fibers. Myelination commences during weeks 16–20.

As previously noted (Chapter 8), the segmented appearance of the adult spinal cord is conferred by the convergence of axon bundles into the mesodermal somites. The gray matter is not segmented.

Ascent of the cord is described in Chapter 8.

APPLIED ANATOMY OF THE IMMATURE SPINAL CORD

Congenital malformations

In *spina bifida cystica* (Fig. 11-6) the meninges, and usually the cord or spinal nerve roots, protrude through un-united (bifid) neural arches at birth. Spina bifida cystica occurs in 1 in 1000 pregnancies in the USA, 0.75 per 1000 in England and 4.3 per 1000 in Ireland and Wales. There are several patterns of inheritance and three anatomical types.

Meningocele 10% of cases. The meningeal cyst contains no nervous elements and there is no neurological deficit. The outlook following surgical repair is good.

Meningomyelocele. Almost 90% of cases. The cyst contains cauda equina (if lumbosacral) or spinal cord (if thoracic or cervical). The infant is often paraplegic at birth and an Arnold–Chiari malformation (protrusion of cerebellum into the vertebral canal, with consequent internal hydrocephalus; see Chapter 24) is nearly always present as well. Surgical repair is possible but the paralysis is permanent.

Myelocele. 1% of cases. The neural folds are open and CSF weeps onto the skin. A cyst often lies deep to the cord. The infant is completely and permanently paraplegic and incontinent.

About half of the cases of meningomyelocele and myelocele have *diastematomyelia* (Gr., *diastema*, a gap), meaning that the cord is forked. One of the forks is usually cystic.

APPLIED ANATOMY OF THE MATURE SPINAL CORD

Spinothalamic tract

Cordotomy is the procedure in which the spinothalamic tract (STT) is destroyed, for relief of intractable pain. In *percutaneous cordotomy*, a needle is introduced to the spinal cord through the side of the neck, in the interval between the atlas and axis. The patient has been sedated, and a local anesthetic is used on the skin and again before the sensitive dura mater is penetrated. Under radiological guidance the needle is inserted into the anterolateral quadrant of the cord.

A stimulating electrode is passed through the needle and used to elicit movements or sensations. If the ipsilateral arm or leg responds, the needle is in the lateral corticospinal tract and must be reintroduced farther forward (Fig. 11-7). Twitching of trapezius or sternomastoid indicates stimulation of the spinal accessory nucleus (Chapter 36). When the needle is in the STT the patient reports tingling on the opposite side of the body. The STT is then destroyed electrolytically. Afterward, the patient is insensitive to pinprick or to heat or cold applied to the other side (Fig. 11-8). Sensitivity to touch is reduced.

Cordotomy is performed to relieve pain from inoperable abdominal and pelvic cancers. It is seldom done for benign conditions because its effect wears off after about a year. The reason for return of pain is unknown, since the STT does not regenerate. Uncrossed spinoreticulothalamic fibers may be responsible, or 'indirect' dorsal column–lemniscal fibers (Chapter 9). The procedure is unsatisfactory for upper limb pain because the level of analgesia commences four to eight segments below the level of injection. (The nociceptive afferents ascend two to three segments in Lissauer's tract

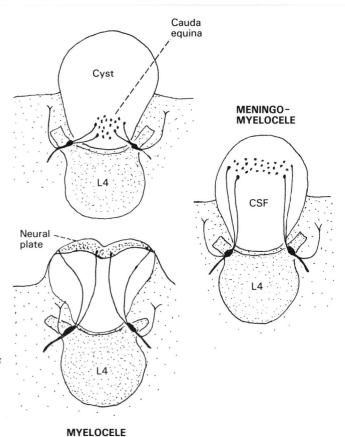

MENINGOCELE

MENINGO-MYELOCELE

MYELOCELE

Fig. 11-6 Varieties of spina bifida cystica. In meningocele the cauda equina is in its normal position in the subarachnoid space; in meningomyelocele the cauda equina is in the cystic protrusion.

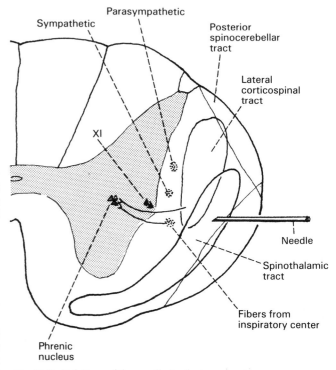

Fig. 11-7 Relations of the needle tip during percutaneous cordotomy. XI, nucleus of spinal accessory nerve.

before entering the gray matter, and the second-order axons ascend while crossing.)

The internal anatomy of the STT has been worked out from postoperative testing, which indicates the arrangement shown in Fig. 11-9. (The tactile component is sometimes called the anterior spinothalamic tract and the pain and temperature component the lateral spinothalamic tract; in the brain stem the two are then known as the spinal lemniscus.)

Complications
Autonomic fibers descend beside the intermediate gray matter to reach the spinal autonomic centers. If the sympathetic path is interrupted during cordotomy the patient may experience postural hypotension (fall of blood pressure on standing up) because of interruption of the afferent limb of the baroreceptor reflex (Chapter 37) on that side. A Horner's syndrome (Chapter 31) also appears. Interruption of the parasympathetic path to the sacral cord on one side may cause urinary retention for a day or two.

Lesions of the posterior part of the STT may also sever posterior spinocerebellar fibers serving the ipsilateral lower limb, producing incoordination of movement (cerebellar ataxia, Chapter 13).

If bilateral cordotomy is required a surgical approach at T1 level is preferred, to ensure that the phrenic nuclei are not denervated. The phrenic and intercostal nuclei have dual innervation: an automatic supply from the inspiratory center descending beside the gray matter, and a voluntary supply from the pyramidal tract (Chapter 38). Unilateral destruction of the automatic supply is not fatal, but after bilateral destruction *the patient will die when voluntary breathing is suspended during sleep.*

Syringomyelia
This disorder is of uncertain etiology, but is characterized by development of a *syrinx* – a fusiform cyst in or beside the central canal, usually in the cervical region (Fig. 11-10). Symptoms arise from injury to the white commissure. The clinical picture is one of *dissociated sensory loss:* painful and thermal sensitivity is lost in the dermatomes affected, but tactile and proprioceptive sensations are preserved. Typically, the patient has severe infections of the fingers from unattended cuts or burns. The joints may be disorganized, or even dislocated, owing to interruption of the protective reflex from joint capsules (Chapter 4).

Sensory ataxia
The term *ataxia* signifies *incoordination of gait*, expressed as *staggering*. Ataxia has three generic causes:
1 The patient staggers because he cannot perceive the position or movement of his legs; in other words, he lacks conscious proprioception. This is *sensory ataxia*, and it is caused by disease of the spinal cord. He may adopt a stamping gait to procure some awareness, and he uses visual guidance.
2 He staggers because the cerebellum is unable to coordinate the reticulospinal tracts switched on by the locomotor generator (Chapter 15). This is *cerebellar ataxia*, and a common enough cause is alcoholic intoxication. Visual guidance cannot compensate.
3 He staggers because of disease in the inner ear. The two labyrinths normally operate the vestibulospinal tracts (under cerebellar guidance) to keep the center of gravity between the feet. If one labyrinth is out of action the patient will veer toward the affected side (akin to a paddle steamer operating on a single paddle). If both labyrinths are out of action he can compensate by using visual guidance, but he will stagger and fall if he closes his eyes.

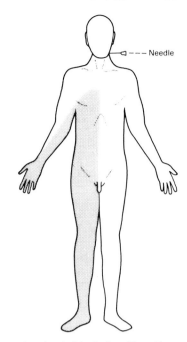
Fig. 11-8 Area of analgesia (shaded) produced by cordotomy.

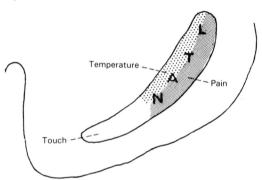
Fig. 11-9 Modality segregation in the spinothalamic tract. L, leg; T, trunk; A, arm; N, neck.

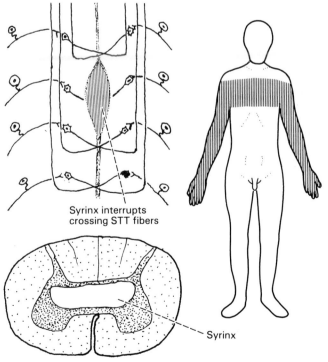
Syrinx interrupts crossing STT fibers
Syrinx
Fig. 11-10 Usual distribution of analgesia in syringomyelia. STT, spinothalamic tract.

Lesions causing sensory ataxia
At cervical or thoracic level, a lesion must include the posterior part of the lateral funiculus, to interrupt fibers ascending from the muscles and joints of the ipsilateral lower limb. In clinical practise, sensory ataxia is usually part of a larger disability produced by multiple lesions. In multiple sclerosis (Chapter 2) plaques of demyelination are scattered in the white matter and often impair the lateral corticospinal tract as well.

Subacute combined degeneration of the cord is a demyelinating disease associated with pernicious anemia. Myelin loss is caused by failure to synthesize methionine. The clinical picture is complicated by 'glove-and-stocking' anesthesia caused by peripheral neuropathy in the longest sensory nerves.

Other causes of sensory ataxia include spinal cord tumor and local vascular disease.

A standard test for sensory ataxia is the *heel-to-knee test*, in which the recumbent patient is asked to place his heel on the opposite knee. He may succeed under visual guidance but he will miss the target if his eyes are closed. (In cerebellar ataxia he will be equally inept whether his eyes are open or closed.) A corresponding test for the upper limb is the *finger-to-nose test*, the patient being asked to place his index finger on the tip of his nose with his eyes closed. This is a test of the integrity of the fasciculus cuneatus.

Motor neuron disease
Motor neuron disease (MND) occurs sporadically throughout the world; its etiology is unknown. Onset is usually between 50 and 70 years of age. If motoneurons alone are affected the disorder is called *progressive muscular atrophy*. Usually the corticospinal tract also degenerates, in which circumstance *amyotrophic lateral sclerosis* is a common term. MND is characterized by wasting, with attendant weakness in the muscles of the upper limbs (especially of the hands and of the shoulder girdle), accompanied (sooner or later) by evidence of corticospinal tract impairment in the lower limbs (Chapter 20). The motor cranial nerves may be involved either initially (*progressive bulbar palsy*) or owing to rostral extension of MND. Fasciculation and fibrillation (Chapter 4) are prominent features in the affected muscles. *The complete absence of sensory symptoms and signs distinguishes MND from other disorders.*

Spinal cord injury
Automobile accidents are the commonest cause of spinal cord injury. Acute flexion of the neck may follow front-end collisions, and acute extension (whiplash) may follow rear-end collision. Either may produce fracture–dislocation above or below vertebra C6, or cause acute prolapse of a cervical intervertebral disc. Direct injury to the spine may produce fracture–dislocation at any level.

Injury to the cord at a thoracic or lumbar segmental level results in *paraplegia* (paralysis of the lower limbs). Injury at cervical level causes *tetraplegia*, in which the extent of upper limb paralysis will depend upon the number of cervical segments involved.

The principal features of complete transection of the cord are: (a) *paralysis of movement* and (b) *loss of all sensation* below the segmental level of injury. In addition, the patient may experience pain from compression of the emerging spinal nerves at the level of vertebral injury ('root pain'). At the initial examination, attention is directed to the possibility of other, life-threatening injuries, for example to the head, larynx, rib cage, or internal organs. Internal injuries may be difficult to detect if sensation has been cut off by a high spinal injury.

Spinal shock
During the first three to four weeks after injury the body below the lesion appears 'dead', although the circulation continues. The limbs are flaccid (floppy), there is no resistance to passive movement at the joints, and reflexes are absent.

Return of spinal function
Muscle tone – defined as the resistance to passive movement of the joints – returns during the second month, and it may become excessive. Tendon reflexes reappear and may become abnormally brisk.

Spastic paraplegia is the final state. The paralyzed lower limbs show increased muscle tone, exaggerated tendon

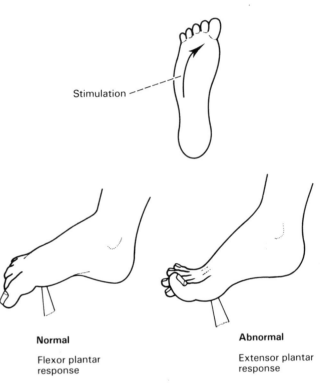

Stimulation ---

Normal

Flexor plantar response

Abnormal

Extensor plantar response

Fig. 11-11 Plantar reflex, showing the Babinski sign – an extensor plantar response to a stimulus applied to the sole.

reflexes, Babinski sign, and ankle clonus. All of these features indicate injury to the pyramidal tract. Their genesis is discussed in Chapter 20. The *Babinski sign* (extensor plantar response) consists of dorsiflexion of the great toe and fanning of the other toes, in response to a noxious stimulus applied to the sole of the foot, such as a nail file dragged along the sole (Fig. 11-11). The normal response is plantar flexion of the toes.

Ankle clonus is a rhythmic plantar flexion of the ankle (5–10 per second) in response to sustained passive dorsiflexion.

Sensory levels
The transition from anesthetic to normal skin is abrupt. Reference levels for the trunk are given below:

Upper limit of anesthesia	Upper limit of cord injury	Upper limit of vertebral injury
Nipples	T5	T4
Xiphisternal joint	T7	T6
Umbilicus	T10	T8
Groin	L1	T11

At the sternal angle, C4 dermatome meets T2 dermatome. Between these two, the level of injury must be sought in the upper limbs (Chapter 8).

Autonomic functions

The autonomic pathway to the sacral cord is interrupted by a lesion at any segmental level. During the stage of spinal shock the bladder and rectum are atonic. Urine dribbles away from a distended bladder (*overflow incontinence*) unless a catheter is introduced to prevent stagnation with its attendant risks of urinary infection and backpressure on the kidneys. After four to eight weeks the bladder empties reflexly every four to six hours (*automatic bladder*), and daily reflex emptying of the rectum can be induced by stimulating the anal canal. However, automatic emptying does not develop if the conus is directly injured.

Although sexual sensation is abolished, procreation is not impossible for paraplegics. If the conus is intact, penile erection can be induced by manipulation. The ejaculation reflex will follow if the cord is intact up to T10 (Chapter 41).

Conus syndrome

Direct injury to the conus terminalis destroys many or all of the sacral–segmental neurons. Necrosis of the intermediolateral cell column paralyzes bladder and rectum (Chapter 40) and causes impotence (Chapter 41). Necrosis of anterior and posterior gray horns causes weakness of movement in the feet (see Fig. 8-20) and loss of sensation in the buttocks, but not in the back of the lower limbs, because of sensory overlap there.

Conus syndrome may be caused by injury to vertebra L1 or prolapse of the L1/L2 intervertebral disc. It is occasionally caused by surgeons, during abdominal operations close to the aorta (nephrectomy, adrenalectomy, sympathectomy or aortic grafts), by injury to the artery of Adamkiewicz.

Hemisection of the cord (Fig. 11-12)

In this rare but well-known condition conduction is blocked on one or other side of the spinal cord to the midline, for instance by a tumor or fractured vertebra. *On the ipsilateral side* there is spastic weakness (interruption of the lateral corticospinal tract), and loss of position, kinesthetic and vibration sense. *On the contralateral side* there is loss of pain and temperature sensation (interruption of spinothalamic fibers, after crossing). Tactile sensation is preserved because it is mediated in part by the contralateral (unaffected) posterior funiculus. The condition is known as the *Brown-Séquard syndrome*.

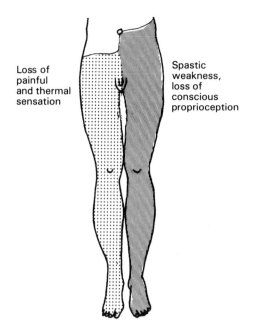

Loss of painful and thermal sensation

Spastic weakness, loss of conscious proprioception

Fig. 11-12 Brown-Séquard syndrome, lesion at segment T10, on patient's left side.

Readings

Ashby, P., Verrier, M. and Lightfoot, E. (1974) Segmental reflex pathways in spinal shock and spinal spasticity in man. *J. Neurol. Neurosurg. Psychiatry*, 37: 1352–1360.

Cope, T.C., Nelson, S.G. and Mendall, L.M. (1980) Selectivity in synaptic changes caudal to acute spinal cord transection. *Neurosci. Lett.*, 20: 289–294.

Dimitrijevic, M.R. and Nathan, P.W. (1970) Studies of spasticity in man. 4. Changes in flexion reflex with repetitive cutaneous stimulation in spinal man. *Brain*, 93: 743–768.

FitzGerald, M.J.T. (1978) *Human Embryology: A Regional Approach.* Hagerstown: Harper & Row.

Harris, W.A. (1981) Neural activity and development. *Annu. Rev. Physiol.*, 43: 689–710.

Ischia, S., Luzzani, A., Ischia, A. and Maffezzoli, G. (1984) Bilateral percutaneous cervical cordotomy: immediate and long-term results in 36 patients with neoplastic disease. *J. Neurol. Neurosurg. Psychiatry*, 47: 141–147.

Kalsbeck, W.D., McLaurin, R.L., Harris, B.S.H. and Miller, J.D. (1980) The national head and spinal cord injury survey. *J. Neurosurg. (Suppl)*: S19–S31.

Karfunkel, P. (1974) The mechanisms of neural tube formation. *Int. Rev. Cytol.*, 38: 245–271.

Kurtzke, J.F. (1982) Motor neurone disease. *Br. Med. J.*, 284: 141–142.

Lemire, R.J. (1975) *Normal and Abnormal Development of the Human Nervous System.* Hagerstown: Harper & Row.

Meier, C. (1976) Some observations on early myelination in the human spinal cord. Light and electron microscope study. *Brain Res.*, 104: 21–32.

Merrit, J.L. (1981) Management of spasticity in spinal cord injury. *Mayo Clin. Proc.*, 56: 614–622.

Okado, N. (1980) Development of the human cervical spinal cord with reference to synapse formation in the motor nucleus. *J. Comp. Neurol.*, 191: 495–513.

O'Rahilly, R. and Gardner, E. (1979) The initial development of the human brain. *Acta Anat. (Basel)*, 104: 123–133.

Padget, D.H. (1970) Neuroschisis and human embryonic development. *J. Neuropathol. Exp. Neurol.*, 29: 192–216.

Peach, B. (1965) The Arnold–Chiari malformation: morphogenesis. *Arch. Neurol.*, 12: 527–535.

Rodriguez, M. and Dinapoli, R.P. (1980) Spinal cord compression with special reference to metastatic epidural tumors. *Mayo Clin. Proc.*, 55: 442–448.

Rokos, J. (1975) Pathogenesis of diastematomyelia and spina bifida. *J. Pathol.*, 117: 155–161.

Rokos, J. (1979) The pathogenesis of spina bifida and related malformations. *Recent Adv. Neuropathol.*, 10: 225–245.

Rowland, L.P. (1984) Motoneuron diseases and amytrophic lateral sclerosis. *Trends Neurosci.*, 7: 110–112.

Scott, R. and Grant, J.C. (1969) Spina bifida cystica: a review of 150 patients. *Scott. Med. J.*, 14: 194–199.

White, R.J. and Albin, M.S. (1970) Spine and spinal cord injury. In *Impact Injury and Crash Protection* (Gurdjian, E.S., Lange, U.A., Patrick, L.M. and Thomas, L.M., eds.), pp. 63–85. Springfield: Thomas.

IV
BRAIN STEM AND CEREBELLUM

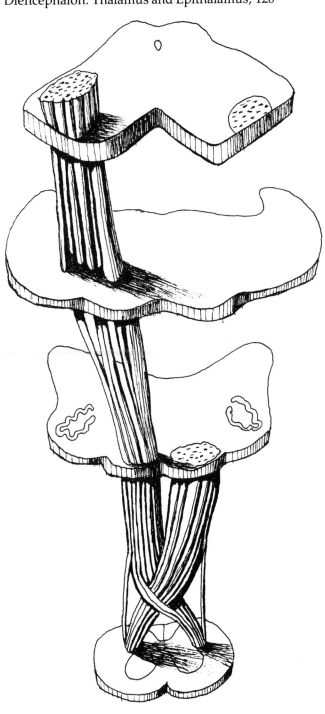

12

Brain Stem

The term 'brain stem', as used here, refers to the medulla oblongata, pons, and midbrain.

SURFACE FEATURES IN VENTRAL VIEW (Fig. 12-1)

Medulla oblongata

The ventral surface of the medulla oblongata shows a *pyramid* on each side of the midline. The pyramid contains the entire corticospinal tract, and the term *pyramidal tract* is synonymous. Most corticospinal fibers cross the midline at the spinomedullary junction, and the *pyramidal decussation* (intersection) fills the anterior median fissure at this level.

Lateral to the pyramid is the *olive*, which contains the inferior olivary nucleus. The rootlets of the hypoglossal nerve are attached between pyramid and olive. Those of the glossopharyngeal, vagus, and cranial accessory are attached behind the olive. The rootlets of the spinal accessory nerve emerge from the side of the spinal cord and run upward to join the cranial accessory. The abducent, facial and vestibulo-cochlear nerves are attached at the pontomedullary junction.

Pons

The ventral surface of the pons is grooved transversely. The attachment of the trigeminal nerve marks the conventional separation of the pons from the middle cerebellar peduncle. The latter is almost entirely composed of transversely running fibers which commence on the contralateral side of the pons.

Midbrain

The ventral part of the midbrain is divided into two *cerebral peduncles*. The longitudinal ridging on the surface of the peduncles is created by corticopontine and corticospinal fibers; the corticospinal fibers create a bulge on each side of the pons as they descend to form the pyramids. The oculomotor nerves emerge on the medial side of the cerebral peduncles.

SURFACE FEATURES IN DORSAL VIEW (Fig. 12-2)

A dorsal view of the brain stem is obtained by removing the cerebellum, which is attached to it by three cerebellar peduncles on each side.

On the dorsal aspect of the medulla the *gracile* and *cuneate tubercles* contain the gracile and cuneate nuclei. Rostral to them are the *inferior cerebellar peduncles* which turn behind the lower pons to enter the cerebellum.

The *middle cerebellar peduncles* enter the cerebellum from the pons. The *superior cerebellar peduncles* leave the cerebellum and plunge into the brain stem at the junction of pons and midbrain. They cross (intersect)

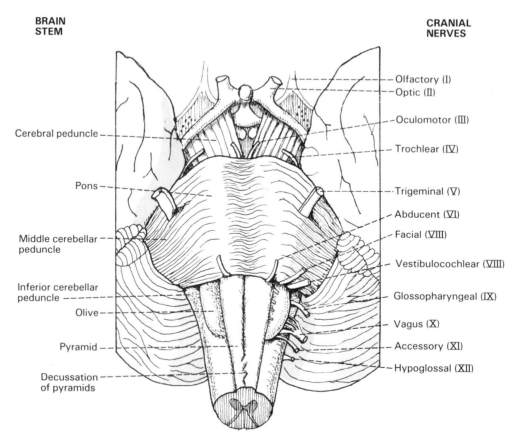

BRAIN STEM

CRANIAL NERVES

Cerebral peduncle

Pons

Middle cerebellar peduncle

Inferior cerebellar peduncle

Olive

Pyramid

Decussation of pyramids

Olfactory (I)
Optic (II)
Oculomotor (III)
Trochlear (IV)
Trigeminal (V)
Abducent (VI)
Facial (VII)
Vestibulocochlear (VIII)
Glossopharyngeal (IX)
Vagus (X)
Accessory (XI)
Hypoglossal (XII)

Fig. 12-1 Brain stem and cranial nerves, from below.

in the lower midbrain en route to the thalamus of the opposite side.

The dorsal part of the midbrain is the *tectum* (L., roof), composed of four *colliculi* (L., little hills). The trochlear nerves emerge below the inferior pair of colliculi and wind around the midbrain.

The *fourth ventricle* is the diamond space bounded by the cerebellar peduncles and roofed by the cerebellum. The pons and upper medulla form its floor, the dividing line between pons and medulla being drawn across the lower borders of the middle peduncles. The fourth ventricle is an expansion of the central canal of the CNS. Cerebrospinal fluid descends the aqueduct of the midbrain to reach it. Although the ventricle is continuous with the central canal of the spinal cord, most of the CSF escapes into the subarachnoid space surrounding the brain and cord, through *median* and *lateral apertures*.

Ventral to the central canal of the brain stem is the *tegmentum*, and in front of this is the *basilar region*.

TRANSVERSE SECTIONS OF THE BRAIN STEM

The eight sections illustrated are taken at the levels indicated in Fig. 12-3.

Spinomedullary junction (Fig. 12-4)

The chief feature is the decussation of the lateral corticospinal tracts, which pass through the base of the anterior gray horns at the uppermost cervical level. At higher levels of the brain stem, motoneurons homologous with those of the cord are confined to the central gray matter.

The ascending and descending tracts enumerated in the cord (Chapters 9, 10) are present in the white matter. However, the posterolateral tract of Lissauer has merged with the (homologous) *spinal root of the trigeminal nerve*. The *spinal nucleus* of the trigeminal replaces substantia gelatinosa and nucleus proprius.

Middle of medulla oblongata (Fig. 12-5)

Most ventral are the pyramids, above the pyramidal decussation. Dorsal to them are the *medial lemnisci*, formed by second-order fibers from the dorsal column nuclei of the opposite side. The intersection of these *internal arcuate fibers* is known as the *sensory decussation*.

Dorsal to the lemnisci are the medial *longitudinal fasciculi*, which run the entire length of the brain stem and end in the cervical part of the cord. These fasciculi form a pathway involved in the coordinated movement of the eyes and head (Chapter 33).

The central gray matter contains three nuclear groups on each side. The *hypoglossal nucleus* gives rise to the hypoglossal nerve which supplies the muscles of the tongue. The *dorsal motor nucleus of the vagus nerve* supplies preganglionic fibers to the vagus. The *nucleus solitarius* extends from mid-medulla to lower pons. At medullary level it receives visceral afferent fibers from the glossopharyngeal and vagus nerves.

Note: Elements of the *reticular formation* seen in this and later sections are considered in Chapters 14 and 15.

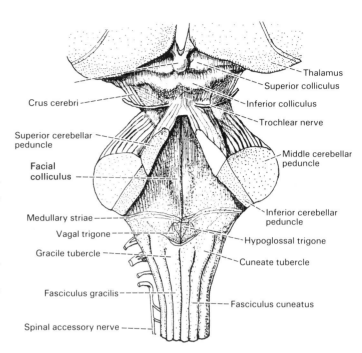

Fig. 12-2 Brain stem, from above, with cerebellum removed.

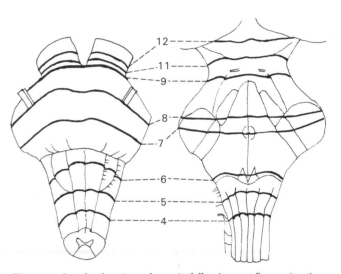

Fig. 12-3 Levels of sections shown in following text figures (section 4 is shown in Fig. 12-4, section 5 in Fig. 12-5, and so on).

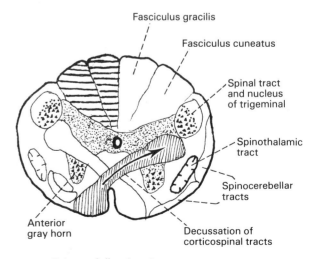

Fig. 12-4 Spinomedullary junction.

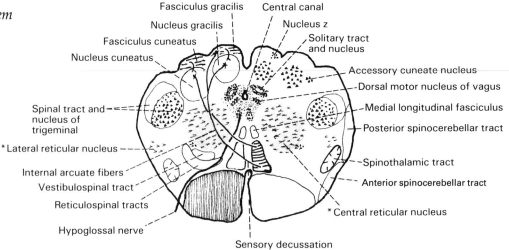

Fig. 12-5 Middle of medulla oblongata. (Nucleus z is slightly rostral to the level indicated here.) The solitary tract occupies the center of the nucleus solitarius. *Indicates an element of the reticular formation.*

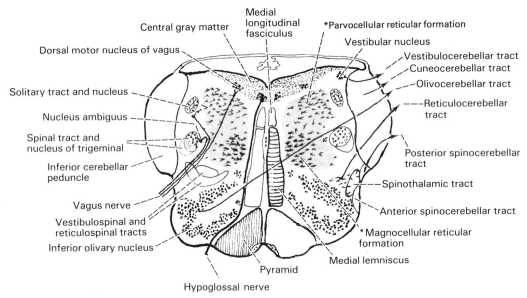

Fig. 12-6 Upper third of medulla oblongata. *Indicates an element of the reticular formation.*

Upper medulla oblongata (Fig. 12-6)

The lateral part of the tegmentum is filled by the *inferior olivary nucleus*. Dorsal to this is the *nucleus ambiguus* which supplies the muscles of the larynx and pharynx. The central gray matter lines the floor of the fourth ventricle. The inferior cerebellar peduncle is a prominent landmark at this level.

Pons

The massive basilar region contains the *pontine nuclei* and the *transverse fibers*. The nuclei receive *corticopontine fibers* from the ipsilateral cerebral cortex, and the transverse fibers are *pontocerebellar* axons passing to the contralateral cerebellar hemisphere. Some of the corticopontine fibers split the corticospinal tract into fascicles but they do not interrupt it.

The medial longitudinal fasciculi at pontine levels contain fibers ascending from the vestibular nuclei to the nuclei controlling the extrinsic muscles of the eyeballs. The *posterior longitudinal fasciculi* occupy the central gray matter. Their largest elements are autonomic fibers descending from the hypothalamus to autonomic nuclei in the brain stem.

The *central tegmental tract* (more properly, central tegmental fasciculus) contains fibers of several kinds. Most numerous are rubro-olivary, running from the red nucleus to the inferior olivary nucleus on the same side.

The medial lemniscus and spinothalamic tract occupy the most ventral part of the tegmentum. They are joined by the *trigeminothalamic tract*, which arises in the trigeminal sensory nuclei and crosses the midline.

Level of facial colliculus (Fig. 12-7)

The facial colliculus is created by the facial nerve as it encircles the abducens nucleus. The *superior olivary nucleus* lies on the central auditory pathway. It contributes to the *lateral lemniscus*, which enters the inferior colliculus of the midbrain.

Level of trigeminal nerve (Fig. 12-8)

The *motor nucleus* of the trigeminal innervates the muscles of mastication. The main *sensory nucleus* receives tactile sensations from the peripheral territory

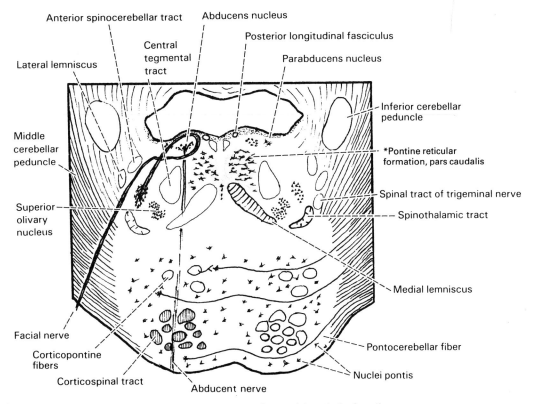

Fig. 12-7 Pons, level of facial colliculus. *Indicates an element of the reticular formation.*

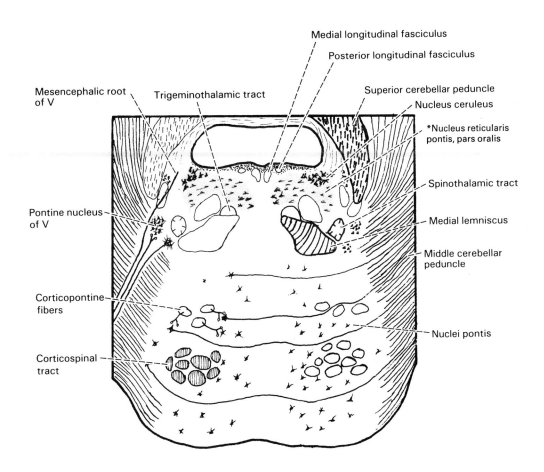

Fig. 12-8 Pons, level of trigeminal nerve (V). *Indicates an element of the reticular formation.*

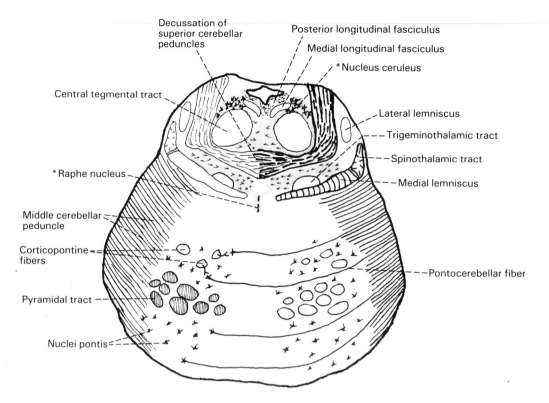

Fig. 12-9 Upper limit of pons. *Indicates an element of the reticular formation.

of the trigeminal (skin of face, mucous membranes of oral and nasal cavities). The *mesencephalic root* of the trigeminal ascends to the midbrain.

Pontomesencephalic junction (Fig. 12-9)

The superior cerebellar peduncles are converging. They decussate here and in the lower midbrain.

Midbrain (mesencephalon)

The named regions in midbrain sections are indicated in Fig. 12-10. The *tectum* is the region dorsal to the central canal. The ventral part of the cerebral peduncle is the *crus cerebri*; it contains corticopontine, corticobulbar and corticospinal fibers. The tegmentum extends from tectum to crus cerebri on each side.

Level of inferior colliculi (Fig. 12-11)

The decussation of the superior cerebellar peduncles is obvious. The medial and trigeminal lemnisci, and the spinothalamic tract, are displaced laterally by the decussation. The lateral lemniscus is entering the inferior colliculus.

    The mesencephalic nucleus of the trigeminal nerve occupies the lateral edge of the central gray matter. The most ventral part of the central gray matter contains the nucleus of the trochlear nerve.

    The most ventral element in the tegmentum is the *substantia nigra*. The substantia nigra comprises a *pars compacta*, filled with pigmented neurons, and a *pars reticulata*, ventrally, having non-pigmented neurons.

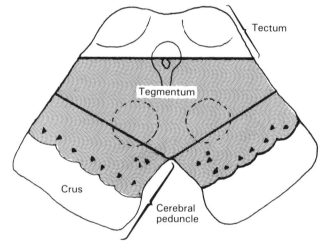

Fig. 12-10 The parts of the midbrain. The tegmentum is the shaded area.

Level of superior colliculi (Fig. 12-12)

The *red nucleus* is a prominent feature of the tegmentum on each side. It is pink in the fresh brain because of a relatively high iron content. It is pierced by the emerging axons of the oculomotor nerve.

    Between the red nucleus and the substantia nigra is the *ventral tegmental area* (VTA) (of Tsai). The VTA contains neurons identical to those of substantia nigra, pars compacta. The pigment is *neuromelanin*, a by-product of the synthesis of *dopamine*. Dopamine is the transmitter substance for both sets of neurons. The nigrostriatal dopaminergic pathway runs from the

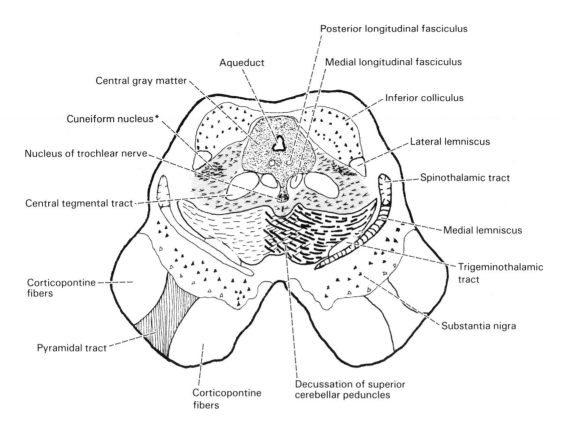

Fig. 12-11 Midbrain, level of inferior colliculi. *Indicates an element of the reticular formation.*

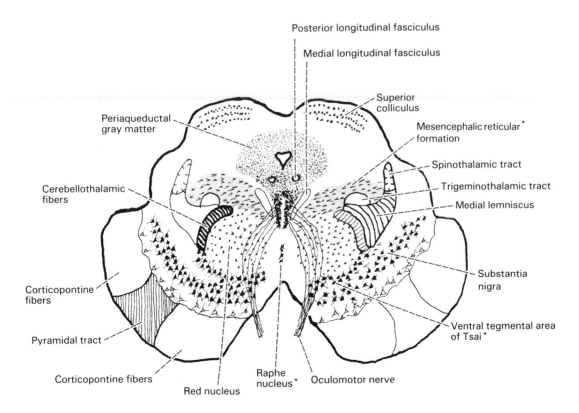

Fig. 12-12 Midbrain, level of superior colliculi. *Indicates an element of the reticular formation.*

substantia nigra to the striatum (a large basal forebrain nucleus). Degeneration of nigrostriatal neurons is associated with Parkinson's disease (Chapter 18). From the VTA, dopaminergic neurons enter the *mesolimbic pathway*, which supplies the limbic structures of the forebrain (Chapter 21). Excess activity in the mesolimbic pathway is thought to be related to the onset of schizophrenia.

The most ventral part of the central gray matter contains the *oculomotor nucleus*. The oculomotor nerve passes through the red nucleus before emerging on the medial side of the cerebral peduncle.

BLOOD SUPPLY OF BRAIN STEM AND CEREBELLUM

The brain stem and cerebellum are supplied by the vertebral and basilar arteries (Fig. 12-13). The two vertebrals unite at the lower border of the pons, to form the basilar. Before uniting, they give off the anterior and posterior spinal arteries, which supply the spinal cord. Each vertebral gives off a posterior inferior cerebellar artery (absent in a quarter of cases). Anterior inferior and superior cerebellar arteries give branches to the side of the brain stem. The *labyrinthine artery* arises from the anterior inferior cerebellar or basilar. A dozen or more *pontine arteries* also arise from the basilar.

The basilar artery gives some branches to the midbrain before dividing into two *posterior cerebral arteries*. The posterior cerebrals and the posterior communicating give further branches to the midbrain.

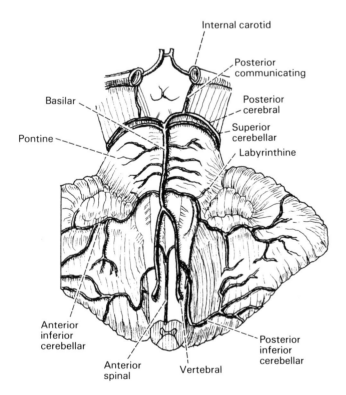

Fig. 12-13 Arterial supply of brain stem.

APPLIED ANATOMY

Brain stem lesions occur quite frequently and may represent an immediate threat to the patient's life or a delayed threat from complications such as aspiration pneumonia. Prompt accurate diagnosis is essential and this can best be achieved with a sound anatomical knowledge and an idea of the common causes of brain stem disease and their clinical behaviour. Patten, 1980

Note: The following account may be read more profitably following study of the cranial nerves in later chapters.

Vascular disorders
Transient ischemic attacks, lasting about 15 minutes, are quite common in the elderly. *Vertebrobasilar ischemia* (brain stem ischemia) is suspected when patients report transient attacks of vertigo or diplopia (double vision), stiffness or numbness in the limbs or face on one side, or tingling sensations around the mouth. Symptoms tend to vary from one episode to the next.

Thrombosis in the vertebrobasilar system usually affects a single lateral or medial branch supplying the brain stem. The result is a lateral or medial wedge-shaped infarct (necrosis). Various eponymous names have been given to these infarcts. The symptomatology is often complex but it arises directly from the regional anatomy.

Lateral and medial medullary syndromes
The effects of right-sided medullary infarcts are listed in Figs. 12-14 and 12-15. The two syndromes are combined following thrombosis of the parent vertebral artery. Thrombosis of the posterior inferior cerebellar artery may be difficult to distinguish from a pure lateral medullary infarct on clinical grounds, because cerebellar ataxia is present in either case.

Lateral and medial pontine syndromes
The effects of lateral and medial infarcts are listed in Figs. 12-16 and 12-17.

Acute hemorrhage into the pons may follow rupture of a medial or lateral branch of the basilar artery. Symptoms are very severe and are bilateral because of edema surrounding the hematoma. The symptom complex includes:
a coma, from disruption of the reticular formation;
b tetraplegia, from injury to both pyramidal tracts;
c pin-point pupils, from bilateral sympathetic paralysis;
d hyperpyrexia (temperature rising to 42°C (106°F) over several days) from injury to heat-losing pathways from the hypothalamus;
e periodic apnea (respiratory arrest) from injury to the pontine respiratory center.

Dorsal and ventral midbrain syndromes
The lateral arteries have larger territories than the medial ones; they extend to the midline. Accordingly, midbrain syndromes are dorsal and ventral. They are listed in Fig. 12-18.

Metabolic disorders of the brain stem may be caused by many drugs. Vertigo, nystagmus, and ataxia are side-effects of anticonvulsant drug therapy. Pyramidal tract signs are common in patients who are comatose from almost any drug overdose. 'Upgoing great toes' are *not* proof of organic disease in a patient first seen in coma.

Other primary brain stem disorders
Multiple sclerosis (MS) has a predelection for the brain stem. MS tends to affect the medial longitudinal fasciculus, the pyramidal and spinocerebellar tracts, the parasympathetic, and the fourth to eight cranial nerves as they pass through the white matter.

MS often presents with an initial brain stem lesion. MS must be suspected in a 20–40-year-old presenting with one

Left   Right

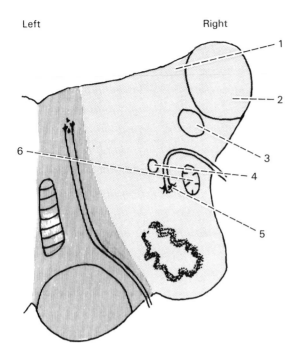

Fig. 12-14 Medullary vascular lesions on right side. A: Lateral medullary (Wallenberg's) syndrome.

On *right* 1 Vertigo, vomiting, nystagmus (vestibular nucleus)
              2 Ataxia of limbs (inferior cerebellar peduncle)
              3 Loss of pain and temperature sensation from face, loss of corneal reflex (spinal tract of trigeminal)
              4 Horner's syndrome (sympathetic)
              5 Dysphagia, hoarseness (nucleus ambiguus)
On *left*   6 Loss of pain and temperature sensation from trunk and limbs (lateral spinothalamic tract)

Note: In this and the later illustrations of vascular lesions, the brain stem sections are viewed from below.

Left   Right

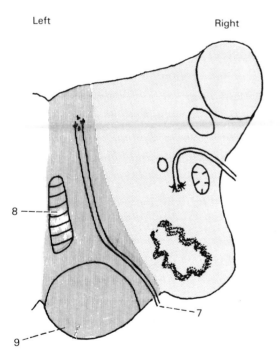

Fig. 12-15 Medullary vascular lesions on right side. B: Medial medullary syndrome.

On *right* 7 Wasting of tongue (hypoglossal)
On *left*   8 Loss of position sense in limbs (medial lemniscus)
              9 Hemiplegia, face spared (pyramid)

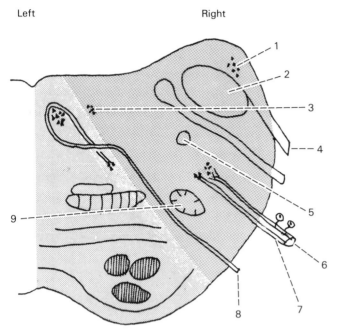

Left   Right

Fig. 12-16 Pontine vascular lesions on right side. A: Lateral pontine (Foville's) syndrome.

On *right* 1 Tinnitus or deafness (cochlear nerve)
2 Ataxia (inferior cerebellar peduncle)
3 Paralysis of conjugate gaze to right (parabducens nucleus)
4 Vertigo, vomiting, nystagmus (vestibular nerve)
5 Horner's syndrome (sympathetic)
6 Anesthesia of face (sensory root of trigeminal)
7 Weakness of jaw muscles (motor root of trigeminal)
8 Facial paralysis (facial nerve)

On *left* 9 Loss of pain and temperature sensation from trunk and limbs (spinothalamic tract)

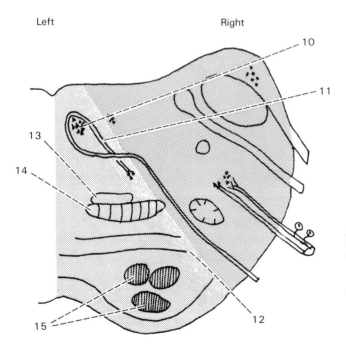

Left   Right

Fig. 12-17 Pontine vascular lesions on right side. B: Medial pontine (Millard–Gubler) syndrome.

On *right* 10 Paralysis of lateral rectus (abducens nucleus)
11 Facial paralysis (facial nerve)
12 Ataxia (transverse fibers of pons)

On *left* 13 Loss of pain and temperature sensation from face (trigeminothalamic tract)
14 Loss of position sense in limbs (medial lemniscus)
15 Hemiplegia (pyramidal tract)

Left   Right

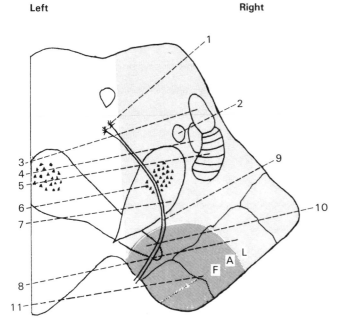

Fig. 12-18   Midbrain vascular lesions, right side. Dorsal midbrain (Claude's syndrome):
On *right* 1 Diplopia, dilated pupil (oculomotor nerve)
            2 Horner's syndrome (sympathetic). Pupil may be dilated or constricted because of 1. Ptosis may be partial (2) or complete (1 + 2)
On *left*   3 Loss of pain and temperature sensation from trunk and limbs (spinothalamic tract)
            4 Loss of pain and temperature sensation from face (trigeminothalamic tract)
            5 Loss of position sense in limbs (medial lemniscus)
            6 Resting tremor (red nucleus)
            7 Ataxia (left dentatothalamic tract, after crossing)
            8 Monoplegia (pyramidal tract, L, leg fibers)
Ventral midbrain (Weber's syndrome):
On *right* 9 Diplopia, dilated pupil (oculomotor nerve)
           10 Ataxia (right dentatothalamic tract, before crossing). This symptom may be absent
On *left* 11 Hemiplegia, mainly upper limb and face (pyramidal tract, A, arm, F, face fibers)
Note: Claude's syndrome plus Weber's syndrome is Benedikt's syndrome.

or more of the following symptoms: diplopia (medial longitudinal fasciculus, trochlear or abducent nerves), spastic weakness or ataxia of a limb, acute retention of urine, pain or numbness in the face, or vertigo. The possibility of a brain stem tumor must be borne in mind, but involvement of more than one part of the brain stem, or remission of a presenting symptom, suggests MS.

Chronic alcoholism may produce lethal disorders of the brain stem, in company with Wernicke's encephalopathy, which is characterized by gross mental confusion and memory loss. Disorders of ocular movement, ataxia, and nystagmus are the chief brain stem features. The brain stem disorders of alcoholism are readily reversed by vitamin B_1 injections. Brain stem disorders may also result from vitamin B_1 deficiency in disease of the small intestine.

Brain stem compression
Because of the outstanding clinical importance of eye signs, consideration of this topic is deferred to Chapter 31.

Readings

Heimer, L. (1983) *The Human Brain and Spinal Cord.* New York: Springer-Verlag.
Nieuwenhuys, R., Voogd, J. and van Huijzen, C. (1981) *The Human Nervous System: A Synopsis and Atlas,* 2nd ed. Berlin: Springer-Verlag.
Patten, J.P. (1980) *Neurological Differential Diagnosis.* London: Harold Stark.

13
Cerebellum

The cerebellum is responsible for the smooth contraction of groups of striated muscles, and for the smooth relaxation of their antagonists. This smoothing action is essential for movements of all kinds, whether automatic (as in postural adjustments) or voluntary. Cerebellar disease is characterized by clumsy, poorly coordinated movements and complete loss of fine motor control.

Phylogenetically, the oldest region of the cerebellum develops in relation to the labyrinth. The oldest region is mainly in the midline (vermal region), and it regulates the postural adjustment of the eyes and of the antigravity musculature that occurs in response to movements of the head. On each side of this, the 'intermediate' cerebellum is richly interconnected with the spinal cord. It regulates automatic movements of relatively slow nature, such as walking. Finally, the lateral parts of the hemispheres, which are uniquely large in the human brain, control highly skilled movements of all kinds, as well as rapid (ballistic) movements of individual body parts.

Each cerebellar hemisphere is primarily involved in controlling movement on the *same* side. The cerebral motor cortex initiates movements on the *opposite* side. The cerebellum exerts its motor control in large part by regulating the activity of the corticospinal tract. Accordingly, the two-way connections with the cerebral cortex cross the midline in the brain stem.

GROSS ANATOMY (Fig. 13-1)

The two hemispheres merge with the *vermis* in the midline. The entire surface of the cerebellum is fissurated, and 80% of the cortex lies on the concealed surfaces of the *folia* (L., leaves).

Roof nuclei (Fig. 13-2)

Buried in the white matter are the paired *roof nuclei* (in the roof of the fourth ventricle). The most medial on each side is the *fastigial* nucleus. The most lateral is the large, wrinkled, *dentate* nucleus. Intermediate in position is the *nucleus interpositus,* made up of the globose and emboliform nuclei.

Phylogeny (Fig. 13-3)

Archicerebellum and vestibulocerebellum

The *archicerebellum* developed in relation to the vestibular apparatus of fishes, and it coordinates movements of the eyes and of the trunk. In mammals, the archicerebellum is represented by the *flocculonodular lobe* and the fastigial nucleus. Both are intimately connected with the nucleus of the vestibular nerve. They have a major function in controlling movements

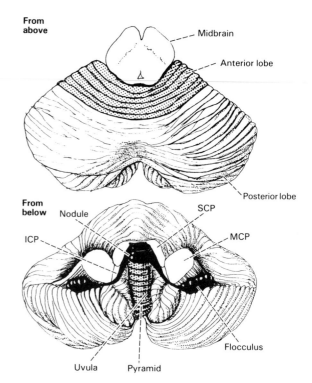

Fig. 13-1 Views of the cerebellum. ICP, MCP, SCP, inferior, middle, and superior cerebellar peduncles. The nodule, uvula, and pyramid belong to the vermis.

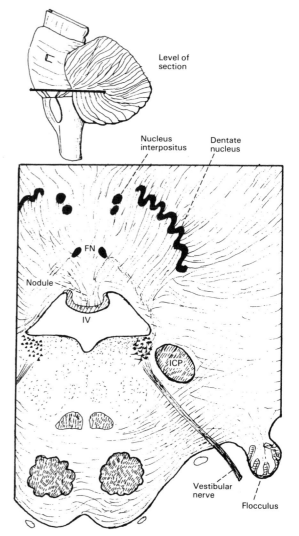

Fig. 13-2 Transverse section at lower border of pons. FN, fastigial nucleus; ICP, inferior cerebellar peduncle; IV, fourth ventricle.

94

of the eyes and trunk in response to changes in the position of the head. Physiological studies have shown that ocular control resides in the full extent of the dorsal vermis as well. The dorsal vermis and flocculonodular lobe are together called the *vestibulocerebellum*.

Paleocerebellum, spinocerebellum

In reptiles, movements of the trunk and limbs are quite elaborate. They are controlled by the *paleocerebellum*, which is represented in the mammals by the *anterior lobe* and the pyramid and uvula. Its effector nucleus is the interpositus. The paleocerebellum receives proprioceptive and exteroceptive information from the trunk and limbs and it is concerned in the control of posture. In mammals, the spinocerebellar tracts have extended their territory to the entire paravermal cerebellum, which is now called the *spinocerebellum*. However, no part of the mammalian cerebellum is entirely devoid of spinal afferents. Effector control of the anterior gray horn in lower mammals is by way of the rubrospinal tracts. In humans, the nuclear interpositus plays mainly upon the trunk area of the opposite motor cortex by way of the thalamus.

Neocerebellum, pontocerebellum

The *neocerebellum* develops in proportion to the emergence of skilled movements. In the human brain it forms 90% of the total cerebellar cortex. It receives 20 million afferents from association areas of the cerebral cortex, via the nuclei pontis. The term *pontocerebellum* is used to acknowledge the huge cerebral input through the middle cerebellar peduncle. The cortico-pontocerebellar input produces the massive basilar region of the pons, pushing the sixth, seventh, and eighth cranial nerves to its lower border. The effector nucleus of the pontocerebellum is the dentate, which projects strongly to the arm and hand areas of the opposite motor cortex via the thalamus.

MICROSCOPIC ANATOMY (Figs. 13-4, 13-5)

Purkinje cells

Cortical structure is uniform throughout the cerebellum. The principal neuron is the *Purkinje cell*, which has the largest dendritic tree of any neuron in the CNS. The Purkinje dendrites all lie in the same vertical plane. They occupy the *molecular layer* of the cortex. *The axons of Purkinje cells constitute the sole output of the cerebellar cortex.* They synapse upon somas and proximal dendrites within the roof nuclei. Their transmitter is GABA, and their function is to produce *selective inhibition* of relay cells in the roof nuclei. They also give recurrent collateral branches capable of inhibiting neighboring Purkinje cells.

Granule cells

The most numerous cell type in the cortex is the *granule cell*. The somas of granule cells are the size of

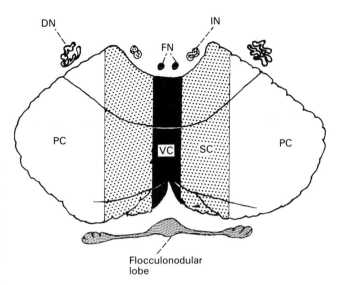

Fig. 13-3 Vestibulocerebellum (VC), spinocerebellum (SC), pontocerebellum (PC). Respective deep nuclei: fastigial (FN), interpositus (IN), dentate (DN).

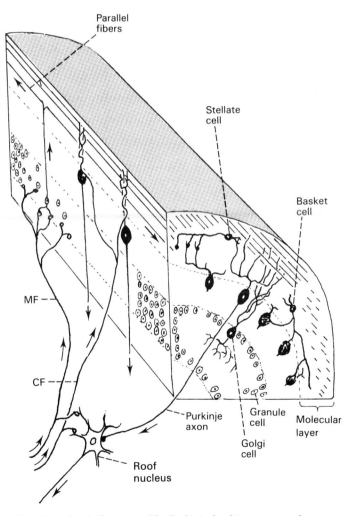

Fig. 13-4 Cerebellar cortex. The Purkinje dendrites are spread at right angles to the plane of the folia – for example, sagittally in the shaded areas of Fig. 13-3. CF, climbing fiber; MF, mossy fiber.

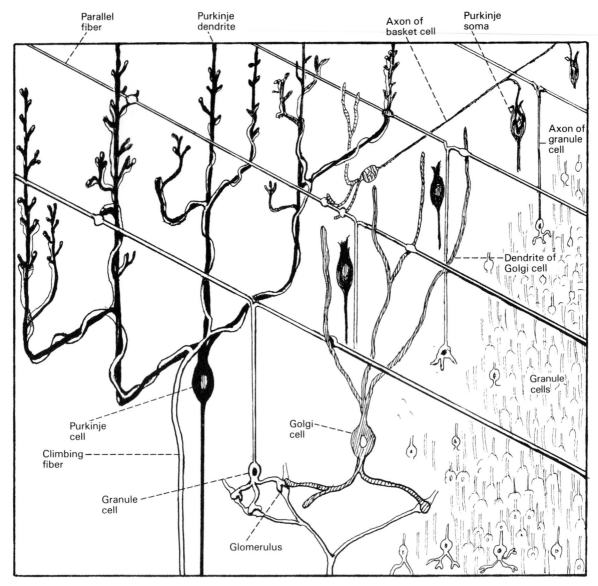

Fig. 13-5 Cerebellar cortex. Schematic.

erythrocytes, and their total number is of the order of 4 × 10^10 – nearly equal to the number of neurons in the two cerebral hemispheres!

The granule cells have small, claw-like dendrites which receive afferents from the vestibular nucleus, spinocerebellar tracts, and pontine nuclei. These afferents are known as *mossy fibers* (Fig. 13-6).

The axons of the granule cells enter the molecular layer and divide in a T-shaped manner to form *parallel fibers*. The parallel fibers run at right angles to the plane of the Purkinje dendrites. The granule cells are the *only* excitatory neurons in the cortex, and their transmitter is glutamate. Because of the geometry, a single granule cell can excite hundreds of Purkinje cells.

Stellate, basket and Golgi cells

All three are GABAergic internuncials. All three are excited by parallel fibers. The somas of the first two occupy the molecular layer, the third the granular layer. The stellate cells inhibit Purkinje dendrites (Fig.

13-7). The basket cells form baskets of inhibitory nerve endings around Purkinje somas and initial axonal segments. Axons of Golgi cells form enormous bushes which synapse (in the main) upon the claw-like dendrites of granule cells.

CEREBELLAR AFFERENTS (Table 13-1)

Several of the *mossy fiber afferents* have already been mentioned. The list comprises direct and indirect afferents from spinal cord and brain stem, and indirect afferents from the cerebral cortex. From a clinical standpoint the most important are the vestibulocerebellar, spinocerebellar, and corticopontocerebellar. The vestibulocerebellar fibers are considered further in Chapter 33. The spinocerebellar contain exteroceptive as well as proprioceptive information, and (in animals) it has been possible to construct somatotopic exteroceptive maps on the spinocerebellar cortex. Corticopontocerebellar afferents include a minority which relay in *arcuate nuclei* on the ventral

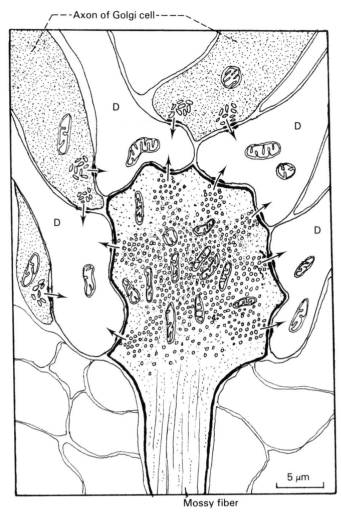

Fig. 13-6 A synaptic glomerulus. The mossy fiber terminal (called a rosette) synapses upon granule-cell dendrites (D) which receive inhibitory synapses from Golgi cells.

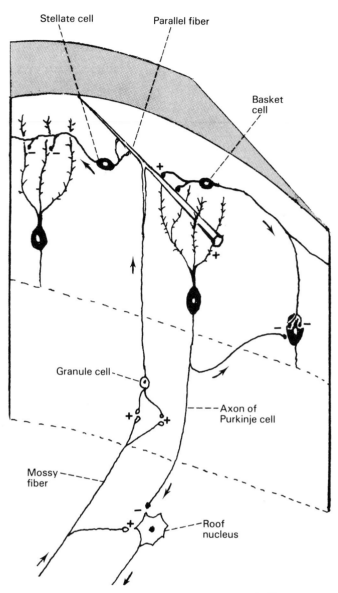

Fig. 13-7 One Purkinje cell shown is excited by parallel fibers. Surround inhibition is produced by parallel-fiber excitation of stellate and basket cells, and by recurrent collaterals of Purkinje cells. +, excitatory transmitter; −, inhibitory transmitter.

surface of the pyramids in the medulla oblongata. They are continued as *external arcuate* fibers which form a variable number of *medullary striae* in the floor of the fourth ventricle (Fig. 13-8).

Climbing fiber afferents are received from the contralateral inferior and accessory olivary nuclei. These nuclei receive descending fibers from the motor cortex and red nucleus. They receive ascending, *spino-olivary* fibers from all segments of the spinal cord, in the form of collaterals from crossed exteroceptive (spinothalamic) and proprioceptive (anterior spinocerebellar) pathways. The inferior olivary nucleus projects to the neocerebellum, the accessory to the spinocerebellum.

Each olivocerebellar fiber gives a single climbing fiber to each of several Purkinje cells. The climbing fibers twine along the Purkinje dendritic trees like ivy (Fig. 13-5).

CEREBELLAR EFFERENTS (Table 13-1)

Vestibulocerebellum

The fastigial nucleus projects to the nucleus of the vestibular nerve, where it controls the vestibulo-ocular and vestibulospinal reflexes. These reflexes elicit postural changes of the eyes and trunk in response to movements of the head (Chapter 33).

Table 13-1 Phylogeny and connections of deep cerebellar nuclei

Roof nucleus	Phylogeny	Afferents		Efferents
		Excitatory	*Inhibitory*	
Fastigial	Archicerebellum ('vestibulocerebellum')	Vestibular nucleus	Purkinje cells	Vestibular nucleus
Globose Emboliform	Paleocerebellum ('spinocerebellum')	Spinal cord	Purkinje cells	Red nucleus, reticular formation
Dentate	Neocerebellum ('pontocerebellum')	Cerebrum via pontine nuclei	Purkinje cells	Motor cortex via thalamus

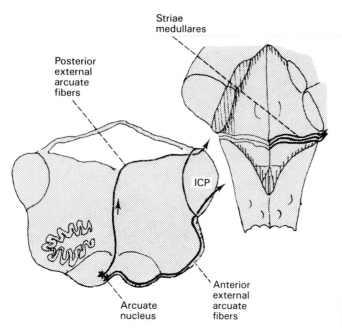

Fig. 13-8 Arcuatocerebellar fibers. ICP, inferior cerebellar peduncle.

Spinocerebellum (Fig. 13-9)

The nucleus interpositus influences anterior horn cells via reticulospinal and corticospinal pathways. Cerebelloreticular fibers modulate the firing of the pontine and medullary reticulospinal tracts. Cerebellothalamic fibers are relayed to the trunk area of the motor cortex. The significance of the substantial input to the opposite red nucleus is not understood.

Pontocerebellum (Fig. 13-10)

The involvement of the lateral cerebellum in skilled movements is reflected in the projection of half a million fibers by the dentate nucleus to the arm and hand areas of the opposite motor cortex, by way of the thalamus. The dentatothalamic tract makes up more than 90% of the superior cerebellar peduncle. Some of its fibers are relayed to other parts of the motor cortex because the lateral cerebellum is also concerned in preprogramming ballistic (fast) voluntary movements of all kinds.

ELECTRICAL ACTIVITY

Mossy fiber effects

A single mossy fiber may excite as many as 8000 Purkinje cells. (There are 15 million Purkinje cells in all.) The enormous *divergence* of mossy fiber input arises because each mossy fiber excites about 20 granule cells, and every granule cell applies a single bouton to each of about 400 Purkinje cells over a distance of 3 mm. Granule cell excitation is not uniform, however, because mossy fibers from particular sources (e.g., spinocerebellar) are themselves excited *in groups*. The result is that the central members of a 'beam' of parallel fibers are excited to threshold while the peripheral members are merely facilitated. The function of the stellate and basket cells seems to be to 'focus the beam' by exerting lateral inhibition upon weakly excited Purkinje dendrites and somas (Fig. 13-7). The Golgi cells are believed to function as 'trip switches', eventually cutting off the granule cells under the core of the excited beam.

Climbing fiber effects

Experimental stimulation of a climbing fiber produces a dramatic response: a single action potential causes the client Purkinje cell to emit four or five spikes. This is not surprising on anatomical grounds since every climbing fiber makes about 300 excitatory contacts at the bases of the dendritic spines (the apices are the property of parallel fibers).

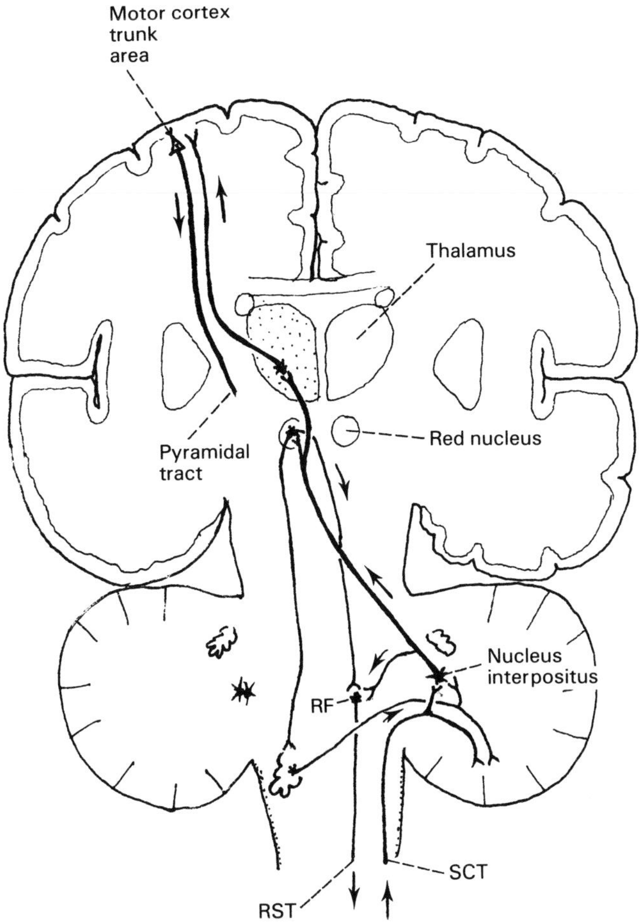

Fig. 13-9 Connections of spinocerebellum. RST, SCT, reticulospinal and spinocerebellar tracts. RF, reticular formation.

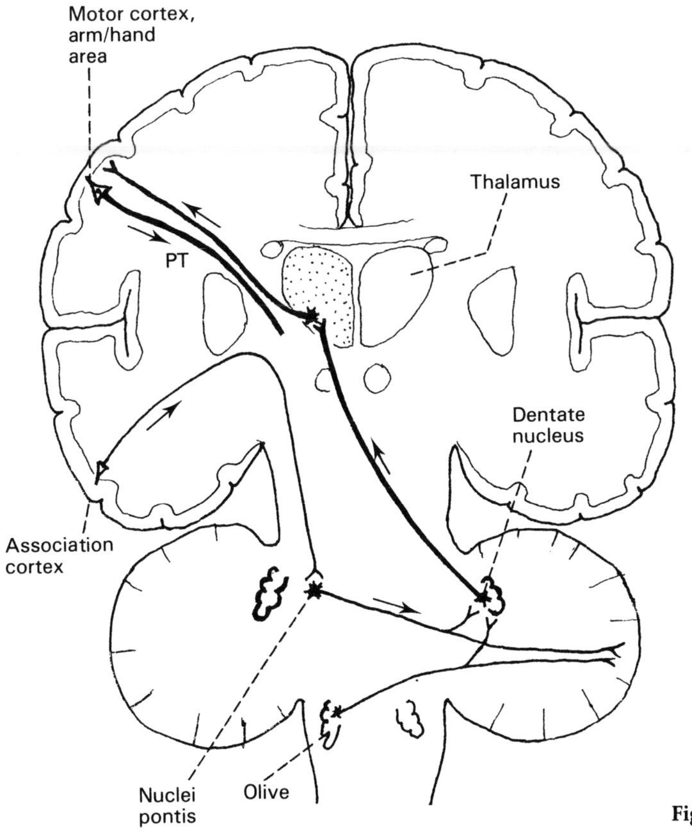

Fig. 13-10 Connections of pontocerebellum. PT, pyramidal tract.

The olive as teacher

It may be very significant that *mossy fibers are facilitated by prior olivocerebellar activity.* 'Imprinting' by the inferior olive may be significant in *motor learning*. The cerebellum is likely to be a repository of *motor programs* – in effect, executive subroutines which are activated by mossy fiber inputs, notably from the cerebral cortex.

A period of 800 ms elapses between a decision to move and the first discharge of impulses along the corticospinal tract. For monkeys, it is known that the dentate nucleus alters its basal firing rate *before* the corticospinal tract is activated, whereas the nucleus interpositus alters its firing rate *after* the movement has commenced. For this reason the neocerebellum is seen as preprogramming the movement, while the spinocerebellum is seen as giving follow-up correction once the movement is under way. Very rapid movements do not allow time for correction, and they are less accurate. In a game of tennis, the first service is less reliable than the slower, second service.

Monoamine-containing fibers in the cerebellum

Brain stem nuclei containing monoaminergic neurons are listed in Chapter 15. Two of them give branches to the cerebellar cortex: the nucleus (locus) ceruleus and the raphe nucleus.

The *nucleus (locus) ceruleus* in the pons, sends fine, beaded axons containing norepinephrine (noradrenaline) to all major parts of the central nervous system gray matter. In the cerebellum, they form a network in the molecular layer of the cortex, where they are capable of increasing the GABA-mediated inhibition of Purkinje cells by the stellate and basket cells there. The nucleus ceruleus is active during arousal (Chapter 14), and its cerebellar effect may be to increase the lateral inhibitory action of stellate and basket cells – in effect, to sharpen the edges of excited beams of Purkinje cells.

A second effect of norepinephrine is to facilitate the release of glutamate from parallel fibers onto 'on-beam' Purkinje cells. This effect would further improve the 'signal-to-noise' ratio ('noise' means spontaneous or weak background neuronal activity).

The *raphe nuclei* in the medulla oblongata give rise to a beaded network of axons containing serotonin. Some of these fibers reach the cerebellar cortex, but their function here is not understood. There is reason to suspect that the effects of serotonin in the cerebellum may be the reverse of those of norepinephrine.

APPLIED ANATOMY

Cerebellar disorders of clinical significance most commonly result from tumors or multiple sclerosis, and less commonly from vascular disease, chronic alcoholic or other drug intoxication, poisoning with heavy metals, or hereditary cerebellar degeneration. Generalized cerebellar malfunction is seen in acute alcoholic intoxication, with staggering gait, clumsy gestures and slurred speech.

The vestibulocerebellum may be attacked by a medulloblastoma, which is a highly malignant tumor arising in the roof of the fourth ventricle in childhood. The cardinal feature is *trunk ataxia*, the inability to stand upright without support. There are usually no physical signs in the recumbent child prior to the onset of raised intracranial pressure. If the nearby vestibular nucleus is involved, the symptoms include those of unilateral inactivation of a labyrinth (Chapter 33).

Unilateral disorder may be caused by tumor, vascular disease, or multiple sclerosis. The symptoms are always on the *same* side. Spinocerebellar and neocerebellar deficits are difficult to differentiate; both divisions are usually involved. Symptoms include difficulty in initiation, execution, and termination of voluntary movements. The clumsy execution is called *cerebellar ataxia*, and it is equally pronounced whether the eyes are open or closed – unlike sensory ataxia (Chapter 11), which is reduced under visual guidance. *Intention tremor* is the coarse tremor that appears when a deliberate movement gets under way (for example, in the heel-to-knee or finger-to-nose test). Lack of proper fixation at the shoulder causes the affected arm to fall away when the arms are pointing forward. Faulty synergic activity may cause *decomposition* of movement; for example, in an oblique movement the shoulder may be abducted and then flexed. Faulty relaxation of antagonists creates difficulty in executing rapid alternating movements, such as pronation–supination. Intricate sequences cannot be executed; thus, there is inability to write if the dominant hand is involved. *Cerebellar dysarthria* is the slow, slurring speech, with uneven volume owing to irregular contraction of the respiratory and laryngeal muscles. *Hypotonia* may be present, due to diminished gamma fusimotor activity.

Several eye signs are described, including nystagmus toward the side of the lesion (Chapter 33), and inability to keep the eyes on a selected target (drifting).

Readings

Allen, G.I. and Tsukahara, N. (1974) Cerebrocerebellar communication systems. *Physiol. Rev., 54:* 957–1006.

Chan-Palay, V. (1979) Recent advances in the morphological localization of gamma-aminobutyric acid receptors in the cerebellum by means of ³H-muscimol. *Prog. Brain Res., 51:* 303–322.

Dolphin, A.C. (1982) Noradrenergic modification of glutamate release in the cerebellum. *Brain Res., 252:* 111–116.

Gilman, S., Bloedel, J.R. and Lechtenberg, R. (1981) *Disorders of the Cerebellum*. Philadelphia: Davis.

Kennedy, P.R., Ross, H.-G. and Brooks, V.B. (1982) Participation of the principal olivary nucleus in neocerebellar motor control. *Exp. Brain Res., 47:* 95–104.

Llinas, R.R. (1975) The cortex of the cerebellum. *Sci. Am., 232:* 56–71.

Nieuwenhuys, R., Voogd, J. and van Huijzen, C. (1981) *The Human Central Nervous System: A Synopsis and Atlas*. Berlin: Springer-Verlag.

Palay, S.L. and Chan-Palay, V. (1974) *Cerebellar Cortex: Cytology and Organization*. Heidelberg: Springer-Verlag.

Rivera-Dominguez, M., Mettler, F.A. and Noback, C.R. (1974) Origin of cerebellar climbing fibers in the rhesus monkey. *J. Comp. Neurol., 155:* 331–340.

Schulman, J.A. (1983) Chemical neuroanatomy of the cerebellar cortex. In *Chemical Neuroanatomy* (Emson, P.C., ed.), pp. 209–228. New York: Raven Press.

Sechtenberg, R. and Gilman, S. (1978) Speech disorders in cerebellar disease. *Ann. Neurol., 3:* 285–290.

Stanton, G.B. (1980) Topographical organization of ascending cerebellar projections from the dentate and interposed nuclei in *Mucacca mulatta*: an anterograde degeneration study. *J. Comp. Neurol., 190:* 699–731.

Strahlendorf, J.C. and Hubbard, G.D. (1983) Serotonergic interactions with rat cerebellar Purkinje cells. *Brain Res. Bull., 11:* 265–269.

14

Reticular Formation: Isodendritic Core

The tegmentum (core) of the brain stem is permeated by a network of branched neurons known as the *reticular formation* (RF). The term is used only with respect to the midbrain, pons, and medulla oblongata, although the polysynaptic net extends rostrally into the thalamus and hypothalamus, and caudally into continuity with the propriospinal network of the spinal cord.

The characteristic neuron is *isodendritic*: its dendrites are long and branch at regular intervals (Fig. 14-1). The dendrites tend to lie across the axis of the brain stem, and their interstices are penetrated by the long ascending and descending fiber systems. The axons of RF neurons travel for at least several millimeters, and some run all the way to the cerebral or cerebellar cortex or to the spinal cord.

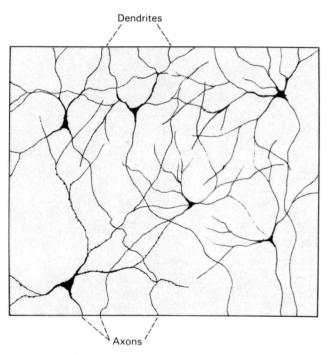

Fig. 14-1 Isodendritic neurons.

The RF has many functions. Some are called non-specific because they are not accompanied by obvious motor or sensory responses. For example, *ascending* RF fibers have an arousal effect on the entire cerebral cortex and are responsible for the waking state, and *descending* RF fibers have a tonic effect on motoneurons (in the waking state) and maintain muscle tone and posture during sitting and standing. Also included in the non-specific group are *aminergic*

neurons whose cell bodies occupy nodal points in the RF network. The axons of these neurons divide prodigiously, permeating all parts of the CNS gray matter. In most regions at least, the amines – norepinephrine (noradrenaline), epinephrine (adrenaline), serotonin, dopamine – do not function as classical neurotransmitters: rather, they *modulate* ongoing nervous activity in a variety of ways.

Other nodal points are known to have specific motor functions. These nodes are called *pattern generators*: they induce patterned (stereotyped) responses in the somatic or autonomic system. The pattern generators are of two kinds. One kind is continuously active and comprises the *vital centers* in the medulla oblongata regulating the cardiovascular and respiratory systems. The second kind is switched on either by 'command centers' in the brain (in or near the motor cortex) or by intense sensory stimulation. Activities organized by the second kind include conjugate eye movements, locomotion (walking and running), mastication, swallowing, vomiting, sneezing, micturition, and defecation.

The aminergic neurons and pattern generators are taken up in Chapter 15.

Excluded from the RF by convention (although not always by their structure) are the dorsal column nuclei, the olivary and pontine nuclei, the red nuclei, and the nuclei of the cranial nerves.

ANATOMY OF THE ISODENDRITIC CORE

The ribbons of isodendritic neurons that make up the reticular core of the brain stem are grouped thus (Fig. 14-2):

1 In the midline are the *raphe* neurons, most of which use serotonin (5-hydroxytryptamine) as transmitter. Some raphe neurons project to the forebrain, others to the spinal cord, and others to the brain stem or cerebellum.

2 The medially placed *nucleus magnocellularis* (L., large-celled) extends from mid-medulla to mid-pons. Its rostral part projects to the midbrain and its caudal part gives rise to the reticulospinal tracts. Its pontine part is called the *nucleus reticularis pontis caudalis*. At its lower end it merges with the *central (ventral) reticular nucleus* of the medulla; this contains the *pressor center*, which maintains peripheral vascular tone (Chapter 37).

3 The laterally placed *nucleus parvocellularis* (L., small-celled) merges with the mesencephalic RF. It contains some large cells. Its pontine part is called the *nucleus pontis oralis*.

In addition to the above, the *paramedian* and *lateral reticular nuclei* of the medulla receive spinoreticular fibers and project to the cerebellum.

The difference between magno- and parvocellular neurons lies in the relative lengths of their axons and dendrites. The parvocellular neurons have shorter neurites; they synapse upon one another and upon magnocellular neurons. The magnocellular neurons send axons to other levels of the neuraxis.

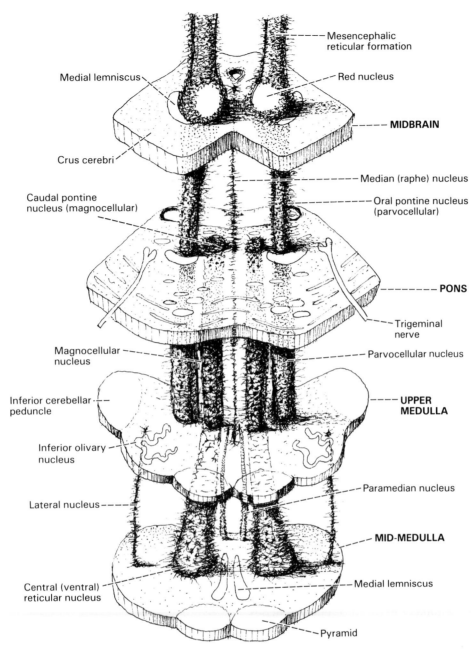

Fig. 14-2 The isodendritic reticular core. Note continuity of central medullary, magnocellular, and caudal pontine nuclei, and of parvocellular, oral pontine, and mesencephalic nuclei.

AFFERENTS TO THE ISODENDRITIC CORE (Fig. 14-3)

1 All of the sensory nuclei of the cranial and spinal nerves contribute fibers to the isodendritic core. Their routes of access to the core are listed in Table 14-1.

Table 14-1 Sensory inputs to the isodendritic core

Sources	Routes of access*
Olfactory	Medial forebrain bundle (16)
Visual	Superior colliculus (29)
Auditory	Superior olivary nuclei (30)
Vestibular	Vestibular nuclei (33)
Visceral	Nucleus solitarius (36)
Cutaneous	Trigeminoreticular (34) and spinoreticular (9) tracts

*Numbers in parentheses refer to chapters giving details.

Stimuli from all of these sources are relayed to the mesencephalic RF and thence to the intralaminar thalamic nuclei, with direct spread from there to many parts of the cerebral cortex.

In contrast to these non-specific inputs to the RF, specific sensory systems penetrate the RF without giving many collaterals to it. Among these are the medial lemniscus, trigeminothalamic tract, and spinothalamic tract. These carry information about the *nature* and *location* of peripheral stimuli and they are somatotopically organized. The spinoreticular and other inputs to the RF convey information about the *intensity* of the stimulus and about its *quality*, that is whether it is pleasurable or aversive. Qualitative interpretation is a function of the limbic cortex (Chapter 21).

103

2 The *descending* reticular formation has separate motor and sensory components, in the functional sense. The motor component (medial and lateral reticulospinal tracts) receives inputs from the premotor cortex, supplementary motor area, red nucleus, and cerebellar roof nuclei (fastigial and interpositus). The sensory component (mainly raphespinal tract) receives afferents from the periaqueductal gray matter of the midbrain and from the spinoreticular tracts.

EFFERENTS FROM THE ISODENDRITIC CORE

Ascending efferents

Ascending efferents run from the pontomedullary RF to the mesencephalic RF, and thence to the intralaminar thalamic nuclei. In addition, many aminergic efferents (Chapter 15) bypass the thalamus and innervate virtually the entire forebrain.

RF and the sleep–wake cycle

Relevant points are as follows (see physiology texts for details). During the first 90 minutes of sleep the electroencephalogram shows a change from the desynchronized (D) low-voltage waves of the waking state to more synchronized (S) waves of higher voltage. At intervals of about 90 minutes S sleep alternates with REM (rapid eye movement) sleep, in which the electroencephalogram is desynchronized ('paradoxical sleep') and dreams occur.

In the cat, the mesencephalic RF shows high rates of discharge during wakefulness and REM sleep, and low rates during S sleep. During the transition from sleep to wakefulness the high level of mesencephalic RF discharge commences about 15 seconds before the cat wakes up.

The pontine and medullary RF show low rates of tonic discharge during sleep, but reticulospinal neurons burst occasionally to produce body twitches, and the parabducens nucleus bursts to produce the rapid eye movements.

Ascending reticular activating system (ARAS)

The ARAS comprises the polysynaptic network ascending the tegmentum and terminating in the intralaminar nucleus of the thalamus. The pontomedullary components are *extrinsic* elements of the system, because they show little variation of activity during the sleep–wake cycle but are intensely responsive to extraneous stimulation from spinal and cranial nerves and project both to midbrain and thalamus. The mesencephalic RF is an *intrinsic* element, because it shows *cyclic activity* in the absence of stimulation from the pontomedullary RF. The cyclic, diurnal changes in mesencephalic RF activity probably derive from the anterior hypothalamus via the medial forebrain bundle (Chapter 16). The anterior hypothalamus (suprachiasmatic region) has strong claims as a rhythm generator, being phylogenetically linked to the optic nerves, and thus to the day–night cycle.

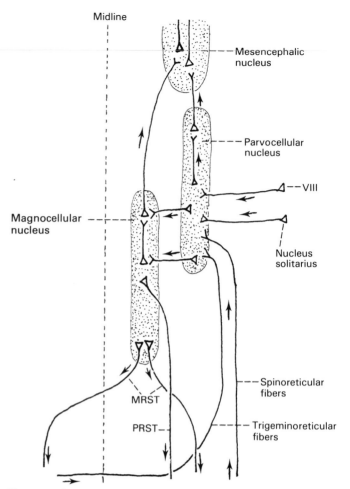

Fig. 14-3 Connections of the magnocellular and parvocellular nuclei. MRST, PRST, medullary and pontine reticulospinal tracts. VIII, acoustic nerve.

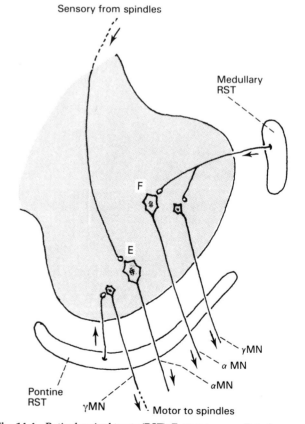

Fig. 14-4 Reticulospinal tracts (RST): E, to extensors; F, to flexors.

In humans, injury to the midbrain tegmentum may be attended by unconsciousness for long periods (weeks or months).

Descending efferents

The *pontine (medial) reticulospinal tract* arises in the caudal pontine nucleus and descends the full length of the cord in front of the anterior gray horn. Its principal action is upon gamma motoneurons supplying extensor muscles (Fig. 14-4). The homonymous (matching) α motoneurons are excited via the gamma loop.

The *medullary (lateral) reticulospinal tract* arises in the medullary part of the magnocellular nucleus. It descends, partly crossed, in the lateral funiculus alongside the anterior gray horn. It synapses upon α and γ motoneurons of flexor muscles.

Both reticulospinal tracts also act upon Ia internuncials in the base of the anterior horn, to cause reciprocal inhibition (Chapter 10).

The reticulospinal tracts maintain postural tone during sitting and standing, in collaboration with the vestibulospinal tracts. The pontine RST is of special importance in sustaining contraction in the erector spinae and lower limb extensors. The basal ganglia seem to have a controlling action on the pontine reticulospinal tracts, since disordered function of the basal ganglia in Parkinson's disease is associated with inability to sustain posture (Chapter 18).

During walking and running, both reticulospinal tracts are played upon by the locomotor generator, a node of the RF located in the midbrain (Chapter 15).

The *raphespinal tract* (Chapter 15) modulates pain transmission in the posterior horn.

Cerebellar efferents

Cerebellar efferents travel from the paramedian and lateral reticular nuclei to the roof nuclei and cortex of the cerebellum.

Readings

Chase, M.H., Enomoto, S., Murakami, T., Nakamura, Y. and Tairo, M. (1981) Intracellular potential of medullary reticular neurons during sleep and wakefulness. *Exp. Neurol., 71:* 226–233.

Dietz, V., Schmidtbleicher, D. and Noth, J. (1979) Neuronal mechanisms of human locomotion. *J. Neurophysiol., 42:* 1212–1221.

Fields, H.L., Vangeas, H., Hentall, I.D. and Zorman, G. (1984) Evidence that disinhibition of brain stem neurones contributes to morphine analgesia. *Nature, 306:* 684–686.

Kuraishi, Y., Harada, Y., Aratani, S., Satoh, M. and Takagi, H. (1983) Separate involvement of the spinal noradrenergic and serotonergic systems in morphine analgesia: the differences in mechanical and thermal algesic tests. *Brain Res., 273:* 245–252.

Le Bars, D. and Chitour, D. (1983) Do convergent neurons in the spinal dorsal horn discriminate nociceptive from non-nociceptive information? *Pain, 17:* 1–19.

Pompeiano, O. (1973) Reticular formation. In *Handbook of Sensory Physiology, Vol. 2, Somatosensory System* (Iggo, A., ed.), pp. 381–488. Bethesda: American Physiological Society.

Ramon-Moliner, E. and Nauta, W.J.H. (1966) The isodendritic core of the brain stem. *J. Comp. Neurol., 126:* 311–336.

Saadé, N.E., Salibi, N.A., Banna, N.R., Towe, A.L. and Jabbur, S.J. (1983) Spinal input pathways affecting the medullary gigantocellular reticular nucleus. *Exp. Neurol., 80:* 582–600.

Scheibel, A. (1980) Anatomical and physiological substrates of arousal. In *The Reticular Formation Revisited* (Hobson, J.A. and Brazier, M.A.B., eds.), pp. 55–66. New York: Raven Press.

Siegel, J.M. (1979) Behavioral functions of the reticular formation. *Brain Res. Rev., 1:* 69–105.

Steriade, M. (1981) Mechanisms underlying cortical activation: neuronal organization and properties of the midbrain reticular core and intralaminar thalamic nuclei. In *Brain Mechanisms and Perceptual Awareness* (Pompeiano, O. and Marsan, C.A., eds.), pp. 327–377. New York: Raven Press.

Vertes, R.P. (1984) Brainstem control of the events of REM sleep. *Prog. Neurobiol., 22:* 241–288.

15
Reticular Formation: Nuclei

The tegmental reticular networks are punctuated by numerous cell aggregates sufficiently condensed to be called nuclei. They fall into two classes: the pattern generators and the monoamine cell groups.

PATTERN GENERATORS

The *pattern generators* play upon the motor nuclei of cranial and spinal nerves to produce sequences of muscular contractions. More than one cranial or spinal nerve may be influenced by a single generator. Although the movement sequence is determined by the generator, the motor activity is modified by feedback of sensory information from the moving parts. The generators are subject to *command centers* – in the supplementary motor area and/or premotor area of the cerebral cortex in the case of striated muscle and in the hypothalamus in the case of smooth muscle. The respiratory and cardiovascular generators are called *oscillators*.

Table 15-1 Brain stem generators

Generator	Function*
Cuneiform nucleus	Walking, running (15)
Ocular generators	Conjugate eye movements (32)
Parabrachial nuclei	Respiratory rhythm (38)
Dorsal respiratory nucleus	Inspiration (38)
Ventral respiratory nucleus	Expiration (38)
Central tegmental nucleus	Pressor area (blood pressure) (37)
Central tegmental nucleus	Depressor area (blood pressure) (37)
Swallowing centre	Deglutition (36)
Area postrema	Vomiting center (36)

*Numbers refer to chapters giving details.

The principal generators are shown in Table 15-1 and Fig. 15-1. They are intimately related to cranial nerves and are described in the chapters listed in the table.

Locomotion

In walking, the pontine and medullary reticulospinal tracts are both active. However, walking movements may continue for a time (in animals) after transection of the cervical cord. At the level of each limb, the motoneurons are linked by internuncials so as to promote rhythmic flexion and extension, and the four spinal centers (one for each limb) are linked by propriospinal neurons so as to promote alternation of fore- and hindlimb movements. All four limbs are under the control of a *locomotor generator* located in the *cuneiform nuclei*, ventral to the inferior colliculi of the midbrain. Following midcollicular transection of the

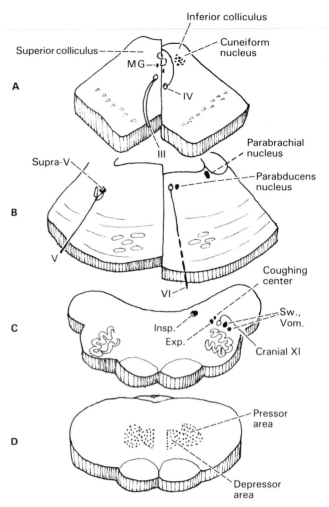

Fig. 15-1 Brain stem generators. A, upper (left) and lower (right) midbrain; B, upper (left) and mid (right) pons; C, upper medulla; D, mid-medulla. Exp., Insp., expiratory and inspiratory centers; MG, midbrain generator (vertical eye movements); Supra-V, supratrigeminal nucleus; Sw, swallowing center; Vom, vomiting center.

brain stem (so-called decerebration) an animal will make walking or galloping motions in response to different intensities of stimulation of the cuneiform nuclei. Since the reticulospinal tracts are active throughout this experiment, they probably mediate the effects on the anterior horns. Human walking may likewise involve the activity of a locomotor generator: we have well-developed cuneiform nuclei. Initiation of a walking pattern is presumed to come from a command center in the cerebral cortex.

MONOAMINE CELL GROUPS

More than two dozen monoamine cell groups are distributed at specific points in the brain stem and hypothalamus. *Catecholamine*-secreting cells can be identified even in unstained sections of human brain by their content of neuromelanin, a byproduct of catecholamine (CA) synthesis (Fig. 15-2). Following exposure of fresh brain slices (animals) to formaldehyde or glyoxylic acid, these and cells secreting *serotonin* (5-HT) can be identified by the fluorescence of their somas and axons in ultraviolet light.

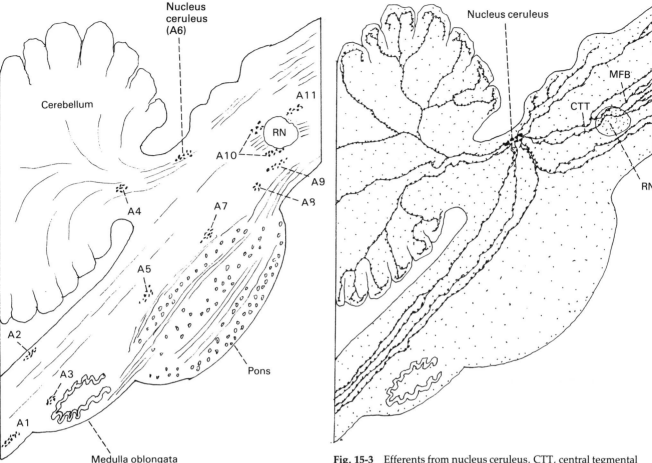

Fig. 15-2 Dopaminergic (A8, A9) and noradrenergic cell groups. RN, red nucleus. (Adapted from Bogerts, 1981.)

Fig. 15-3 Efferents from nucleus ceruleus. CTT, central tegmental tract; MFB, medial forebrain bundle; RN, red nucleus.

Fourteen monoamine cell groups (A1–A14) contain either *norepinephrine* (noradrenaline) or *dopamine*. Nine cell groups (B1–B9) contain serotonin, an indoleamine. Three cell groups (C1–C3) contain epinephrine (adrenaline).

The principal norepinephrine cells are those of the *nucleus ceruleus* in the pons (Fig. 15-3). Norepinephrine neurons are characterized by truly prodigious branching patterns and enormous innervation territories. They number less than 10 000, yet they penetrate every part of the gray matter of the CNS. Their axons have innumerable varicosities, containing dense-cored vesicles similar to those in peripheral sympathetic fibers. The released norepinephrine acts as a modulator of synaptic transmission between other neurons, and its effect is generally inhibitory. However, the inhibition may be directed to inhibitory neurons so that effector neurons may be facilitated.

In the spinal cord, norepinephrine fibers reaching the anterior horn facilitate local reflex arcs. Part of the action of the midbrain locomotor generator is to cause norepinephrine to be released in the anterior horn. Norepinephrine fibers reaching the posterior horn inhibit transmission from primary to secondary afferents (see later).

Norepinephrine fibers in the hypothalamus are described in Chapter 16, those in the forebrain in Chapter 19.

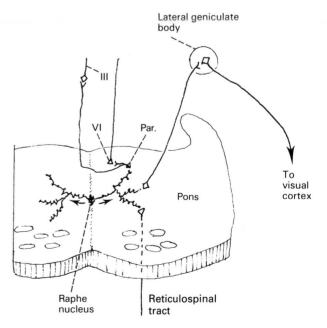

Fig. 15-4 Nuclear groups inhibited by pontine raphe nucleus. Par., parabducens nucleus.

The principal *dopamine* cell groups are in the midbrain and hypothalamus. They are described in Chapters 12, 16, and 18.

The three epinephrine cell groups occupy the medulla oblongata. They project rostrally as far as the hypothalamus.

The *serotonin* cell groups occupy the raphe nuclei of the brainstem. The midbrain raphe nuclei project mainly to the forebrain, the pontine raphe nuclei project locally, and the medullary raphe nuclei project to the spinal cord.

Serotonin and sleep

Pontine raphe neurons exert tonic inhibition on magnocellular neurons of the pontine RF (Fig. 15-4). The inhibition ceases only at the onset of rapid-eye-movement (REM) sleep. Release of the parabducens nucleus causes REM. Release of pontine reticulospinal neurons leads to intermittent twitching of the trunk and limbs. Release of pontogeniculate neurons synapsing in the lateral geniculate nucleus causes characteristic spikes to appear in occipital EEG leads. These 'PGO spikes' (pontine–geniculate–occipital) may have a bearing on the highly visual content of REM-stage dreams. Tryptophan-containing hypnotics (such as milk or malted milk) supply serotonin precursor and prolong S (dreamless) sleep.

GATE CONTROL

The term 'gate control' was introduced (Melzack and Wall, 1965) to describe the manner in which transmission of impulses from nociceptive primary afferents to spinothalamic neurons could be modulated by spinal internuncial neurons. In particular the 'gate' could be 'closed' by inhibitory internuncials exerting presynaptic inhibition on primary afferent terminals and postsynaptic inhibition on spinothalamic relay cells. It is now clear that 'gating' is subject to supraspinal as well as local controls. A significant gate may also exist at thalamic level, but this has received little attention and will not be discussed.

Spinal gate controls

Spinal controls reside chiefly in the substantia gelatinosa (SG), whose synaptology and autopharmacology are extremely complex. It is clear at least that both excitatory and inhibitory SG neurons play upon spinothalamic (STT) relay cells – and upon one another. Excitatory SG neurons predominate in the medial SG and inhibitory neurons in the lateral SG (Fig. 15-5). Their axons run up and down Lissauer's tract and re-enter the gray matter before terminating.

Electrophysiological evidence indicated that SG neurons exert *tonic inhibition* on STT relay cells. Their effect has been demonstrated surgically in monkeys, as shown in Fig. 15-6, where the L1 posterior nerve

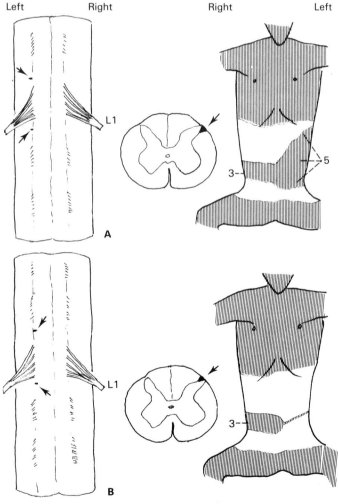

Fig. 15-6 L1 dermatome in the monkey. Posterior view of cord, anterior view of trunk. A, lateral section of Lissauer's tract expands L1 from three dermatomes to five. B, medial section almost obliterates L1 dermatome. (Adapted from Denny-Brown et al., 1973.)

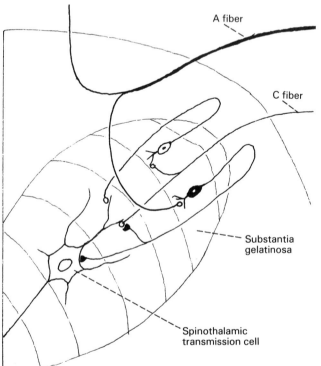

Fig. 15-5 Excitatory (clear) and inhibitory (black) neurons of substantia gelatinosa, with primary afferent sources of stimulation.

roots have been isolated by sectioning three roots above and below them. Behavioral responses to skin scratching indicated that L1 supplied three dermatomes (result expected). If the lateral (inhibitory) part of Lissauer's tract was then cut, the animal immediately responded over *five* dermatomes. On the other hand, if the medial (excitatory) part was cut, the responses tended to disappear altogether.

The expansion of the receptive zone from three to five dermatomes could be produced instead by systemic administration of a small dose of strychnine – a specific antagonist of the inhibitory transmitter glycine. (It is now apparent that other inhibitory SG neurons contain GABA, and still others, enkephalin.)

Since it is known that human intercostal nerves span three dermatomes by *physiological* testing, the 'gate' at spinal level is apparently 'half open' under resting conditions, as the result of competition between excitatory and inhibitory SG neurons for chemical access to STT cells.

Closure at spinal level

1 The simplest example of gate control is 'rubbing the sore spot'. Rubbing the skin excites follicular nerves which, inter alia, synapse upon enkephalinergic neurons in the SG and tend to 'close the gate'. Rubbing is ineffective if naloxone (a specific opiate antagonist) is administered beforehand.
2 *Transcutaneous nerve stimulation* (TNS) is justifiably popular among physiotherapists for treating disorders accompanied by intractable pain, such as rheumatoid arthritis and post-herpetic neuralgia. Electrodes are placed on the skin overlying large nerve trunks, and follicular and other large afferents are stimulated to relieve the chronic, nagging pain; it is simple and effective. TNS can also be used to relieve labor pains (an electrode is placed over the sacrum).
3 Severe pain may be alleviated by placing disc electrodes on the dorsal columns (or on the overlying dura mater), to excite large collaterals synapsing upon inhibitory SG neurons.

Supraspinal gate controls

Multiple supraspinal inputs to the posterior horn and to the caudal trigeminal nucleus are therapeutically more important than purely spinal closure mechanisms. Many details are far from clear, but the following is an acceptable outline.

Two principal supraspinal mechanisms modulate nociceptive transmission at spinal and trigeminal levels: monoaminergic pathways and stress. Two monoaminergic pathways are known: the raphespinal pathway and the ceruleospinal pathway (Fig. 15-7).

The raphespinal pathway

The raphespinal pathway runs from the nucleus raphe magnus (NRM) of the medulla to the caudal trigeminal nucleus and spinal posterior horn. It descends in the spinal tract of the trigeminal nerve and, below this, in Lissauer's tract. Several transmitters are included, the

best known being serotonin. The serotonergic component (20% at most) synapses upon enkephalin neurons in the substantia gelatinosa (which they excite) and directly upon STT relay cells (which they inhibit).

The term *stimulus-produced analgesia* (SPA) is conventionally reserved for the profound analgesia produced by stimulation of the NRM. The same effect can be produced by stimulating the periaqueductal gray matter of the midbrain or the periventricular gray matter of the third ventricle. In each case, SPA is accompanied by elevated serotonin and enkephalin levels in the spinal CSF, into which these transmitters diffuse from the posterior horn.

Inputs to the NRM. Two important sources of excitation of the NRM are (a) the central gray matter at higher levels and (b) spinoreticular and trigeminoreticular afferents.

The *periaqueductal gray matter* (PAG) of the midbrain, and the periventricular gray matter of the hind end of the third ventricle (PVG) contain neurons that descend to synapse upon NRM neurons. This descending pathway is not enkephalinergic, but the PAG and PVG contain opiate receptors.

Diffuse noxious inhibitory control (DNIC) is the term used to describe the protection afforded one part of the

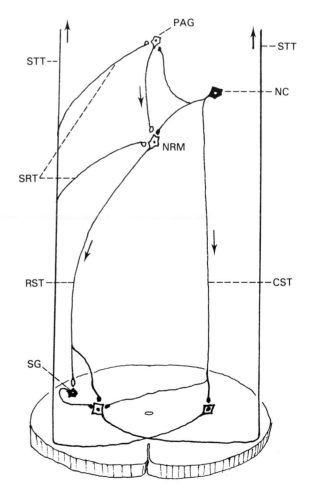

Fig. 15-7 Two supraspinal gate controls: the raphespinal tract (RST) from the nucleus raphe magnus (NRM), and the ceruleospinal tract (CST) from the nucleus ceruleus (NC). PAG, periaqueductal gray matter; SG, substantia gelatinosa; SRT, spinoreticular tract; STT, spinothalamic tract.

body by noxious stimulation elsewhere. For example, painful stimulation in the trigeminal area relieves pain from the upper and lower limbs, and vice versa. Veterinarians know that if the muzzle of a horse is tightly squeezed, a laceration of fore- or hind-foot can be stitched without danger of reprisal. 'Biting on a bullet' may be a human equivalent. The spino/trigeminothalamic relay neurons stilled by such exercises are 'wide dynamic range' (synonyms: polymodal, convergent) neurons, responding naturally to mechanical as well as noxious stimulation. A counterpart is the relief of toothache afforded by applying ice to the hand. The relevance to acupuncture is obvious, in the sense that the traditionally selected points for needle insertion are without anatomical logic (for example, piercing the first interdigital cleft of the foot to relieve headache). In animals, DNIC effects are much reduced by destruction of the NRM (but not abolished, perhaps because spino/trigeminoreticular fibers synapse also in the nucleus ceruleus).

The ceruleospinal pathway

At least as powerful as the raphespinal system is a noradrenergic pathway descending in the lateral funiculus from the nucleus ceruleus. In contrast to the raphespinal path, it is opiate-indifferent. It appears to function by means of direct inhibitory synapse upon spinothalamic relay cells. Alpha receptors are involved. Curiously, there is antagonism between this pathway and the raphespinal, both at PAG and NRM levels (Fig. 15-7).

Stress-induced analgesia

It is well known that severe injury may not be perceived under *extreme* conditions (the soldier in the heat of battle and the martyr entering the flames). In *physical exertion* all kinds of somatic sensation are dampened by pyramidal tract fibers synapsing upon inhibitory internuncials in the posterior horn and trigeminal equivalent. In *emotional stress* the arcuate nucleus of the hypothalamus (Chapter 16) responds to limbic excitation by releasing β endorphin from fibers that descend to the PAG.

FURTHER NOTES ON SPINAL CORD MONOAMINERGIC FIBERS

Noradrenergic fibers descend to the cord from several brain stem aminergic nuclei. In the anterior horn, the fibers are excitatory to motoneurons.

Dopaminergic fibers descend from the midbrain and hypothalamus, and terminate in all parts of the spinal gray matter. Their numbers are small and their function is not known.

Serotonergic fibers descending from medullary cell groups also spread to all parts of the gray matter. Their effects on visceral and somatic motoneurons have not yet been clarified.

Readings

Basbaum, A.I. (1984) Anatomical substrates of pain and pain modulation and their relationship to analgesic drug action. In *Analgesics: Neurochemical, Behavioral and Clinical Perspectives* (Kuhar, M. and Pasternak, G., eds.), pp. 97–123. New York: Raven Press.

Basbaum, A.I. and Fields, H.L. (1984) Endogenous pain control systems: brainstem spinal pathways and endorphin circuitry. *Annu. Rev. Neurosci., 7:* 309–338.

Basbaum, A.I., Moss, M.S. and Glazer, E.J. (1983) Opiate and stimulation-produced analgesia: the contribution of the monoamines. In *Advances in Pain Research and Therapy, Vol. 5* (Bonica, J.J., Lindblom, U. and Iggo, A., eds.), pp. 323–340. New York: Raven Press.

Bogerts, B. (1981) A brainstem atlas of catecholaminergic neurons in man, using melanin as a natural marker. *J. Comp. Neurol., 197:* 63–80.

Bowker, R.M., Westlund, K.N., Sullivan, M.C., Wilbar, J.F. and Coulter, J.D. (1983) Descending serotonergic, peptidergic and cholinergic pathways from the raphe nuclei: a multiple transmitter complex. *Brain Res., 288:* 33–48.

Denny-Brown, D., Kirk, E.J. and Yanagisawa, N. (1973) The tract of Lissauer in relation to sensory transmission in the dorsal horn of spinal cord in the Macaque monkey. *J. comp. Neurol., 151:* 175–199.

Drugan, R.C., Moye, D.B. and Maier, S.F. (1982) Opioid and monopioid forms of stress-induced analgesia: some environmental determinants and characteristics. *Behav. Neurol. Biol., 35:* 251–264.

Dubner, R. and Bennett, G.J. (1983) Spinal and trigeminal mechanisms of nociception. *Annu. Rev. Neurosci., 6:* 381–418.

Fields, H.L. (1981) An endorphin-mediated analgesia system: experimental and clinical observations. In *Neurosecretion and Brain Peptides* (Martin, J.B., Reichlin, S. and Bick, K.L., eds.), pp. 199–212. New York: Raven Press.

Forno, L.S. and Norville, R.L. (1981) Synaptic morphology in the human locus ceruleus. *Acta Neuropathol. (Berlin), 53:* 7–14.

Héry, F. and Ternaux, J.P. (1981) Regulation of release processes in central serotonergic neurons. *J. Physiol. (Paris), 77:* 287–301.

Le Bars, D. and Besson, J.M. (1981) The spinal site of action of morphine in pain relief: from basic research to clinical applications. *Trends Pharmacol. Sci., 2:* 323–325.

Le Bars, D., Dickenson, A.H. and Besson, J.M. (1983) Opiate analgesia and descending control systems. In *Advances in Pain Research and Therapy, Vol. 5* (Bonica, J.J., Lindblom, U. and Iggo, A., eds.), pp. 341–372. New York: Raven Press.

Melzack, R. and Wall, P.D. (1965) Pain mechanisms: a new theory. *Science, 150:* 971–978.

Moore, R.Y. (1980) The reticular formation: monoamine neuron systems. In *The Reticular Formation Revisited* (Hobson, J.A. and Brazier, M.A.B., eds.), pp. 67–82. New York: Raven Press.

Moore, R.Y. and Bloom, F.E. (1978) Central catecholamine neuron systems: anatomy and physiology of the dopamine systems. *Annu. Rev. Neurosci., 1:* 129–169.

Neff, N.H. (1984) Biogenic amines: an overview. In *Dynamics of Neurotransmitter Function* (Hanin, I., ed.), pp. 5–10. New York: Raven Press.

Nobin, A. and Björklund, A. (1973) Topography of the monoamine neuron systems in the human brain as revealed in fetuses. *Acta Physiol. Scand., Suppl. 388:* 1–40.

Pearson, J., Goldstein, M., Markey, K. and Brandeis, L. (1983) Human brain stem catecholamine neuronal anatomy as indicated by immunocytochemistry with antibodies to tyrosine hydroxylase. *Neuroscience, 8:* 3–32.

Saavedra, J.P., Pasik, T. and Pasik, P. (1983) Immunocytochemistry of serotonergic neurons in the central nervous system of monkeys. In *Neural Transmission, Learning and Memory* (Caputto, R. and Marsen, C.A., eds.), pp. 81–96. New York: Raven Press.

Schofield, S.P.M. and Everitt, B.J. (1981) The organization of catecholamine containing neurons in the brain of the rhesus monkey. *J. Anat., 132:* 391–418.

Wall, P.D. (1980) The role of substantia gelatinosa as a gate control. In *Pain* (Bonica, J.J., ed.), pp. 225–243. New York: Raven Press.

Willis, W.D. (1984) The raphe–spinal system. In *Brainstem Control of Spinal Function*, pp. 141–214. New York: Academic Press.

Willis, W.D., Gerhart, K.D., Willcockson, W.S., Yezurski, R.P., Wilcox, T.K. and Cargill, C.L. (1984) Primate raphe- and reticulospinal neurons: effects of stimulation in periaqueductal gray or VPL$_c$ thalamic nucleus. *J. Neurophysiol., 51:* 467–480.

Yaksh, T.L., Hammond, D.L. and Tyce, G.M. (1981) Functional aspects of bulbospinal monoaminergic projections in modulating processing of somatosensory information. *Fed. Proc., 40:* 2786–2794.

Yaksh, T.L. (1981) Spinal opiate analgesia: characteristics and principles of action. *Pain, 11:* 293–346.

16
Diencephalon: Hypothalamus

The hypothalamus is the gray matter flanking the third ventricle below the thalamus. It is phylogenetically very ancient, being the most rostral part of the reticular formation and linking the most primitive parts of the forebrain – the olfactory and limbic lobes – with the caudal neuraxis. It has very important functions in homeostasis and in survival. Its homeostatic functions include the regulation of the body temperature and the circulation of the blood. Its survival functions include the regulation of food and water intake, the sleep–wake cycle, sexual behavior patterns, and defense mechanisms against attack.

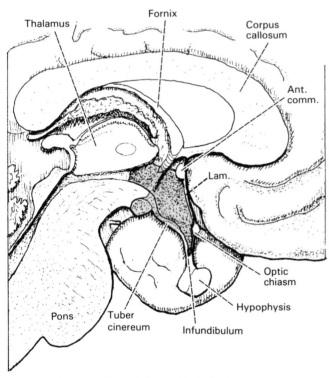

Fig. 16-1 Position of hypothalamus (shaded). Ant. comm., anterior commissure; Lam., lamina terminalis.

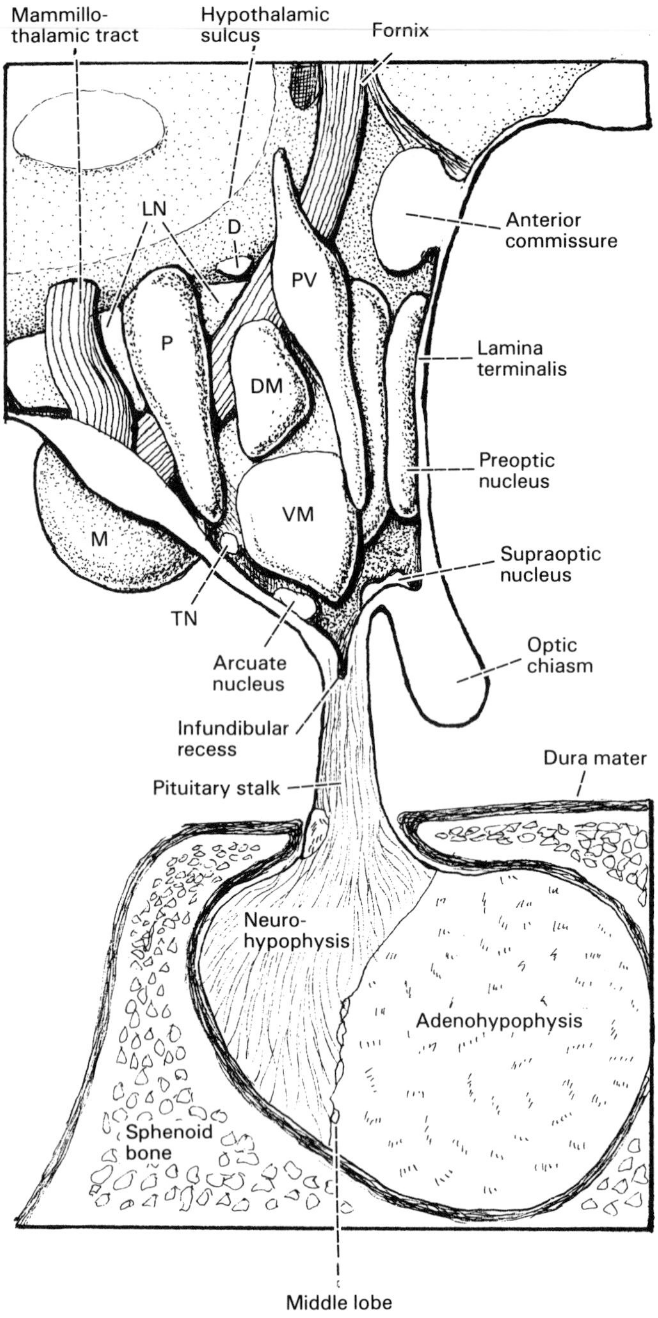

Fig. 16-2 Hypothalamic nuclei and hypophysis. D, dorsal nucleus; DM, dorsomedial nucleus; LN, lateral nucleus; M, mammillary body; P, posterior nucleus; PV, paraventricular nucleus; TN, tuberal nucleus; VM, ventromedial nucleus.

Boundaries (Fig. 16-1)

The hypothalamus is bilateral. It extends up to the hypothalamic sulcus, forward to the anterior commissure and back to include the mammillary bodies. In its floor are the optic chiasm, infundibulum, and tuber cinereum.

Subdivisions (Fig. 16-2, Table 16-1)

In the sagittal plane there are anterior, intermediate, and posterior regions. In the coronal plane there are

Table 16-1 Hypothalamic nuclei

Anterior	Intermediate	Posterior
Preoptic	Arcuate	Mammillary
Supraoptic	Tuberal	Posterior
Paraventricular	Lateral	
Anterior	Dorsal	
	Dorsomedial	
	Ventromedial	
	Posterior periventricular	
	Infundibular	

112

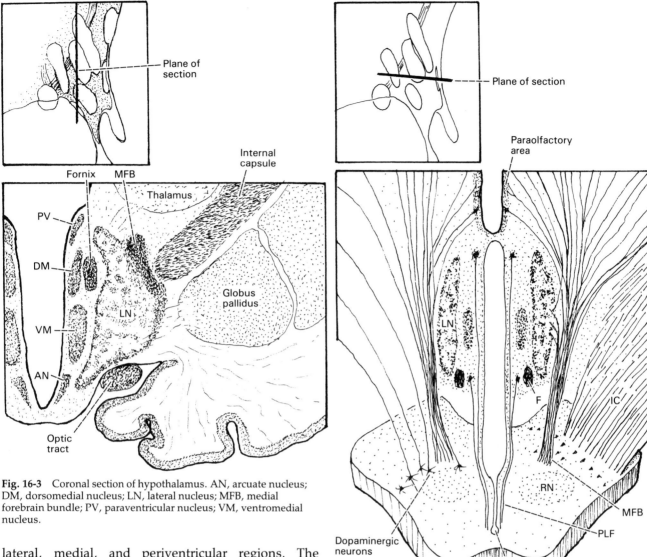

Fig. 16-3 Coronal section of hypothalamus. AN, arcuate nucleus; DM, dorsomedial nucleus; LN, lateral nucleus; MFB, medial forebrain bundle; PV, paraventricular nucleus; VM, ventromedial nucleus.

lateral, medial, and periventricular regions. The numerous nuclei vary in size between individuals and often shade into one another; hence, there is a common preference for the term 'area' rather than nucleus.

Fig. 16-4 Horizontal section of hypothalamus with midbrain added. F, fornix; IC, internal capsule; LN, lateral nucleus; MFB, medial forebrain bundle; PLF, posterior longitudinal fasciculus; RN, red nucleus.

Connections

Two-way system

The *medial forebrain bundle* evolved as a linkage between basal forebrain and brain stem. It passes alongside the hypothalamus (Fig. 16-3), and many of its fibers enter or leave the lateral nucleus (Fig. 16-4). It is limited caudally by the red nucleus. In the *ventral tegmental area* of the midbrain (between red nucleus and substantia nigra) it receives fibers of the ascending reticular system (ARAS). Entering from its rostral end are fibers from olfactory and limbic nuclei.

One-way systems (Fig. 16-5)

Entering the hypothalamus:
1 The *fornix* is the main projection from the hippocampus. The postcommissural fornix (behind the anterior commissure) terminates in the arcuate nucleus and mammillary body on each side.

2 The *stria terminalis* arises in the amygdala. It arches around the thalamus within the C formed by the fornix. It terminates in its own *bed nucleus* and in the ventromedial nucleus of the hypothalamus.
3 The *mammillary peduncle* runs from the midbrain tegmentum to the mammillary body.

Leaving the hypothalamus:
4 The *posterior longitudinal fasciculus* runs from autonomic centers in anterior and posterior hypothalamic areas to autonomic nuclei in the brain stem and spinal cord. A few fibers ascend the fasciculus from the nucleus solitarius and reticular formation.
5 The *mammillotegmental tract* runs from mammillary body to midbrain tegmentum.
6 The *mammillothalamic tract* runs from the mammillary body to the anterior nucleus of the thalamus.
7 The *hypothalamohypophyseal tract* runs from the supraoptic and paraventricular nuclei of hypothalamus to the neurohypophysis (see later).

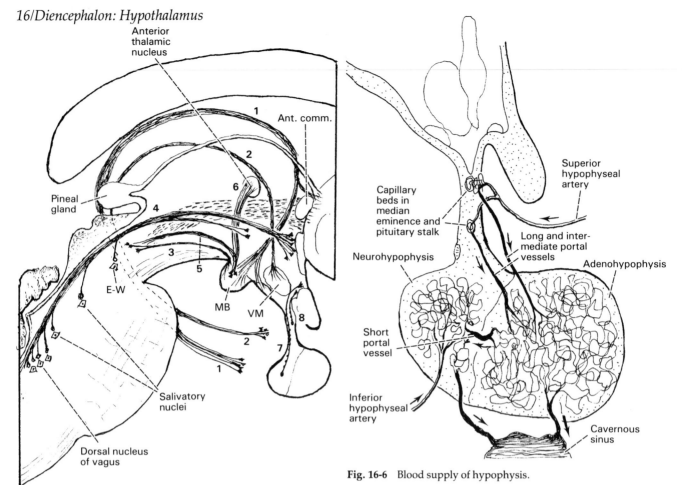

Fig. 16-5 Afferent and efferent hypothalamic pathways (see text). Ant. comm., anterior commissure; E-W, Edinger-Westphal nucleus (III nerve); MB, mammillary body; VM, ventromedial nucleus.

8 The *tuberoinfundibular tract* runs from the hypophysiotropic area of hypothalamus to the median eminence and pituitary stalk (see later).

BLOOD SUPPLY OF THE HYPOPHYSIS (Fig. 16-6)

The capillary beds of the median eminence and pituitary stalk are supplied by superior hypophyseal branches of the internal carotid artery. The beds are drained by *long* and *intermediate portal veins* which form a second capillary bed in the adenohypophysis and provide its entire blood supply. The adenohypophyseal bed drains into the cavernous sinus. *Short portal veins* also link the bed to that of the neurohypophysis, and the blood flow here is probably anteroposterior.

The capillary bed of the neurohypophysis is supplied directly from an inferior hypophyseal branch of the internal carotid.

FUNCTIONAL ANATOMY

Endocrine hypothalamus

Magnocellular neurons

From the *magnocellular neuroendocrine cells* of the supraoptic and paraventricular nuclei, the hypothalamohypophyseal tract descends to the neurohypophysis, giving branches to the pituitary stalk on the way (Fig. 16-7). Secretory granules 120–180 nm in diameter

Fig. 16-6 Blood supply of hypophysis.

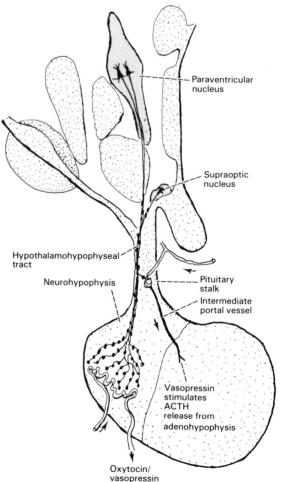

Fig. 16-7 Hypothalamohypophyseal tract.

114

are synthesized on the ribosomes of the cell body and packaged in Golgi complexes. Some granules in both nuclei contain vasopressin and the rest contain oxytocin. Both are peptides, linked to a precursor protein, neurophysin. The granules undergo rapid transport and accumulate in the nerve endings (Figs. 16-8, 16-9). Following depolarization of the neuroendocrine cells the granules exocytose into the pericapillary spaces. The capillaries are outside the blood–brain barrier (Chapter 24) and are fenestrated, permitting easy passage of the hormones into the blood.

Nearly half the volume of the neurohypophysis is composed of axonal swellings. The largest are the Herring bodies, which may be as big as erythrocytes. Their secretory granules are slightly larger and longer-lived (half-life of more than two weeks) than those of the small swellings. The Herring bodies are thought to provide a ready source of granules for release from the small swellings. There is no recycling of neurohormones at the nerve endings. The granule membranes are retrieved from the axolemma by endocytosis and digested in autophagic vacuoles; some membrane material may be reutilized.

Vasopressin is the antidiuretic hormone (ADH), which continuously stimulates water uptake by the distal tubules of the kidneys. Disease of the hypothalamus may result in *diabetes insipidus*, in which condition several gallons of dilute urine are excreted daily and are replenished by copious drinking. Hypophysectomy in patients suffering from cancer or chronic pain produces only a temporary (days) diabetes insipidus, provided the capillary bed in the pituitary stalk remains intact. The normal function of ADH released into the adenohypophysis is to stimulate release of adrenocorticotropic hormone (ACTH, corticotropin).

Oxytocin belongs to the efferent limb of the *milk ejection reflex*. The afferent limb is provided by sensory nerve endings in the female nipple and areola. During suckling, spinoreticular fibers relay via the posterior longitudinal fasciculus to the supraoptic and paraventricular nuclei. Liberated oxytocin causes contraction of the myoepithelial cells surrounding the lactiferous ducts.

Oxytocin has a moderate action on uterine muscle during labor, in response to spinoreticular stimulation by the genital tract.

Note Some branches of the magnocellular neurons are directed not to the hypophysis but to the limbic system (septum and amygdala, Chapter 22), and to autonomic nuclei in the brain stem (dorsal motor nucleus of vagus) and spinal cord (lateral horn). Vasopressin may have a memory function in the limbic system, which also contains some vasopressin-secreting neurons. In the autonomic nuclei the two neuron types seem to have some function in the control of blood pressure and (via the sympathetic) in regulation of heat loss.

Parvocellular neurons

From the *parvocellular neuroendocrine cells* of the *hypophysiotropic area*, a bundle of axons passes to the

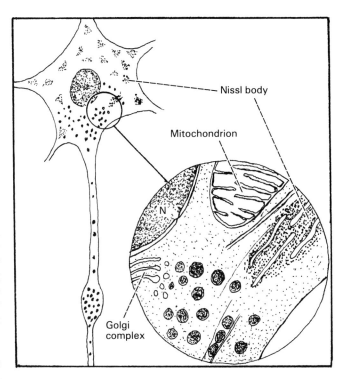

Fig. 16-8 Synthesis of granules in neuroendocrine cells. N, nucleus.

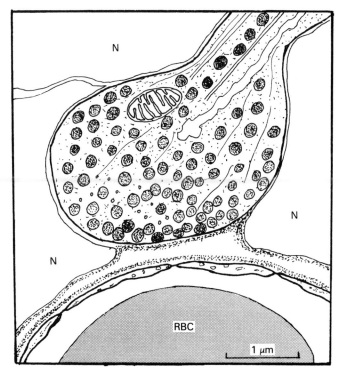

Fig. 16-9 Neurosecretory granules in nerve ending. N, neuroglia (pituicytes); RBC, erythrocyte.

median eminence and pituitary stalk. The hypophysiotropic area is a crescentic band of cells, mostly periventricular, extending from the preoptic area to the arcuate nucleus (Fig. 16-10). The bundle of axons is called the *tuberoinfundibular tract*, and their terminals

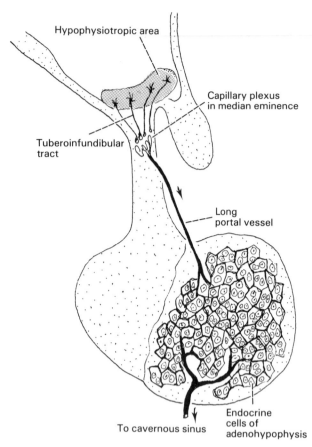

Hypophysiotropic area

Capillary plexus
in median eminence

Tuberoinfundibular
tract

Long
portal vessel

To cavernous sinus

Endocrine
cells of
adenohypophysis

Fig. 16-10   Tuberoinfundibular tract.

abut on fenestrated capillaries draining into the long portal veins.

The parvocellular neuroendocrine cells synthesize seven established releasing/inhibiting factors (Table 16-2).

Release of the various factors into the capillary bed is regulated by the action of neurons reaching the median eminence from several sources. Most numerous are dopaminergic fibers from cells in the arcuate nucleus. Dopamine is the prolactin inhibitory factor. In addition, the dopaminergic endings inhibit FSHRF and LHRF liberation by means of axo-axonic synapses on these neuroendocrine cells. Estrogen-containing contraceptives act in part upon estrogen receptors on the somatodendritic trees of the dopaminergic neurons. The normal cyclic release of FSHRF and LHRF is probably controlled by axons reaching the median eminence from the anterior hypothalamic area, where several biorhythms originate.

Table 16-2   Releasing factors (RF) and inhibitory factors (IF) synthesized in hypophysiotropic nuclei

Releasing/inhibiting factors	Nuclei of origin
Thyrotropin RF (TRF)	Dorsomedial
Growth hormone RF (GRF)	Ventromedial
Growth hormone IF (somatostatin)	Periventricular
Luteinizing hormone RF (LRF)	Preoptic
Follicle-stimulating hormone RF (FSHRF)	Arcuate
Corticotropin RF (CRF)	Contained within supraoptic and paraventricular nuclei
Prolactin IF	Arcuate

Other central transmitters/modulators released in the median eminence include: norepinephrine and epinephrine (from brain stem aminergic neurons), acetylcholine (from the basal forebrain), and GABA produced locally. They have complex effects, both direct and indirect, upon the axons of the tuberoinfundibular tract.

Tanycytes

Tanycytes are specialized ependymal cells found in the walls of the third ventricle. Long processes extend from their bases and place end feet on capillaries in the median eminence. Tanycytes are thought to transfer metabolites from CSF to median eminence or vice versa. Some end feet receive synaptic contacts from dopaminergic fibers; these may cause the cells to change their shape so as to control access of neurohormones to the capillary bed.

Autonomic centers

Stimulation of the anterior hypothalamic area produces parasympathetic effects: slowing of heart, constriction of pupils, salivation, and intestinal peristalsis. Stimulation of the posterior hypothalamic area produces sympathetic effects: increase in heart rate and blood pressure, pupillary dilatation, and intestinal stasis. Axons from both areas project via the posterior longitudinal fasciculus to autonomic nuclei in the brain stem and spinal cord. The hypothalamic centers are played upon by fibers from the forebrain, notably from limbic areas.

Temperature control

The *anterior hypothalamic area* contains a center which acts to prevent a rise in body temperature. The center responds to information from thermoreceptors in skin and mucous membranes, and from heating of the hypothalamic blood stream, by activating heat loss mechanisms: cutaneous vascular dilatation, sweating, panting, and appropriate behavioral activities.

The *posterior hypothalamic area* contains a center which promotes heat conservation and heat production. This center responds to activity of cold-sensitive peripheral nerve endings, and to cooling of the blood. Heat is conserved by cutaneous vasoconstriction, piloerection, and behavioral responses. Heat is produced by increased metabolic activity and by shivering.

Eating

Eating habits have obvious social and cultural components, mediated by the neocortex and by limbic areas of the brain. The hypothalamus provides a baseline for feeding activities, in the form of interplay between the lateral and ventromedial nuclei. Together, they are called the *appestat*. Stimulation of the lateral hypothalamic nucleus (the feeding center) causes an experimental animal to eat, whereas destruction of both lateral nuclei causes a refusal to eat. Conversely, stimulation of the ventromedial nucleus (the satiety center) inhibits the urge to eat, and bilateral lesions result in overeating.

Animal experiments suggest that the feeding center is tonically active, being suppressed after meals by the satiety center. The satiety center contains neurons responsive to a rise in the level of glucose in the blood. These *glucostats* receive inhibitory inputs relayed from vagal nerve fibers (Chapter 36) whose afferent endings in the liver discharge in response to a rise in glucose concentration in the portal vein. Efferent vagal fibers respond by promoting the release of insulin from the pancreas.

Drinking

Stimulation of the *lateral nucleus* induces polydypsia (excessive drinking). Lesioning may induce adypsia, with severe dehydration. There is reason to believe that the *zona incerta* (ZI) is affected by these experiments, rather than the lateral nucleus proper. The ZI is a ribbon of cells extending from the anterior hypothalamus to the rostral end of the midbrain (see Fig. 17-4). It is intimately connected to the lateral nucleus.

Osmoreceptors – neurons sensitive to increased osmolarity of the blood – are found in several areas of the hypothalamus, including the lateral nucleus and the vasopressin-secreting nuclei. Peripheral volume receptors are also important: in the resting state, 80% of the blood occupies the venous side of the circulation, and filling of the veins exerts an inhibitory action on the lateral hypothalamus through tonic stimulation of stretch receptors in the walls of veins. These *volume receptors* are comparable in structure to the arterial baroreceptors, although they are less elaborate.

Extracellular hypovolia, for example after hemorrhage or diarrhea, induces vasoconstriction of peripheral vessels, including those in the kidneys (Fig. 16-11). Activation of the renin–angiotensin system is considered important in inducing drinking, because angiotensin instilled into the anterior hypothalamus causes vigorous drinking even in normovolemic animals. At the same time, angiotensin increases sodium retention by stimulating the release of aldosterone from the suprarenal cortex.

Fear and rage

The *ventromedial and lateral nuclei* are concerned in avoidance reactions to threatening stimuli (fear response) and in aggressive reactions (rage response).

Rage may be produced experimentally either by destruction of both ventromedial nuclei or by stimulation of the lateral nuclei. However, this latter response can be abolished by prior removal of the amygdalas from the temporal lobes. Removal of the two amygdalas results in a placid animal which can be rendered aggressive by subsequent destruction of the ventromedial nucleus. In this situation the lateral hypothalamus is apparently freed from inhibitory controls.

Reward and punishment

Stimulation of the ventromedial nucleus in humans produces an unpleasant feeling and an avoidance reaction. Stimulation of the preoptic area, or of the septal area above it, produces a glow of pleasure – a 'good feeling'.

Sleeping and waking

Sleeping and waking are cyclical activities, and the anterior hypothalamic area seems to be concerned in maintaining the normal rhythm. Bilateral lesions of the anterior hypothalamus may result in prolonged periods of wakefulness in animals, and rarely in human patients. By contrast, bilateral lesions of the posterior hypothalamic area may result in 'rousable hypersomnolence' resembling normal sleep. If the adjacent medial forebrain bundle is included in a posterior lesion, or if the bundle is selectively injured on both sides, profound coma follows.

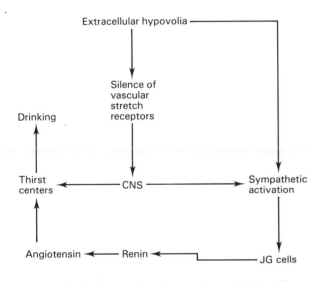

Fig. 16-11 Mechanisms involved in stimulating drinking. JG, juxtaglomerular. (After Plum and van Uitert, 1978.)

APPLIED ANATOMY

Neurological lesions confined to the hypothalamus are rare. To elicit hypothalamic dysfunction a lesion must be bilateral. The commonest single cause is a craniopharyngioma, a tumor of embryologic (Rathke's pouch) origin declaring itself in the first or second decade.

Hypothalamic lesions may injure pathways, specific nuclei, or both. Neural pathways are especially vulnerable to posterior lesions. Damage to the two medial forebrain bundles results in profound, unrousable coma. Damage to the posterior longitudinal fasciculi interrupts the heat-production and heat-dissipating pathways to the neuroaxis. Various autonomic dysfunctions have also been described.

Neural pathways may also be interrupted by expanding tumors in the intermediate area, through which course the fornix and stria terminalis. Interruption of both pillars of the fornix may produce a classical Korsakoff syndrome (Chapter 22), with loss of short-term memory and preservation of intermediate and long-term memory. Injury to the striae terminales may be accompanied by changes of mood.

Endocrine pathways are readily damaged by midline lesions because the hypothalamohypophyseal and tubero-infundibular tracts lie close to the third ventricle. Diabetes insipidus follows a lesion of the final common pathway for antidiuretic hormone secretion, in the interval between the two nuclei concerned and the median eminence (where some of the secretion enters the blood stream). Lesions in the interval between the hypophysiotropic area and the median eminence result in varying degrees of hypopituitarism.

Bilateral nuclear lesions may affect the anterior, intermediate, or posterior areas, but only rarely the lateral areas, because these are further apart. The effects conform to those produced by destructive lesions in animals.

Readings

Anderson, G.H., Li, E.T.S. and Glanville, N.T. (1984) Brain mechanisms and the quantitative and qualitative aspects of food intake. *Brain Res. Bull.*, 12: 167–173.

Buijs, R.M. (1983) Vasopressin and oxytocin – their role in neurotransmission. *Pharmacol. Ther.*, 22: 127–141.

Buijs, R.M. and Van Heerikhuize (1982) Vasopressin and oxytocin release in the brain: a synaptic event. *Brain Res.*, 252: 71–76.

Defandini, R. and Zimmerman, E.A. (1978) The magnocellular neurosecretory system of the mammalian hypothalamus. In *The Hypothalamus. Research Publications: Association for Research in Nervous and Mental Disease*, Vol. 56. (Reichlin, S., Baldessarini, R.J. and Martin, J.B., eds.), pp. 137–152. New York: Raven Press.

Everitt, B.J., Herbert, J. and Keverne, E.B. (1983) The neuroendocrine anatomy of the limbic system: a discussion with special reference to steroid responsive neurons, neuropeptides and monoaminergic systems. In *Progress in Anatomy*, Vol. 3 (Navaratnam, V. and Harrison, R.J., eds.), pp. 235–260. Cambridge: Cambridge University Press.

Fitzsimons, J.T. (1970) The renin–angiotensin system in the control of drinking. In *The Hypothalamus* (Martini, L., Motta, M. and Fraschini, F., eds.), pp. 195–212. New York & London: Academic Press.

Flament-Durand, J. and Desclin, L. (1970) The hypophysiotropic area. In *The Hypothalamus* (Martini, L., Motta, M. and Fraschini, F., eds.), pp. 245–258. New York & London: Academic Press.

Ganong, W.F. (1979) Neural centers regulating visceral function. In *The Nervous System* (Ganong, W.F., ed.), pp. 163–183. Los Altos: Lange.

Grossman, S.P. (1984) A reassessment of the brain mechanisms that control thirst. *Neurosci. Behav. Rev.*, 8: 95–104.

Jackson, I.M.D. (1978) Extrahypothalamic and phylogenetic distribution of hypothalamic peptides. In *The Hypothalamus. Research Publications: Association for Research in Nervous and Mental Disease*, Vol. 56. (Reichlin, D., Baldessarini, R.J. and Martin, J.B., eds.), pp. 217–232. New York: Raven Press.

Kawata, M., Hashimoto, K., Takahara, J. and Sano, Y. (1982) Immunohistochemical demonstration of the localization of corticotrophin releasing factor-containing neurons in the hypothalamus of mammals including primates. *Anat. Embryol. (Berl.)*, 165: 303–313.

Kawata, M. and Sano, Y. (1982) Immunohistochemical identification of the oxytocin and vasopressin neurons in the hypothalamus of the monkey. *Anat. Embryol. (Berl.)*, 165: 151–167.

Langevin, H. and Iversen, L.-L. (1980) A new method for the microdissection of the human hypothalamus, with mapping of cholinergic, GABA, and catecholamine systems in twelve nuclei and areas. *Brain*, 103: 623–638.

Leonard, B.E. (1984) GABA and endocrine regulation. *Neurochem. Int.*, 6: 17–22.

Nauta, W.J.H. and Haymaker, W. (1969) *The Hypothalamus* (Haymaker, W., Anderson, E. and Nauta, W.J.H., eds.), pp. 136–202. Springfield: Thomas.

Nujima, A. (1983) Glucose-sensitive afferent nerve fibres in the liver and their role in food intake and blood glucose regulation. *J. Auton. Nerv. Syst.*, 9: 207–220.

Plum, F. and van Uitert, R. (1978) Neuroendocrine diseases and disorders of the hypothalamus. In *The Hypothalamus. Research Publications: Association for Research in Nervous and Mental Disease*, Vol. 56 (Reichlin, D., Baldessarini, R.J. and Martin, J.B., eds.), pp. 415–474. New York: Raven Press.

Silverman, A.-J. and Pickard, G.E. (1983) The hypothalamus. In *Chemical Neuroanatomy* (Emson, P.C., ed.), pp. 295–336. New York: Raven Press.

Smith, P.H. and Davis, B.J. (1983) Morphological and functional aspects of pancreatic islet innervation. *J. Auton. Nerv. Syst.*, 9: 53–56.

Sofroniew, M.V. (1983) Morphology of vasopressin and oxytocin neurones and their central and vascular projections. *Prog. Brain Res.*, 60: 101–114.

Theodosis, D.T. (1983) Intracellular membrane movements associated with hormone release in magnocellular neurons. *Prog. Brain Res.*, 60: 273–279.

17
Diencephalon: Thalamus and Epithalamus

THALAMUS

The thalamus is composed of some three dozen nuclear groups. It is integrated into the motor, sensory, and limbic systems and into the reticular formation.

Subdivisions (Fig. 17-1, Table 17-1)

Anatomical

The Y-shaped *internal medullary lamina* divides the thalamus into anterior, mediodorsal, and lateral cell groups. The lateral group has dorsal and ventral tiers, each containing three nuclei. Below the hindmost member of the dorsal tier (the pulvinar) lie the medial and lateral geniculate nuclei.

Functional

1 *Specific nuclei* are reciprocally connected to localized areas of the cerebral cortex. They are said to be 'cortically dependent', because they degenerate when the target area of cortex is removed.

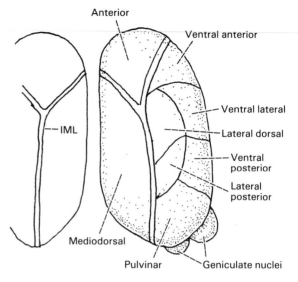

Fig. 17-1 Thalamus from above, with nuclear subdivisions. IML, internal medullary lamina.

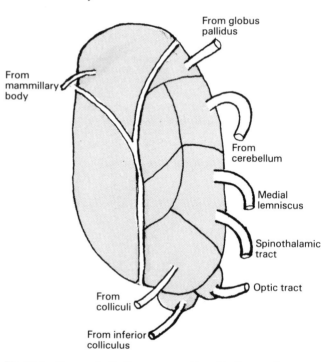

Fig. 17-2 Diagram indicating sources of input to the specific thalamic nuclei.

2 *Non-specific nuclei* project to wide areas of the cortex and influence their level of activity. They are not cortically dependent because they give abundant sustaining collaterals to one another.
3 *Association nuclei* have reciprocal linkages with association areas of the cerebral cortex (Table 17-1).

Specific nuclei (Fig. 17-2)

The *anterior nucleus* belongs to the limbic system (Chapter 22).

The *ventral anterior nucleus* (VA) is involved in the programing of movements controlled by the basal ganglia (Chapter 18).

The *ventral lateral nucleus* (VL) contains a spatial map of similar shape to that in the ventral posterior nucleus

Table 17-1 Thalamic nuclei and their chief connections: all receive afferents from the cerebral cortex

Nuclei	Afferents	Efferents
Specific		
Anterior	Mammillary body	Cingulate cortex
Ventral anterior	Globus pallidus	Premotor cortex, intra-laminar
Ventral lateral	Cerebellar roof nuclei	Motor cortex
Ventral posterior	Medial lemniscus Spinothalamic tract Trigeminothalamic tract	Somesthetic cortex
Medial geniculate	Inferior colliculus	Auditory cortex
Lateral geniculate	Superior colliculus	Visual cortex
Non-specific		
Intralaminar	Reticular formation	Widespread to cortex
Reticular	Thalamic efferents	Thalamic nuclei, reticular formation
Association		
Mediodorsal	Frontal cortex, amygdala, etc.	Frontal cortex, orbital cortex
Dorsal lateral	Ventral anterior, intralaminar	Parietal cortex
Dorsal posterior	Pulvinar, intra-laminar	Parietal cortex
Pulvinar	Colliculi, intra-laminar	Parietal, occipital, superior temporal cortex

(see later): localized stimulation of VL produces movement of a contralateral body part. VL has point-to-point interconnections with the homunculus (Chapter 20) in the motor cortex.

The globus pallidus is the output nucleus of the basal ganglia. It projects mainly to VA, and less to VL. The cerebellar roof nuclei project mainly to VL, less to VA. The fastigial nucleus gives a small projection to the trunk cells of VL; the nucleus interpositus gives a medium projection to trunk and proximal limb cells; the dentate gives a massive projection (half a million fibers) to proximal and distal limb cells.

The *ventral posterior nucleus* is known as the *ventrobasal complex*. It comprises a lateral nucleus (VPL), receiving the medial lemniscus and spinothalamic tract, and a medial nucleus (VPM), receiving

corresponding inputs from the face in the trigeminothalamic tract (Fig. 17-3). The ventrobasal complex contains modality-specific cell groups projecting to homunculi in the somesthetic cortex (Chapter 20).

Painful and thermal information from the contralateral body surface is segregated from tactile and proprioceptive information. It enters the posterior ends of the VPL and VPM, an area sometimes called the posterior thalamic nucleus. This nucleus projects mainly to the second somatic sensory cortex (SII) at the foot of the postcentral gyrus.

The *medial geniculate nucleus* is the specific thalamic nucleus for hearing (Chapter 30).

The *lateral geniculate nucleus* is the specific thalamic nucleus for vision (Chapter 29).

Nonspecific nuclei (Fig. 17-4)

The chief *intralaminar nuclei* are the *centromedian* and *parafascicular*. They receive afferents from the ascending reticular activating system (ARAS, Chapter 14) and project to wide areas of the cerebral cortex. Intralaminar stimulation produces the EEG arousal pattern in animals; the pattern builds up slowly during several seconds and outlasts the stimulus by half a minute. The intralaminar nuclei modulate the responsivity of the cortex to specific thalamocortical inputs.

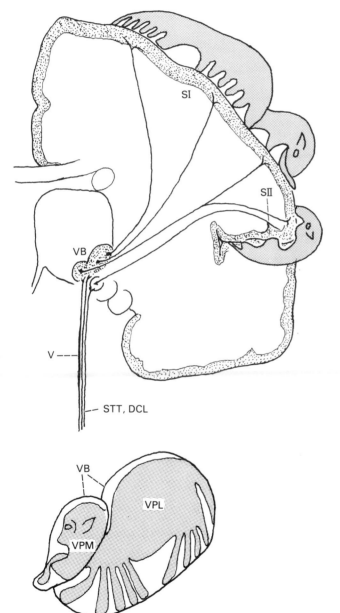

Fig. 17-3 Simunculi (monkey) in ventrobasal complex (VB) and in primary and secondary somatic sensory areas. DCL, dorsal column–lemniscal pathway; STT, spinothalamic tract; V, trigeminothalamic; VPL, ventral posterior lateral nucleus; VPM, ventral posterior medial nucleus; SI, first somatic sensory cortex; SII, second somatic sensory cortex.

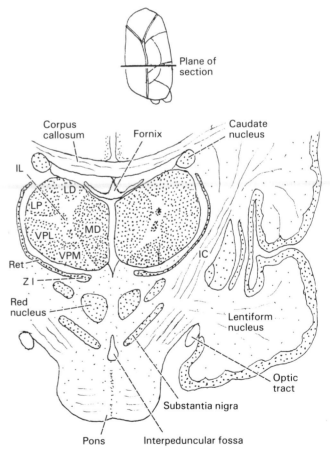

Fig. 17-4 Frontal section of brain base. IC, internal capsule; IL, internal medullary lamina; LD, lateral dorsal nucleus; LP, lateral posterior nucleus; MD, mediodorsal nucleus; Ret., reticular nucleus; S, subthalamic nucleus; VPL, ventroposterolateral nucleus; VPM, ventroposteromedial nucleus; ZI, zona incerta.

In human patients, intralaminar stimulation may produce painful sensations of very unpleasant nature over large areas of the body. The natural sources of painful information to the intralaminar nuclei are spinoreticulothalamic fibers, which also synapse in the mediodorsal nucleus. The intralaminar and mediodorsal terminations are concerned with arousal and with the qualitative (affective) aspects of painful stimuli. The 'where' and 'how much' aspects are handled by the spinothalamic tract and posterior nucleus.

The centromedian nucleus also receives fibers from the globus pallidus and ventral striatum (Chapter 18).

The *reticular nucleus* is perforated by all corticothalamic and thalamocortical fibers, and all give collaterals to it. The nucleus contains many GABAergic neurons which backtrack to the specific thalamic nuclei. The inhibitory screen is itself inhibited by GABAergic fibers from the intralaminar nucleus; this would be expected in view of the function of the ARAS. In addition, the frontal lobe of the brain seems able to operate a selective gating mechanism through excitatory thalamoreticular fibers from the mediodorsal nucleus (see later).

The zona incerta lies beside the ventral part of the reticular nucleus. The zona is functionally a hypothalamic structure concerned with regulation of water intake (Chapter 16).

So-called 'nuclei of the midline' have been thought to underlie the ependyma of the third ventricle. Their existence has recently been called into question.

Association nuclei

The massive *mediodorsal nucleus* (MD) has point-to-point interconnections with the prefrontal cortex (Fig. 17-5). It is also connected to the anterior temporal, visual association, and secondary olfactory cortex, to the hypothalamus, and to the fornix.

In relation to its size, the mediodorsal nucleus is the least understood part of the brain. Its rich connections with the frontal lobe imply important functions in cognitive (thinking, judgment) functions and in affective (emotional) behavior.

Surgical disconnection of the frontal lobe from the MD (frontal leukotomy) produces alterations of mood with a tendency to euphoria and to inappropriate social behavior. Lesions of the MD itself may result in *Korsakoff's psychosis*, characterized by difficulty in remembering new information. Such lesions may interrupt a pathway from fornix to frontal cortex (Chapter 22).

The MD projects excitatory fibers to the entire reticular nucleus. At least in theory, the MD may operate 'minigates' by exciting all but a selected group of reticular neurons, permitting selective access of motor or sensory impulse streams to the cerebral cortex.

The *lateral dorsal* and *lateral posterior* nuclei and the *pulvinar* nuclei are also poorly understood. They receive afferents from adjacent thalamic nuclei (thus, lateral dorsal from anterior, lateral posterior from ventrobasal, pulvinar from geniculate nuclei). The lateral dorsal and lateral posterior project to the superior parietal cortex and the pulvinar to wide

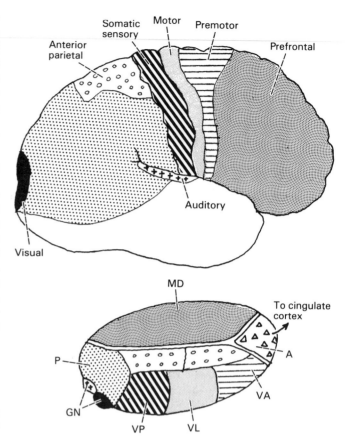

Fig. 17-5 Interconnections between thalamus and cerebral cortex. A, anterior nucleus; GN, geniculate nuclei; MD, mediodorsal nucleus; P, pulvinar; VA, VL, VP, ventral anterior, ventral lateral and ventral posterior nuclei.

cortical areas around the posterior end of the lateral sulcus (Fig. 17-5).

The pulvinar is especially mysterious in view of its large size in the primate brain. It receives auditory and visual information and it projects to auditory and visual association areas. The involvement of the pulvinar in 'blindsight' is described in Chapter 29.

Non-thalamic projections to the cortex

Although the thalamus (Gr., meeting place) is well-named, not all projections to the cerebral cortex relay there. Aminergic cell groups in the brainstem send myriads of beaded axons to the cortex by way of the internal capsule. Other fibers run direct to the cortex from basal forebrain nuclei. Details are in Chapter 19.

Thalamic peduncles (Figs. 17-6, 17-7)

The reciprocal connections between thalamus and cortex travel in the *thalamic peduncles* (radiations). The anterior peduncle passes through the anterior limb of the internal capsule to reach the frontal cortex and cingulate gyrus. The superior peduncle passes through the posterior limb to reach the premotor, motor, and somatic sensory cortex. The posterior peduncle is retro- and sublenticular, reaching the parietal, occipital and temporal cortex. The inferior peduncle descends to reach the orbital and anterior temporal cortex and amygdala.

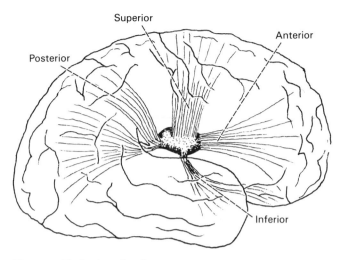

Fig. 17-6 Thalamic peduncles.

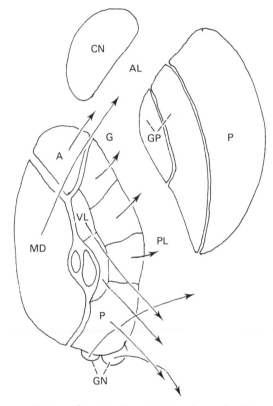

Fig. 17-7 Horizontal section through internal capsule. AL, anterior limb; G, genu; PL, posterior limb. Caudate nucleus (CN) and lentiform nuclei (P, putamen; GP, globus pallidus) are shown. A, anterior nucleus; MD, mediodorsal nucleus; VL, ventral lateral nucleus; GN, geniculate nuclei. Arrows indicate thalamic radiations.

EPITHALAMUS

The epithalamus includes the pineal gland, habenula, and stria terminalis. The latter two belong to the limbic system (Chapter 22).

Pineal gland

The pineal gland is an endocrine gland synthesizing *melatonin*, an amine hormone with an obscure relationship to gonadal function. Melatonin is synthesized in *pinealocytes*, which are paraneurons (see later). The pinealocytes contain the specific secretory granules and they lie in a rich capillary bed outside the blood–brain barrier (see 'Circumventricular organs' in Chapter 24).

Melatonin is derived by a two-step transformation of serotonin, the enzymes being unique to the pineal. In rats melatonin production is governed by an oscillator, the *suprachiasmatic nucleus* in the anterior hypothalamus, which is inhibited by light via unmyelinated axons traveling from the retina. Melatonin production is ten times higher during the night, when rats are active. The suprachiasmatic nucleus acts through the sympathetic system: it sends fibers all the way to T1 segment, whence preganglionic fibers travel to the superior cervical ganglia. Postganglionic fibers reach the gland from both sides, and norepinephrine promotes melatonin synthesis by activating β receptors on the surface of pinealocytes.

Paraneurons

Many cell types in the body are intermediate in character between neurons and endocrine cells. Criteria for paraneurons include (a) origin from neurectoderm, (b) scarcity or absence of neurites, and (c) ability to synthesize transmitters and/or hormonal peptides, which are released from appropriate vesicles and/or secretory granules.

Release of active substance

Modes of release of active substance vary from one paraneuron type to another. Some paraneurons use more than one mode. Examples of release modes (numbers refer to chapters) are:
1 Into synaptic clefts: olfactory and gustatory cells (27), hair cells of inner ear (30, 33), carotid body glomus cells (37), small intensely fluorescent (SIF) cells in sympathetic ganglia (6), Merkel cells in skin (5).
2 Into capillary beds: adrenomedullary cells (6), pinealocytes.
3 Into intercellular spaces: gastrointestinal 'paracrine' cells (39).

Pinealocytes as paraneurons

Pinealocytes satisfy the three criteria above. Phylogenetically, they are derived from photoreceptor cells of amphibia and fishes. The photoreceptors closely resemble retinal cones (Chapter 28); they are linked by a *pineal nerve* to the midbrain tectum and hypothalamus. In human fetuses a possibly comparable nerve strand links the pineal to the posterior commissure.

APPLIED ANATOMY

From the third decade onward, calcareous deposits ('pineal sand') accumulate in astrocytes within the pineal. Pineal calcification is often detectable on plain X-ray films of the skull. A shift of the pineal to one side may denote a space-occupying intracranial lesion on the other side. However, a normal pineal may lie slightly to the left because the right cerebral hemisphere tends to be wider than the left hemisphere at this level.

Tumors or cysts arising in or near the pineal may be associated with obesity and hypogonadism, probably as a result of pressure on the hypothalamus. Compression of the midbrain may obstruct the aqueduct or paralyze upward gaze (Chapter 32).

Readings

Albe-Fassard, D. and Besson, J.M. (1973) Convergent thalamic and cortical projections – the non-specific system. In *Handbook of Sensory Physiology, Vol. 2, Somatosensory System* (Iggo, A., ed.), pp. 489–560. Berlin, Heidelberg & New York: Springer-Verlag.

Bovie, J. (1979) An anatomical reinvestigation of the termination of the spinothalamic tract in the monkey. *J. Comp. Neurol., 186:* 343–370.

Carmel, P.W. (1969) Efferent projections of the ventral anterior nucleus of the thalamus in the monkey. *Am. J. Anat., 128:* 159–184.

Crosby, E.C., Humphrey, T. and Lauer, E.W. (1962) Diencephalon. In *Correlative Anatomy of the Nervous System*. New York: Macmillan.

Dewulf, A. (1971) *Anatomy of the Normal Human Thalamus.* Amsterdam, London & New York: Elsevier.

Goldman-Rakic, P.S. (1981) Development and plasticity of primate frontal association cortex. In *The Organization of the Cerebral Cortex* (Schmidt, F.O., Worden, F.G., Adelman, G. and Dennis, S.G., eds.), pp. 69–97. Cambridge, Massachusetts: M.I.T. Press.

Hansen, J.T. and Karasek, M. (1982) Neuron or endocrine cell? The pinealocyte as a paraneuron. In *The Pineal and its Hormones*, pp. 1–9. New York: Alan R. Liss.

Houser, C.R., Vaughn, J.E., Barber, R.P. and Roberts, E. (1980) GABA neurons are the major cell type of the nucleus reticularis thalami. *Brain Res., 200:* 341–354.

Jones, E.G. (1983) The thalamus. In *Chemical Neuroanatomy* (Emson, P.C., ed.), pp. 257–294. New York: Raven Press.

Kenshalo, D.R., Giesler, G.J., Leonard, R.B. and Willis, W.D. (1980) Responses of neurons in primate ventral posterior lateral nucleus to noxious stimuli. *J. Neurophysiol., 43:* 1594–1614.

Klein, D.C. (1978) Pineal gland as model of neuroendocrine control systems. In *The Hypothalamus* (Research Publications: Association for Research in Nervous and Mental Disease, Vol. 56) (Reichlin, S., Baldessarini, R.J. and Martin, J.B., eds.), pp. 303–328. New York: Raven Press.

Markowitsch, H.J. (1982) Thalamic mediodorsal nucleus and memory: a critical evaluation of studies in animals and man. *Neurosci. Behav. Rev., 6:* 351–380.

Markowitsch, H.J., Irle, E. and Streicher, M. (1982) The thalamic mediodorsal nucleus receives input from thalamic and cortical regions related to vision. *Neurosci. Lett., 32:* 131–136.

Massion, J. (1976) The thalamus in the motor system. *Appl. Neurophysiol., 39:* 222–238.

Mehler, W.R. (1971) Idea of a new anatomy of the thalamus. *J. Psychiat. Res., 8:* 203–217.

Narabayashi, H. and Ohya, E. (1978) Parkinsonian tremor and nucleus ventralis intermedius of the thalamus. *Prog. Clin. Neurophysiol., 5:* 165–182.

Pollin, B. and Rokyta, R. (1982) Somatotopic organization of nucleus reticularis thalami in chronic awake cats and monkeys. *Brain Res., 250:* 211–221.

Reiter, R.J. (ed.) (1983) *Pineal Research Reviews*, Vol. 1. New York: Alan R. Liss.

Steriade, M. (1981) Mechanisms underlying cortical activation: neuronal organization and properties of the midbrain reticular core and intralaminar thalamic nuclei. In *Brain Mechanisms and Perceptual Awareness* (Pompeiano, O. and Marsan, C.A., eds.), pp. 327–377. New York: Raven Press.

Steriade, M., Parent, A., Ropert, N. and Kitsikis, A. (1982) Zona incerta and lateral hypothalamic afferents to the midbrain reticular core of the cat – an HRP and electrophysiological study. *Brain Res., 238:* 13–28.

Strick, P.L. (1976) Anatomical analysis of ventrolateral thalamic input to primate motor cortex. *J. Neurophyiol., 39:* 1020–1031.

V
CEREBRAL HEMISPHERES

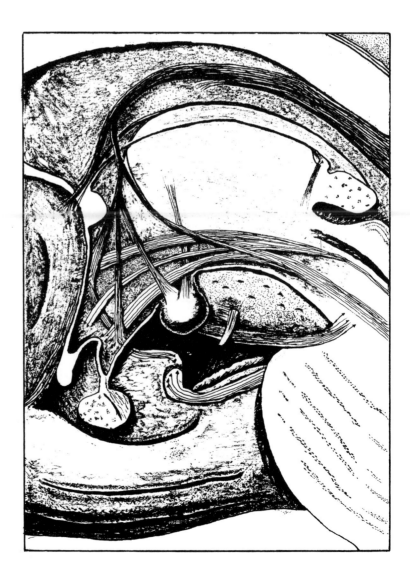

18
Basal Ganglia

Definition

The term 'basal ganglia' originally denoted the nuclear groups that develop in the basal (inferior) part of the cerebral hemispheres. These are the caudate and lentiform nuclei, the claustrum and the amygdala. However, these nuclei do not constitute a functional entity. A more meaningful use of the term has been sought in the context of clinical disorders subsumed under the old title 'extrapyramidal disease'.

The certain involvement of the substantia nigra and of the subthalamic nucleus in 'extrapyramidal' disorders has extended the conventional use of the term 'basal ganglia' to the brain stem. Today, four nuclear groups are so designated: the caudate, the lentiform, the subthalamic, and the substantia nigra. All four are known to be involved in the control of movement. Some elements of the limbic system have been added, notably the nucleus accumbens.

Striatum and pallidum (Figs. 18-1, 18-2)

The striatum comprises the caudate nucleus and the outer part – the *putamen* – of the lentiform. The caudate and putamen are identical in structure and they are linked anteriorly by strands (striae) of gray matter.

The inner part of the lentiform nucleus is known as the globus pallidus, or simply as the pallidum (Fig. 18-3). It is pallid (pale) because of an abundance of myelinated fibers.

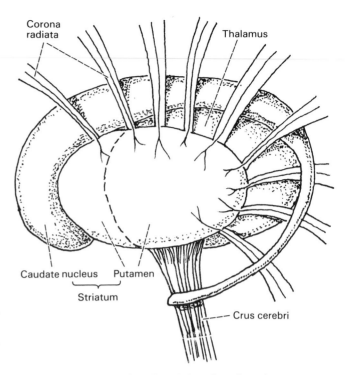

Fig. 18-2 Enlargement from Fig. 18-1, to show the striatum.

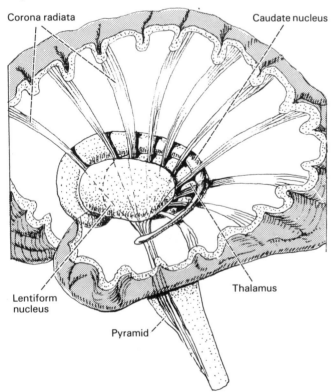

Fig. 18-1 Lateral view of corpus striatum. Most of corona radiata removed.

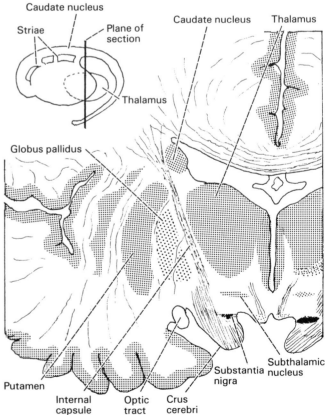

Fig. 18-3 Coronal section in the plane indicated above.

126

Substantia nigra

The substantia nigra (Chapter 12) is made up of a dorsal strip of pigmented (black) neurons called the *pars compacta* (or substantia nigra proper) and a ventral strip called the *pars reticulata*. The pars reticulata is characterized by an *absence* of pigment; it is in fact an extension of the pallidum.

Diseases of the basal ganglia give rise to motor disorders known as *dyskinesias* (Gr., difficulty of movement).

THE BASIC CIRCUIT

The basic circuit comprises five elements (Fig. 18-4):

1 From all parts of the cerebral cortex, axons stream into the striatum. The largest input is from the sensorimotor cortex. The inputs from other cortical areas are from neurons with no other destination. The significance of the prefrontal, posterior parietal, occipital and temporal contributions is enigmatic; they may be involved in imprinting motor programs in the striatum (see later). Disorders of cognitive functions (such as judgment, calculation, and appraisal of sensory information) are not characteristic of dyskinetic states in general, at least in the earlier stages.

2 The structure of the striatum is immensely complex. Most striatal neurons are short-axon internuncials. The most important appear to be excitatory cholinergic and inhibitory GABAergic internuncials, both of which lack dendritic spines.

The largest projection from the striatum is from inhibitory, GABAergic, spiny neurons which project to all parts of the pallidum (and to the substantia nigra proper).

3 The neurons of the pallidum are spiny and their axons are myelinated. The axons run to the thalamus in the *pallidothalamic tract* (Fig. 18-5). During prenatal development the crus cerebri displaces some of these axons, creating a loop – the *ansa lenticularis* (L., *ansa*, handle) – beneath the crus. The rest perforate the internal capsule as the *lenticular fasciculus*. The two strands unite medially in the *thalamic fasciculus*, which synapses in the ventral anterior (VA), and ventral lateral (VL), nuclei of the thalamus. Like the striopallidal fibers, the pallidothalamic fibers are inhibitory and GABAergic.

4 From VA and VL, excitatory fibers run to the premotor, supplementary motor, and primary motor areas of the cerebral cortex.

5 The motor cortex gives rise to the bulk of the pyramidal tract, which generates contralateral movements in response to thalamocortical stimulation.

Selective disinhibition

At rest, the striatum is almost silent while the pallidum is discharging at a high rate. Just before a contralateral movement begins the general level of pallidal firing increases. Although the pallidal effect is inhibitory, thalamocortical fibers fire to initiate a movement. An

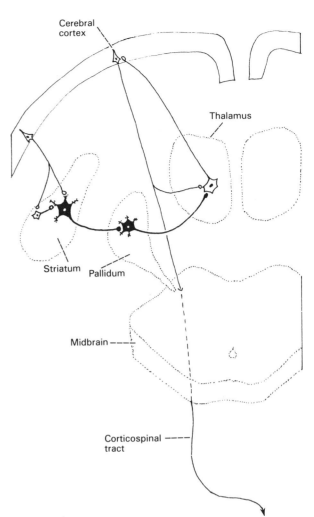

Fig. 18-4 The cortico-strio-pallido-thalamo-cortical loop.

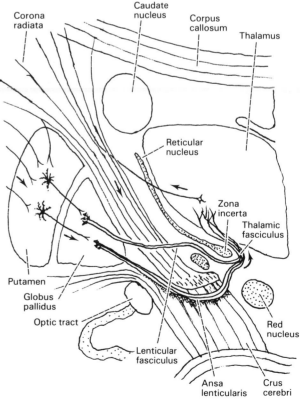

Fig. 18-5 Pallidothalamic fibers.

attempt to resolve the paradox is shown in Fig. 18-6, where it is shown that thalamocortical neurons are *selectively disinhibited*.

Before the movement begins, the cerebellum plays on the ventral lateral nucleus (through the dentatothalamic tract) to ensure smooth cooperation of pyramidal tract fibers selected by the striopallidal complex.

When the movement gets under way, pyramidal tract activity is reinforced by positive feedback from collaterals synapsing upon thalamocortical neurons (Fig. 18-4). At the same time, the pyramidal tract is influenced (unless the movement is very fast) by the cerebellar nucleus interpositus on receipt of feedback from the muscles.

Nigrostriatal pathway

The dopaminergic neurons of the substantia nigra synapse almost exclusively in the striatum, upon cholinergic and GABAergic neurons (Fig. 18-7). They also give a small projection to the reticular formation and spinal cord.

The nigrostriatal pathway is tonically active. It maintains a constant level of firing, regardless of movement. Its mode of action in the striatum is not understood – some neurons there are excited by dopamine, others are inhibited, and there are at least two kinds of dopamine receptor on striatal neurons. If dopamine stores are depleted in a monkey (by giving reserpine) the *pallidum* ceases its resting discharge and the animal becomes akinetic (cannot move). The inference is that striopallidal neurons are released by reserpine and exert tonic inhibition on the pallidum.

The normal function of the nigrostriatal pathway may be to have a tonic braking effect upon the striopallidal neurons. It may achieve this by inhibiting cholinergic or striopallidal neurons directly, or by facilitating internuncial GABAergic neurons. (Some of its action may be upon substance-P-containing neurons or enkephalin-containing neurons in the striatum, whose functions are unknown.)

How is the nigrostriatal pathway controlled? The somas and dendrites of pars compacta neurons are studded with GABAergic boutons (Fig. 18-8) derived from the pallidum and pars reticulata (Fig. 18-7). The pars reticulata also contains glycinergic (inhibitory) neurons projecting to the VA/VL and to the ipsilateral superior colliculus (Fig. 18-7).

The firing rate of nigrostriatal neurons is never more than moderate (in health) because the surrounding GABAergic boutons have presynaptic receptors activated by dopamine released from nigral dendrites into the extracellular fluid (Fig. 18-9).

Ventral striatum and ventral pallidum (Fig. 18-10)

The substantia nigra gives a small contribution to the nucleus accumbens and adjacent small nuclei (known together as the *ventral striatum*) and to the substantia innominata and amygdala (*ventral pallidum*). The ventral striatum and ventral pallidum belong to the limbic system (Chapter 31). The nucleus accumbens sends GABAergic fibers to the substantia nigra and to the pallidum. In animals, dopamine depletion of the accumbens is followed by akinesia.

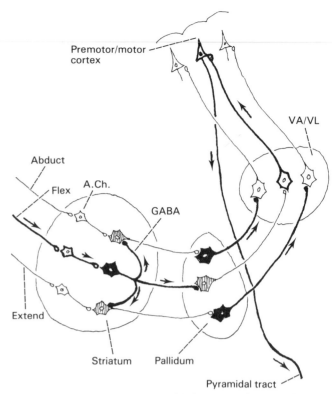

Fig. 18-6 Selective disinhibition of thalamocortical neurons by the striatum. A.Ch., cholinergic internuncial; GABA, GABAergic neuron; VA/VL, ventral anterior and ventral lateral nuclei of the thalamus. (Based on Penney and Young, 1983.)

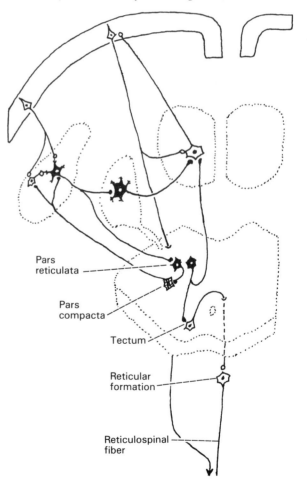

Fig. 18-7 The cortico-strio-pallido-thalamo-cortical loop (as shown in Fig. 18-4), with nigral connections added.

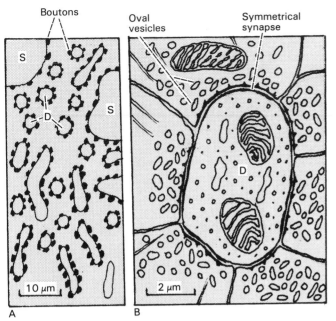

Fig. 18-8 A, dendrites (D) and somas (S) of dopaminergic neurons are studded with GABAergic boutons. B, one dendrite surrounded by inhibitory-type boutons. (Adapted from Ribac et al., 1981.)

Functional considerations

The exact role of the basal ganglia in movement is far from clear. One speculation is that the striatum contains *learned motor programs* imprinted there by the multiplicity of cortical inputs. In Parkinson's disease, patients may have to rely instead on the premotor cortex. These patients find it hard to initiate movements learned in early life (such as standing up and turning around) and in carrying them through. 'Freezing' of movement is a particular source of annoyance. (See also 'Premotor cortex' and 'Supplementary motor area' in Chapter 20.)

APPLIED ANATOMY

Parkinson's disease (paralysis agitans) usually begins in the fifth decade. *The cardinal pathologic feature is a degeneration of nigrostriatal neurons.* At autopsy, neuromelanin cannot be seen in midbrain slices.

Clinically, the cardinal signs are akinesia, rigidity, and tremor. *Akinesia* is a difficulty in initiating movements, in carrying them through (freezing), or in terminating them. *Rigidity* affects postural muscles in particular. Postures become difficult to maintain, and the patient slumps when seated in a chair. *Resting tremor* (not always present) affects the muscles of the fingers ('pill-rolling'), the forearms (pronation–supination tremor) and the head (nodding). The tremor disappears during movement, unlike the intention tremor of cerebellar disease (Chapter 13).

Chorea is an intermittent twitching of individual muscles occurring regardless of movement. Sydenham's chorea is a disorder of children; Huntington's chorea is a rare, hereditary disorder of adults. At postmortem, the striatum in Huntington's disease is severely depleted of cholinergic and GABAergic neurons.

Athetosis is characterized by continuous, writhing movements of the limbs and trunk which may continue even during sleep. Voluntary movement may be impossible. It is most often seen as a congenital disorder following asphyxia during labor. The basal ganglia show extensive degeneration.

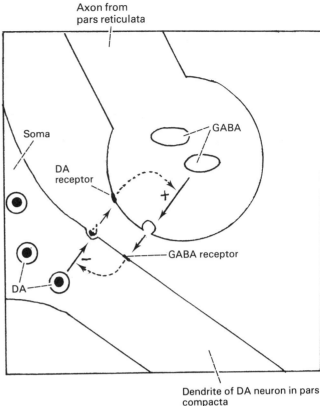

Fig. 18-9 Interactions of GABA and DA (dopamine) in the substantia nigra.

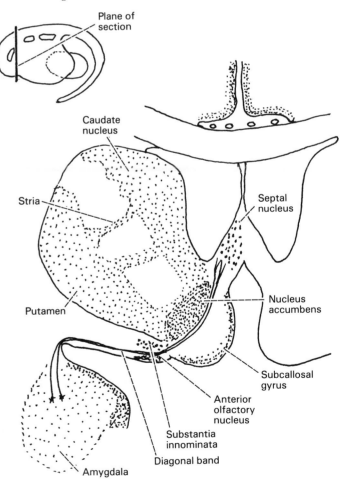

Fig. 18-10 The ventral striatum and ventral pallidum.

Hemiballismus is produced by a lesion (usually vascular) of the subthalamic nucleus. It is manifested by uncontrollable flailing movements of one or both limbs on the contralateral side.

Drug treatments of Parkinson's disease and chorea produce opposite effects. Levodopa is used in Parkinson's disease: it crosses the blood–brain barrier and is converted to dopamine by surviving nigrostriatal neurons. Its beneficial effects usually wear off within five years because 80% of nigrostriatal neurons are already dead before symptoms commence, and the rest die progressively. Levodopa is especially useful for akinesia. Anticholinergic drugs preceded levodopa, and they are more effective for tremor. Overdosage with either tends to produce choreiform movements. On the other hand, chorea is relieved by cholinergic or antidopaminergic agents, and overdosage tends to produce Parkinsonism.

Both conditions can be ascribed to faults in the loop depicted in Fig. 18-4. *In Parkinson's disease the striatum is overactive* and the circuit lacks flexibility. The cholinergic interneurons in the striatum develop spontaneous, rhythmic bursting (causing rhythmic *tremor*), which can be relieved by anticholinergic drugs or by surgical destruction downstream – of the pallidum, posterior VL (the ventral intermediate nucleus) or even of the motor cortex or pyramidal tract.

Rigidity in Parkinson's disease has two possible explanations at present: (a) disinhibition of tectoreticular neurons, resulting in excessive reticulospinal excitation of anterior horn cells; (b) overactivity of the motor thalamus, with reverberation from collaterals of the pyramidal tract.

In Huntington's chorea it is the pallidum that is overactive. VA and VL are suppressed and the motor cortex produces unwanted movements. GABA-mimetic (imitative) drugs are useless because they enhance the pallidothalamic effects.

The function of the subthalamic nucleus is not understood. It receives excitatory fibers from the motor cortex and inhibitory fibers from the pallidum and substantia nigra. It projects inhibitory (GABA) fibers to all parts of the pallidum. Excitation from the cortex should have the same effect as striatal excitation: disinhibition of the motor thalamus.

Hemiballism can be controlled either by GABA-mimetic drugs such as diazepam, or by dopamine antagonists. The reason for the latter's efficacy is obscure, although there is evidence of dopaminergic hyperactivity in these patients, as shown by an increase of the major dopamine metabolite, homovanillic acid, in the CSF.

Readings

Barnes, C. (1983) The basal ganglia in extrapyramidal dysfunction. *Brain Res. Bull., 11:* 271–275.

Becker, R.E. and Lal, H. (1983) Pharmacological approaches to treatment of hemiballism and chorea. *Brain Res. Bull., 11:* 187–189.

Beckstead, R.M. (1983) Long collateral branches of substantia nigra pars reticulata axons to thalamus superior colliculus and reticular formation in monkey and cat. *Neuroscience, 10:* 767–779.

Braak, H. and Braak, E. (1982) Neuronal types in the striatum of man. *Cell Tissue Res., 227:* 319–342.

Carpenter, M.B., Carleton, S.C., Keller, J.T. and Conte, P. (1981) Connections of the subthalamic nucleus in the monkey. *Brain Res., 224:* 1–29.

Commissiong, J.W., Gentleman, F. and Neff, N.H. (1979) Spinal cord dopaminergic neurones: evidence for an uncrossed nigrospinal pathway. *Neuropharmacology, 18:* 565–568.

Cooper, I.S. (1969) Cryogenic neurosurgery. *GP, 39:* 96–109.

Creese, I. (1982) Dopamine receptors explained. *Trends Neurosci., 5:* 40–43.

DiFiglia, M., Pasik, P. and Pasik, T. (1982) A Golgi and ultrastructural study of the monkey globus pallidus. *J. Comp. Neurol., 212:* 53–75.

Dunnett, S.B., Björklund, A. and Steveni, U. (1983) Dopamine-rich explants in experimental parkinsonism. *Trends Neurosci., 6:* 266–269.

Foley, J. (1983) The athetoid syndrome. A review of a personal series. *J. Neurol. Neurosurg. Psychiatry, 46:* 289–298.

Fonnum, F. (1984) Glutamate: a neurotransmitter in mammalian brain. *J. Neurochem., 42:* 1–11.

Graybiel, A.M. and Ragsdale, C.W. (1979) Fiber connections of the basal ganglia. *Prog. Brain Res., 51:* 239–283.

Graybiel, A.M. and Ragsdale, C.W. (1983) Biochemical anatomy of the striatum. In *Chemical Neuroanatomy* (Emson, P.C., ed.), pp. 427–504. New York: Raven Press.

Grofova, I., Denian, J.M. and Kitai, S.T. (1982) Morphology of the substantia nigra pars reticulata projection neurons intracellularly labeled with HRP. *J. Comp. Neurol., 208:* 352–368.

Groves, P.M., Wilson, C.J., Young, S.J. and Rebec, G.V. (1975) Self-inhibition by dopaminergic neurons. *Science, 190:* 522–529.

Hassler, R.G. (1984) Role of the pallidum and its transmitters in the therapy of Parkinsonian rigidity and akinesia. In *Advances in Neurology*, Vol. 40 (Hassler, R.G. and Christ, J.F., eds.), pp. 1–14. New York: Raven Press.

Hassler, R. and Chung, Y.-W. (1984) Identification of eight types of synapses in the pallidum externum and internum of squirrel monkey. *Acta Anat., 118:* 65–81.

Heimer, L., Switzer, R.D. and Van Hoesen, G.W. (1982) Ventral striatum and ventral pallidum: components of the motor system? *Trends Neurosci., 4:* 83–86.

Hornykiewicz, O. (1981) Biochemical determinants of Parkinson's disease. In *Handbook of Biological Psychiatry*, Part 4 (Van Praag, ed.), pp. 584–593. New York: Dekker.

Iansek, R. (1980) The effects of reserpine on motor activity and pallidal discharge in monkeys: implications for the genesis of akinesia. *J. Physiol., 301:* 457–466.

Jones, D.L. and Mogenson, G.J. (1980) Nucleus accumbens to globus pallidus GABA projection: electrophysiological and iontophoretic applications. *Brain Res., 188:* 93–105.

Marsden, C.D. (1980) The enigma of the basal ganglia and movement. *Trends Neurosci., 2:* 284–287.

Marsden, C.D. (1982) Neurotransmitters and CNS disease. *Lancet, 2:* 1141–1147.

Marsden, C.D. (1984) Motor disorders in basal ganglia diseases. *Human Neurobiol., 2:* 245–250.

Narabayashi, H. (1980) Clinical analysis of akinesia. *J. Neural Transmission, Suppl. 16:* 129–136.

Parent, A., De Bellefeuille, L. and Mackay, A. (1984) Organization of the primate internal pallidum as revealed by fluorescent retrograde tracing of its afferent projections. In *Advances in Neurology*, Vol. 40 (Hassler, R.G. and Christ, J.F., eds.), pp. 15–20. New York: Raven Press.

Parnevelas, J.G. and McDonald, J.K. (1983) The cerebral cortex. In *Chemical Neuroanatomy* (Emson, P.C., ed.), pp. 505–550. New York: Raven Press.

Pasik, P., Pasik, T. and DiFiglia, M. (1979) The internal organization of the neostriatum in mammals. In *The Neostriatum* (Divac, I. and Oberg, R.G.E., eds.), pp. 5–36. Oxford & New York: Pergamon Press.

Penney, J.B. and Young, A.B. (1983) Speculations on the functional anatomy of basal ganglia disorders. *Annu. Rev. Neurosci., 6:* 73–94.

Poirier, L.J., Sourkes, T.L. and Bedard, P.J. (eds.) (1979) *The Extrapyramidal System and its Disorders.* New York: Raven Press.

Powell, E.W. and Leman, R.B. (1976) Connections of the nucleus accumbens. *Brain Res., 105:* 389–403.

Ribak, C.E., Vaughn, J.E. and Barber, R.P. (1981) Immunocytochemical localization of GABAergic neurones at the electron microscopical level. *Histochem. J., 13:* 555–582.

Staines, W.A., Nagy, J.I., Vincent, S.R. and Fibiger, H.C. (1980) Neurotransmitters contained in the efferents of the striatum. *Brain Res., 194:* 391–402.

Cerebral Cortex: General

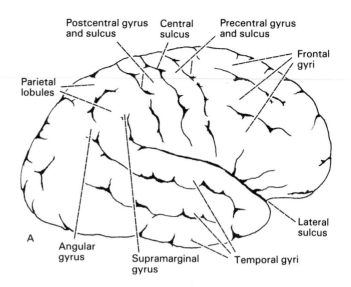

The cerebral cortex is the gray matter at the surface of the cerebral hemispheres. Its average thickness is three millimeters and it contains some 5×10^{10} neurons.

GROSS ANATOMY

Sulci and gyri

The chief sulci (fissures) and gyri (convolutions) are shown in Figs. 19-1 and 19-2. Most of the sulci are variable in extent. Sulci delimiting functionally distinct areas of the cerebral cortex include the central, postcentral, cingulate, rhinal, and collateral. The calcarine sulcus contains primary visual cortex in its walls. More than half the surface of the cerebral cortex occupies the walls of sulci.

Lobes (Fig. 19-3)

On the lateral surface, four major lobes of the brain are defined by (a) the central sulcus (Rolandic fissure), (b) the lateral sulcus (Sylvian fissure), (c) a line drawn from the parieto-occipital fissure to the pre-occipital notch, and (d) a line drawn from the horizontal part of the lateral fissure to join line c.

Association fibers (Fig. 19-4)

Within each hemisphere the gyri are linked by association fibers. Short association (arcuate) fibers connect adjacent gyri. Long association fibers, such as the superior and inferior *longitudinal fasciculi* and the *uncinate fasciculus*, link different lobes of the brain. The *cingulum* underlies the cingulate cortex; it contains short and long association fibers and passes into the parahippocampal gyrus.

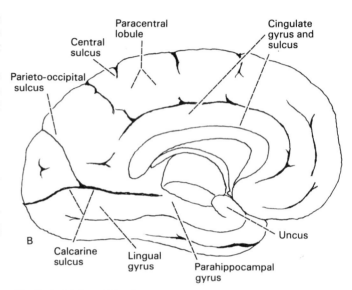

Fig. 19-1 Major sulci and gyri. A, lateral surface of right hemisphere; B, medial surface of left hemisphere.

Commissures (Figs. 19-5, 19-6)

The *cerebral commissures* are two-way connections between matching areas of the left and right hemispheres. Most important are the corpus callosum (Chapter 25) and the anterior commissure. The bulk of the *corpus callosum* passes above the lateral ventricles and basal ganglia. It is the largest fiber bundle in the entire brain. The *anterior commissure* passes through the upper part of the lamina terminalis. In primitive forms it links olfactory parts of the brain, but in mammals it extends to interconnect large areas of the temporal lobe.

Phylogeny

The cerebral cortex, or pallium, appears in three stages. The first or *archipallium*, and the second or

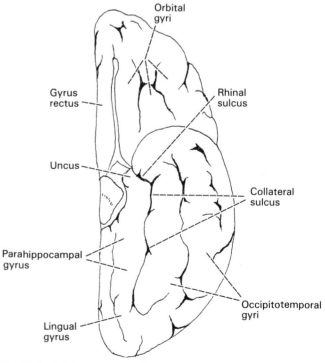

Fig. 19-2 Sulci and gyri on inferior surface of left hemisphere.

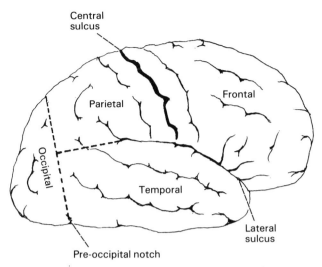

Fig. 19-3 Lateral view of the lobes of the right hemisphere.

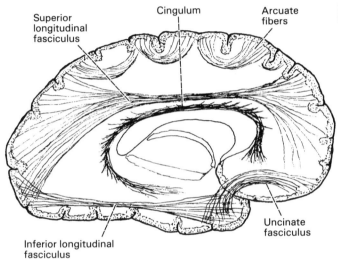

Fig. 19-4 Medial view of the left hemisphere, showing association fibers.

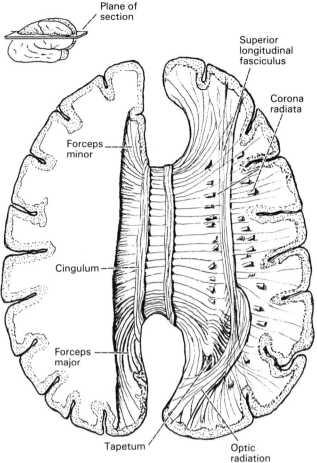

Fig. 19-5 Corpus callosum, viewed from above. (Some of the terms are explained in later chapters.)

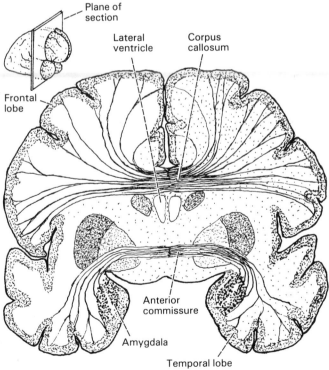

Fig. 19-6 Coronal section through anterior commissure. (The amygdala is in fact a little posterior to the plane of section.)

paleopallium, both contribute to the 'smell' brain (rhinencephalon) of the vertebrates. The *neopallium* is already present in reptiles; it expands greatly in the mammals to form the bulk of the cortex.

HISTOLOGY

A *laminar organization* is obvious in a vertical section taken from any part of the cortex. In the archi- and paleopallium the cortex contains three laminae (layers) for the most part. The trilaminar cortex is called *allocortex*. The cortex of the neopallium is six-layered and is called *isocortex* in this context (Table 19-1).

The allocortex is considered in Chapters 21 and 27. The cortex of the cingulate gyrus and of the insula (Chapter 21) is six-layered but has certain allocortical characters as well. It is sometimes referred to as *mesocortex*.

The general isocortex outside the primary motor and sensory areas is termed *homotypic* (meaning typical of its kind). Within the primary motor and sensory areas it is *heterotypic* (atypical) in that the six laminae are less

133

Table 19-1 Cortical subdivisions based on laminar structure

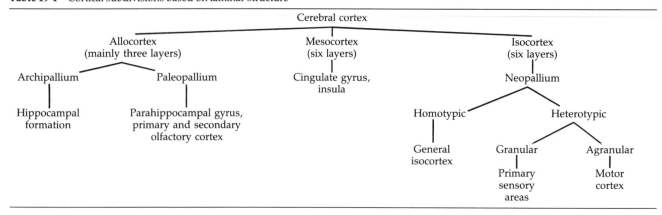

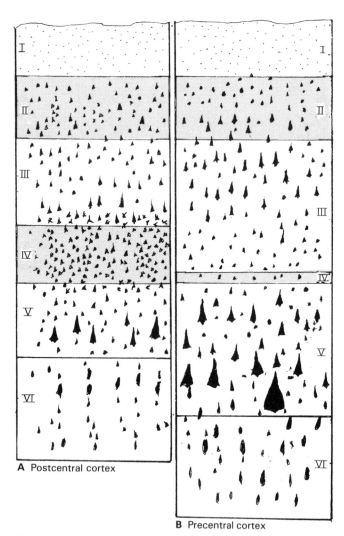

Fig. 19-7 A, granular, and B, agranular cortex.

At the microscopic level the organization of cortical neurons is manifestly laminar, but at the functional level it is vertical, or *columnar*. The columnar organization is only obvious in the primary sensory cortical areas, but physiological studies and histological tracing methods have demonstrated this arrangement in all parts of the isocortex. A few of the major cell types will be described before their organization is examined.

Cell types

Although the variety of neuronal types is very large, cortical neurons are broadly divisible into *pyramidal neurons*, which project to other parts of the cortex or to subcortical structures; and *local circuit neurons*, which are confined within the cortex.

Pyramidal neurons (Fig. 19-8)

The somas are pyramidal in shape, the dendrites are spiny, and the axon acquires a myelin sheath before entering the white matter. A single *apical dendrite* radiates branches towards the pial surface of the brain. Several *basal dendrites* come off the basal angles of the soma and radiate branches tangentially. The axon gives off several *recurrent collaterals* into the gray matter. All pyramidal neurons are excitatory and all appear to use glutamate as transmitter.

Local circuit neurons (Fig. 19-9)

Most local circuit neurons are *stellate cells*, having star-like dendritic radiations. *Spiny* stellate cells in lamina IV receive thalamocortical afferents and give rise to dozens of axonal branches which form axospinous synapses upon the dendrites of pyramidal cells. The spiny stellates are excitatory, and they are most numerous in the primary visual cortex.

Smooth (aspinous) stellate cells receive boutons from other local circuit neurons and from the recurrent collaterals of pyramidal neurons. The largest aspinous neurons are called *basket cells*; their axons run across the cortex for several millimeters and enclose the somas of pyramidal cells. They resemble the basket cells of the cerebellar cortex, and they are powerfully inhibitory, using GABA as transmitter.

easily defined. The heterotypic character derives from the number of granule (stellate) cells in lamina IV. The stellate cells are the principal targets of afferents from the specific (cortically dependent) thalamic nuclei. In the primary sensory cortical areas (somatic, visual, auditory) lamina IV is very obvious and its cells are small; hence the term *granular* applied to these areas (Fig. 19-7). In the primary motor cortex, on the other hand, stellate cells are scarce in lamina IV; hence the term *agranular* for this area.

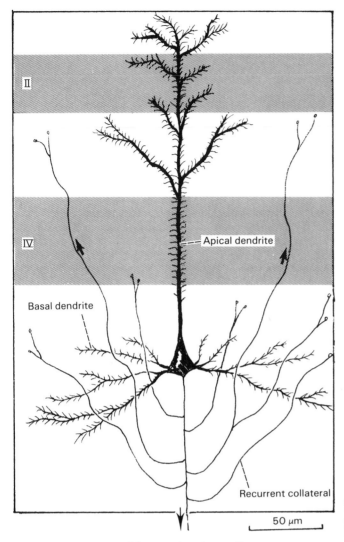

Fig. 19-8 Large pyramidal neuron from lamina V.

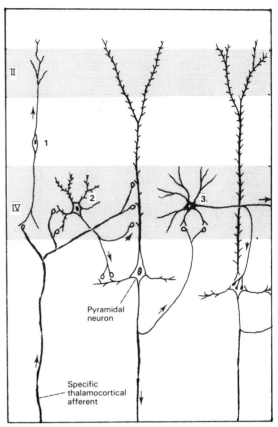

Fig. 19-9 Three local circuit neurons: 1, bipolar; 2, spiny stellate; 3, smooth stellate.

Bipolar neurons project to lamina II. Their transmitters include vasoactive intestinal polypeptide (VIP) and cholecystokinin (CKK). In experimental cortical brain slices, these peptides cause glycogen breakdown. They may also be concerned in the regulation of regional blood flow during cortical activity (Chapter 24).

Notes Some of the smallest pyramidal neurons are local circuit neurons; that is, they do not leave the cortex. Some of the largest spiny stellates send association fibers to other parts of the cortex.

ORGANIZATION OF THE ISOCORTEX

The cellular laminae (Fig. 19-10)

I The *plexiform layer* contains a dense network of axons and dendrites. Some of the axons are terminals of nonspecific thalamocortical fibers. Others belong to a small number of *horizontal cells* (of Cajal) which are numerous before birth. The apical dendrites of pyramidal cells reach this layer.

II The *outer granular layer* is composed of small stellate cells and small pyramidal cells.

III The *outer pyramidal layer* contains small and

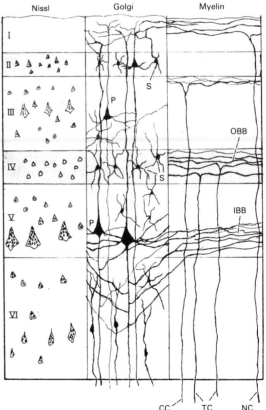

Fig. 19-10 Laminar structure of isocortex. CC, corticocortical; IBB, OBB, inner and outer bands of Baillarger; NC, nonspecific thalamocortical fibers; P, pyramidal cells; S, stellate cells; TC, specific thalamocortical fibers. Labels at top indicate staining methods.

medium pyramidal cells which (with those of lamina II) give rise to corticocortical axons, both association and commissural.

IV The *inner granular layer* contains spiny and aspinous stellate cells.

V The *inner pyramidal layer* contains large pyramidal cells whose axons supply a wide range of subcortical neurons in the basal ganglia, brain stem, and spinal cord.

VI The *multiform layer* contains a variety of cell types. The predominant type is a modified pyramidal neuron called a *fusiform cell*, whose axon runs to the thalamus.

The fibrous laminae (Fig. 19-10)

Myelin stains reveal intracortical laminae made up of thalamocortical afferents and collateral branches of pyramidal and local circuit neurons. Most obvious are the two *bands of Baillarger*. The outer band occupies lamina IV. It is created by afferents from the specific thalamic nuclei. It is prominent in the granular cortex of primary sensory areas. The inner band is produced by myelinated collaterals from large pyramidal cells, and it also contains the basal dendrites of these cells.

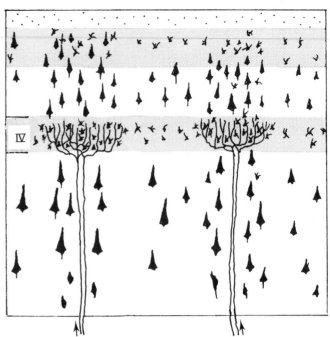

Fig. 19-11 The columnar organization is structured around thalamocortical afferents to lamina IV.

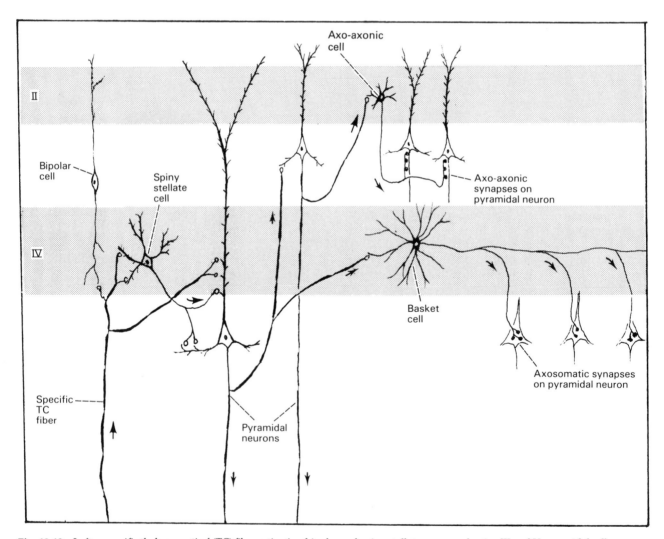

Fig. 19-12 Left: a specific thalamocortical (TC) fiber activating bipolar and spiny stellate neurons; lamina III and V pyramidal cells are activated by spiny stellates and by recurrent pyramidal-cell collaterals. Right: weakly active lamina III neurons are silenced by axo-axonic cells. Peri-columnar inhibition is exerted by basket cells.

Columnar organization of the isocortex

A given cortical cell column, or *module*, is organized around one or two thalamocortical fibers terminating in lamina IV (Fig. 19-11). The number of neurons in a column is about ten thousand and the column width is 0.3–0.5 mm. The thalamocortical fibers synapse mainly upon spiny stellate cells, which in turn powerfully excite the several hundred pyramidal cells contained within the module.

The lateral spread of excitation within a module is carried out by pyramidal cells. Recurrent axon collaterals of lamina III pyramidal cells synapse upon apical and basal dendrites of their neighbors. Spread is aided by occasional dendrodendritic contacts – some synaptic, others electrotonic (nexuses).

The spread of excitation to other columns of similar function is by means of recurrent collaterals of lamina V pyramidal cells; some of these run for several millimeters within the inner band of Baillarger.

Under experimental conditions, activation of a particular column by a peripherally applied stimulus is characteristically accompanied by inhibition of its neighbors. This *surround inhibition* is executed by the basket cells. The margins of an active module are 'sharpened' by inhibition of weakly active pyramidal cells; several small GABA internuncials are involved, notably the axo-axonic cell, which has a powerful veto at the level of the initial segment, especially in lamina III (Fig. 19-12).

In addition to specific thalamocortical effects, the activity of cortical cell columns is modified by corticocortical afferents, most of which enter the cortex in the intervals between modules. Commissural afferents arise from medium and large pyramidal cells in matching contralateral areas; they terminate in laminae II and IV. Association fibers arise in laminae II and III and terminate in lamina II of the same hemisphere. Non-specific thalamocortical afferents terminate in all layers but mainly in lamina I, where they 'arouse' the great majority of pyramidal cell apical dendrites.

Monoaminergic fibers in the cerebral cortex

The cortex is pervaded by fine, varicose axons arising in monoaminergic neurons in the brainstem and basal forebrain.

Noradrenergic fibers

From the nucleus ceruleus in the pons, noradrenergic (NA) fibers ascend to the cortex via the central tegmental tract and internal capsule. Unlike the specific sensory and motor pathways to the cortex, the NA fibers bypass the thalamus. They pass in front of the corpus callosum and enter the frontal cortex; then they pass backward within the gray matter to reach all cortical areas. They are found in all cortical laminae and they traverse the cortical cell columns. They form innumerable en passant synapses upon cortical neurons. These fibers have four possible functions:

1 Moderately active cortical neurons are inhibited by norepinephrine while sensory transmission is unaffected. By improving the 'signal-to-noise ratio' they may enhance sensory perception and have a role in sensory attention.

2 Norepinephrine causes biochemical changes in neurons consistent with a role in learning. Animals depleted of cortical norepinephrine perform poorly in avoidance tasks.

3 Norepinephrine liberation causes contraction of cerebral capillaries by acting on pericytes. Such action may direct capillary flow toward active neurons.

4 The presence of norepinephrine seems to be required for plastic changes (Chapter 26) to take place in the cortex under experimental conditions.

Serotonergic fibers

From the raphe region of the midbrain, serotonergic fibers accompany the NA fibers to all parts of the cortex. They are less profuse than the NA fibers. Serotonin has a general inhibitory effect on cortical neurons which may relate to a function in inducing sleep. Serotonergic neurons are inhibited by LSD, and LSD's hallucinogenic effects may be related to this.

Dopaminergic fibers

From the ventral tegmental area of Tsai (between red nucleus and substantia nigra) dopaminergic fibers pass to the limbic cortex (Chapter 21).

Cholinergic fibers

From limbic nuclei in the forebrain (notably the basal nucleus of the amygdala) cholinergic fibers are

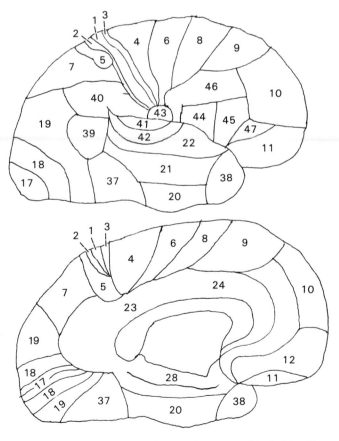

Fig. 19-13 Brodmann's cytoarchitectural map (simplified). Not all of the areas have been numbered.

extensively distributed in the cortex, especially to lamina I. Some cholinergic neurons are also found in the deeper layers of the cortex. The function of acetylcholine in the cortex is uncertain. It is mainly excitatory. Severe loss of basal nucleus cholinergic neurons accompanies Alzheimer's disease, a common form of senile dementia.

BRODMANN'S MAP

On the basis of cytoarchitectural studies (number and thickness of cortical laminae, cell types) Brodmann divided the cortex into 47 different areas. Most of them are shown in Fig. 19-13. Other workers have carried out more detailed cortical mapping. Area 19, for example, may contain as many as ten subsections, each having a specific architecture and a distinct visual function.

Some conventional terms are related to Brodmann's areas in Table 19-2.

Table 19-2   Conventional terms and Brodmann equivalents

Conventional terms	Brodmann's areas
Frontal polar	10
Orbitofrontal	47, 11
Supplementary motor	Medial 6
Premotor	Lateral 6
Motor	4
Somesthetic	3, 1, 2
Somesthetic association	5
Sensorimotor or Rolandic	4, 3, 1, 2
Primary visual	17
Visual association	18, 19
Primary auditory	41, 42
Auditory association	21, 22
Temporal polar	38
Inferotemporal	20

A further term, *prefrontal*, denotes the entire frontal cortex rostral to the premotor area.

Readings

Braak, H. (1980) *Architectonics of the Human Telencephalic Cortex.* Berlin, Heidelberg & New York: Springer-Verlag.

Brodmann, K. (1904) Beiträge zur histologischen Localization der Grosshirnrinde. *J. Psychol. Neurol., 6:* 275–400.

Crosby, E.C., Humphrey, T. and Lauer, E. (1962) White matter of the hemisphere. In *Correlative Anatomy of the Nervous System*, pp. 394–409. New York: Macmillan.

Cuello, A.C. and Sofroniew, M.V. (1984) The anatomy of the CNS cholinergic neurons. *Trends Neurosci., 7:* 74–78.

Dykes, R.W. (1983) Parallel processing of sensory information: a theory. *Brain Res. Rev., 6:* 47–115.

Jones, E.G. and Friedman, D.P. (1982) Projection pattern of functional components of thalamic ventrobasal complex on monkey somatosensory cortex. *J. Neurophysiol., 48:* 521–544.

Jones, E.G., Friedman, D.P. and Hendry, S.H.C. (1982) Thalamic basis of place- and modality-specific columns in monkey somatosensory cortex: a correlative anatomical and physiological study. *J. Neurophysiol., 48:* 545–568.

Juliano, S.L., Hand, P.J. and Whitsel, B.L. (1981) Patterns of increased metabolic activity in somatosensory cortex of monkeys (*Macaca fascicularis*) subjected to controlled cutaneous stimulation: a deoxyglucose study. *J. Neurophysiol., 46:* 1260–1284.

Lindvall, O. and Björklund, A. (1984) General organization of cortical monoamine systems. In *Monoamine Innervation of Cerebral Cortex* (Descarries, L., Reader, T.R. and Jasper, H.H., eds.), pp. 9–40. New York: Alan R. Liss.

McKenna, T.M., Whitsel, B.L. and Dreyer, D.A. (1982) Anterior parietal cortical topographic organization in macaque monkey: a re-evaluation. *J. Neurophysiol., 48:* 289–317.

Molliver, M.E., Grzanna, R., Lidov, H.G.W., Morrison, J.H. and Olschowska, J.A. (1982) Monoamine systems in the cerebral cortex. In *Cytochemical Methods in Neuroanatomy*, pp. 255–277. New York: Alan R. Liss.

Morrison, J.H. and Magistretti, P.J. (1983) Monoamines and peptides in cerebral cortex. *Trends Neurosci., 6:* 146–150.

Morrison, J.H., Magistretti, P.J., Benoit, R. and Bloom, F.E. (1984) The distribution and morphological characteristics of the intracortical VIP-positive cell: an immunohistochemical analysis. *Brain Res., 292:* 269–282.

Mountcastle, V.B. (1978) An organizing principle for cerebral function: the unit module and the distributed system. In *The Mindful Brain* (by Edelman, G.M. and Mountcastle, V.B.). Cambridge, Massachusetts: MIT Press.

Peters, A. and Jones, E.G. (1984) *The Cerebral Cortex, Vol. 1, Cellular Components.* New York: Plenum Press.

Porter, R. (1981) Internal organization of the motor cortex for input–output arrangements. In *Handbook of Physiology, Section 1: The Nervous System, Vol. 2, Motor Control, Part 2* (Brooks, V.B., ed.), pp. 1063–1081. Bethesda: American Physiological Society.

Powell, T.P.S. (1981) Certain aspects of the intrinsic organisation of the cerebral cortex. In *Brain Mechanisms and Perceptual Awareness* (Pompeiano, O. and Marsan, C.A., eds.), pp. 1–19. New York: Raven Press.

Shaw, G.L., Harth, E. and Scheibel, A.B. (1982) Cooperativity in brain function: assemblies of approximately 30 neurons. *Exp. Neurol., 77:* 324–358.

Somogyi, P., Freund, T.F. and Cowey, A. (1982) The axo-axonic interneuron in the cerebral cortex of rat, cat and monkey. *Neuroscience, 11:* 2577–2607.

Szentagothai, J. (1977) The neuron network of the cerebral cortex: a functional interpretation. *Proc. R. Soc. Lond. B., 201:* 219–248.

Vogt, C. and Vogt, O. (1919) Allgemeinere Ergebnisse unserer Hirnforschung. *J. Psychol. Neurol., 25:* 279–461.

Woolsey, C.N., Erickson, T.C. and Gilsen, W.E. (1979) Localisation in somatic and sensory motor areas of human cerebral cortex as determined by direct recording of evoked potentials and electrical stimulation. *J. Neurosurg., 51:* 476–506.

20
Sensorimotor Cortex and Pyramidal Tract

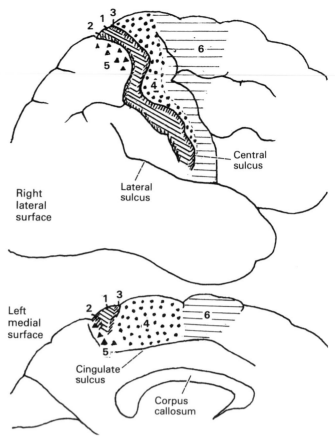

Fig. 20-1 Brodmann's areas 1–6.

The sensorimotor cortex is so called because of the close interrelationship between sensation and movement, especially during exploratory activities of the hands. The somatic sensory cortex is coextensive with the postcentral gyrus and corresponds to Brodmann's areas 3, 1, and 2. The motor cortex corresponds to Brodmann's area 4. *The pyramidal tract arises from areas 1 to 5* (Fig. 20-1).

SOMATIC SENSORY (SOMESTHETIC) CORTEX

Stimulation of the human postcentral gyrus gives rise to tingling sensations referred to the contralateral side of the body. A sensory homunculus (manikin) can be constructed by such stimulation (Fig. 20-2). The hands, face, lips, and tongue have large representations in the cortex, proportionate to their peripheral innervation densities. At the lower end of the gyrus a second, much smaller homunculus can be constructed, this time with bilateral representation of body parts. This second somatic sensory area (SII) occupies the *medial* surface of the parietal operculum (cover) of the insula (Fig. 20-3).

The tongue has the largest representation of any body part, in relation to its size (Fig. 20-4). The representation is slightly larger in the dominant hemisphere (Chapter 25), in accordance with the latter's role in speech.

Modality segregation

In monkeys, area 3 of the primary somesthetic cortex responds to stimulation of slowly adapting cutaneous receptors, whereas rapidly adapting cutaneous receptors relay to area 1. Articular receptors relay to area 2. It is possible to construct a separate 'simunculus' (in monkeys) for each of these areas, and a fourth one for the anterior limit of area 3 (called 3a), which is excited by afferents from muscle spindles. Each area comprises sets of modality-specific cortical cell columns. In area 2, however, joint-specific columns are interspersed with higher-level cutaneous columns showing 'feature extraction' – for example, columns responding only to edges drawn across the skin.

It is usual to call the primary cortex SI in mammals although only area 3 exists below the primates.

Connections

Afferents

SI receives afferents from the ventrobasal complex of the thalamus (Fig. 20-5). Modality segregation there

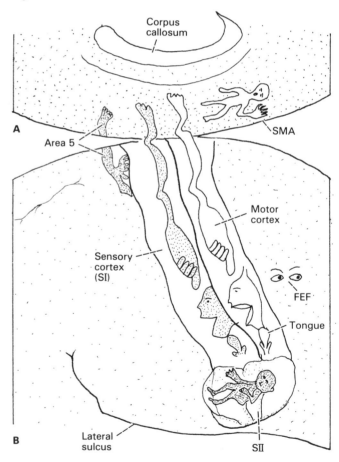

Fig. 20-2 Motor and sensory homunculi. A, medial surface; B, lateral surface. FEF, frontal eye field; SMA, supplementary motor area. The multiple homunculi that exist within SI are not represented. The tongue representations are raised in order to depict SII, which is under cover of the parietal operculum. (Adapted from Penfield and Jasper, 1954.)

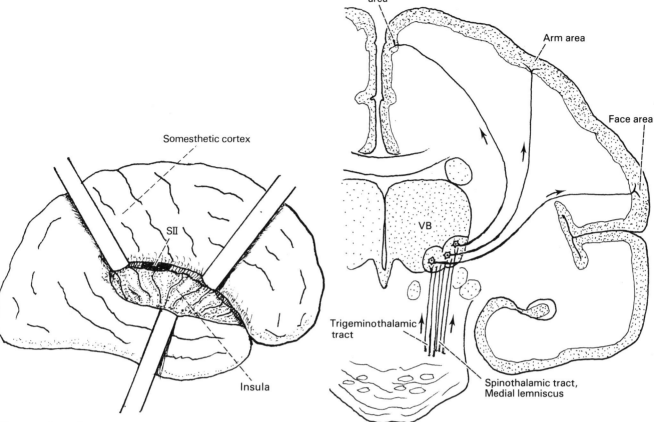

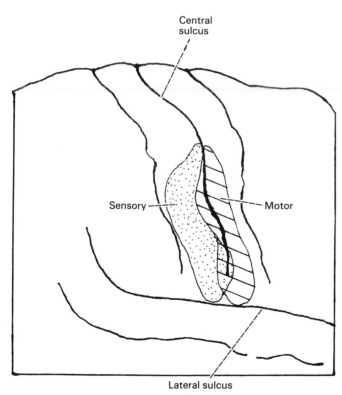

Fig. 20-3 Frontal, parietal and temporal opercula retracted to show the insula. SII (in black) is on the undersurface of the parietal operculum.

Fig. 20-5 Thalamocortical projections from the ventrobasal complex (VB) of the thalamus to the primary sensory cortex.

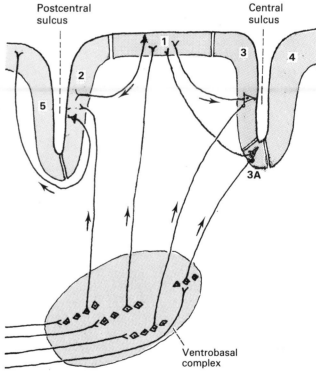

Fig. 20-4 The tongue representations completely overlap those of the face. (Adapted from Picard and Olivier, 1983.)

Fig. 20-6 Sagittal section including central and postcentral sulcus, and the ventrobasal complex of the thalamus. Sensory modalities are segregated in the thalamus as well as in the somesthetic cortex. Numbers refer to Brodmann's areas.

141

takes the form of sagitally disposed cellular rods (Fig. 20-6). Thickly myelinated fibers project from the rods to area 3 where they synapse upon a multitude of spiny stellate cells, as well as directly upon lamina V pyramidal cells. Finer myelinated fibers synapse in areas 1 and 2. *Area 4* sends corticocortical fibers to SI; these may account for sensations sometimes felt when area 4 is stimulated. Matching areas of the two sides are interconnected through the *corpus callosum*. In the monkey (at least) the hand areas are not interconnected, perhaps reflecting their relative independence.

Efferents

There are three kinds of efferents from SI: association, commissural, and projection. Association fibers pass to areas 5 and 4 (Fig. 20-6). Area 5 is sometimes called the *supplementary sensory area*. The cell columns there have peripheral receptive fields covering several dermatomes; many are multimodal, and some show feature extraction, such as responding to movement across the skin in one direction only. Area 4 receives axons from areas 1, 2, and 3.

Commissural fibers pass to matching areas of the opposite SI.

Projection fibers pass to the thalamic ventrobasal complex, striatum, and pyramidal tract.

Second somatic sensory area (SII)

The function of SII is not known. It occupies the undersurface of the parietal operculum of the insula and the uppermost part of the insula itself. Removal of SII in patients may relieve intractable pain, perhaps because spinothalamic fibers are relayed there from the posterior thalamic nucleus. It is reciprocally connected with SI and contralateral SII, and projects to the supplementary motor area.

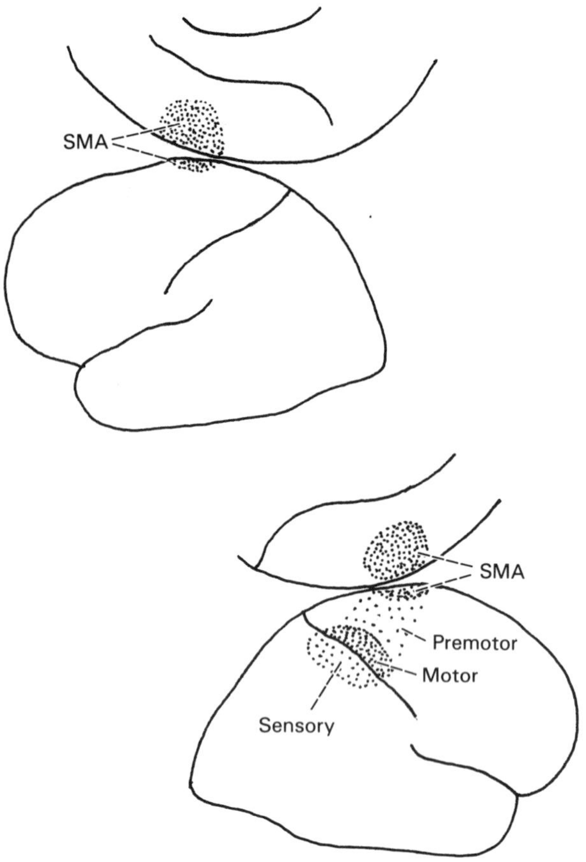

Fig. 20-7 Areas of increased cortical blood flow during voluntary movements of the left fingers. SMA, supplementary motor area.

PRIMARY MOTOR CORTEX (AREA 4, MI)

Area 4 is the thickest part of the cortex (4.5–5.0 mm, as against 3.5 mm for area 3). Unique to it are the *giant cells of Betz*, in lamina V. Betz cells provide 3% of pyramidal tract fibers, which number one million. Area 4 reaches the upper border of the cingulate sulcus on the medial surface of the hemisphere. Laterally, it terminates just above the lateral sulcus.

Connections

1 The largest single input is from the ventrolateral (VL) nucleus of thalamus which receives from the pallidum and from the deep cerebellar nuclei. The VL fibers have extensive direct synapses on basal pyramidal dendrites in lamina V.

2 The principal corticocortical afferents are from areas 5 and 6. Area 5 has composite sensory data from skin, muscles and joints. Area 6 includes the premotor cortex on the lateral brain surface and the supplementary motor area (SMA) on the medial surface (Fig. 20-7). The premotor cortex projects mainly to the

reticular formation, through which it acts upon the anterior horn cells of axial and proximal limb muscles. The two premotor areas act together to maintain postures such as sitting and standing, and to stabilize the shoulders and trunk during reaching movements of the hands. Postural functions are governed in turn by the basal ganglia through the large input received by the premotor cortex from the ventral anterior nucleus of the thalamus (Chapter 18).

The SMA, too, receives afferents from the ventral anterior nucleus of the thalamus. It projects to area 4, striatum, red nucleus and reticular formation. Of particular interest is the fact that the SMA becomes active even if the intended movement is not performed. The SMA is evidently involved in the *planning* (conception) of movements. It seems to be required also for their initiation (see 'Applied anatomy'.)

3 The outputs from area 4 are very numerous. Its projections fibers form the bulk of the pyramidal tract. Other projection fibers supply the basal ganglia, subthalamic nucleus, pontine nuclei, and reticular formation.

PYRAMIDAL TRACT

The pyramidal tract (PT) is of major clinical importance because it spans the entire length of the CNS and is frequently involved in vascular and neoplastic disorders. The PT is present only in mammals. Its myelination commences during the sixth month of gestation; all of its fibers are myelinated 18 months after birth.

Origin

About 80% of the neurons of the human PT arise in area 4. Some 10% arise in area 6 (premotor and SMA) and the rest in areas 3, 1, 2, and 5. All arise from pyramidal cells in lamina V and all are excitatory (glutamate).

The motor homunculus in area 4 closely resembles the sensory homunculus of SI. The largest representations (face, tongue, and fingers) control small motor units capable of fine gradations of movement.

Course

The PT descends in the corona radiata to the internal capsule, where it occupies the posterior limb (Fig. 20-8). It continues through the middle of the crus cerebri and the basilar pons and forms the pyramid of the medulla oblongata.

In the lower third of the medulla about 75% (the number varies) of the fibers decussate and continue as the lateral corticospinal tract (CST). About 15% continue as the anterior CST. About 10% enter the lateral CST without decussating (Fig. 20-9). The anterior CST fades away at upper thoracic levels. Its fibers cross in the white commissure and supply motoneurons serving deep muscles of the neck.

Distribution

Before leaving the cortex, PT neurons give off *recurrent collaterals*. Some reach laminae II and III and excite corticocortical pyramidal cells (including callosal neurons). Others excite neighboring PT neurons within their cell column. Still others exert pericolumnar inhibition by exciting basket cells.

The subcortical distribution of PT neurons lying in front of the central sulcus (the motor component) is to movement-related nuclei. That of PT neurons behind the central sulcus (the sensory component) is to sensory relay nuclei. However, segregation is not rigid: some sensation can be obtained upon electrical stimulation of the motor cortex, and sometimes movements can be elicited by stimulating the somesthetic cortex. These effects cannot be fully accounted for by coincidental stimulation of association neurons passing from one area to the other.

The targets of pyramidal tract fibers are numerous. Some of the target cells receive collateral branches, some receive terminals, and some receive both.

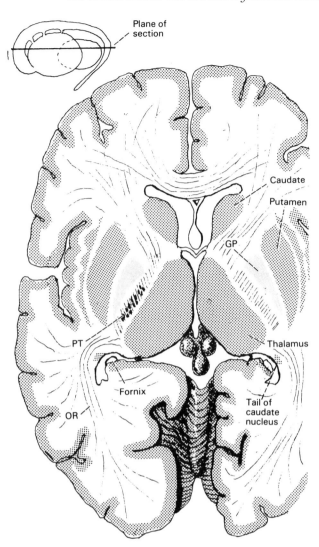

Fig. 20-8 Horizontal section through internal capsule. GP, globus pallidus; OR, optic radiation; PT, pyramidal tract.

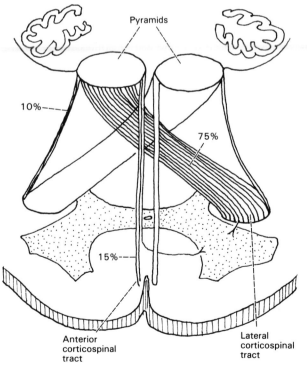

Fig. 20-9 Corticospinal fibers at spinomedullary junction.

Motor component

The motor component arises almost exclusively from areas 4 and 6 and its chief targets are:

1 SI
2 Striatum
3 VL thalamus
4 Red nucleus
5 Inferior olive
6 Pontine nuclei
7 Reticular formation
8 Motor cranial nerve nuclei
9 Ia internuncials
10 α and γ motoneurons
11 Renshaw cells

1 Collaterals to SI may give rise to the *sense of effort* during voluntary movements.
2 Striatal collaterals are additional to other corticostriatal fibers arising in lamina V (Chapter 18).
3 Thalamic collaterals are additional to corticothalamic fibers arising in lamina VI. The collaterals provide positive feedback to area 4 via VL (Chapter 18).
4 and 5 The rubro-olivocerebellar loop greatly facilitates the corticopontocerebellar system and may be involved in motor learning (Chapter 13).
6 PT inputs to the pontine nuclei inform the cerebellum about the intended movement.
7 PT collaterals are thought to exert tonic excitation of inhibitory reticulospinal fibers acting on α motoneurons. When the PT is out of action, αMNs are abnormally excitable (see 'Applied anatomy').
8 Motor cranial nerve nuclei V, VII, X (to larynx and pharynx), spinal XI (to sternomastoid and trapezius) and XII are activated monosynaptically. Cortical control of the ocular motor nuclei (III, IV, VI) is the business of the frontal eye fields (Chapter 32), not of the PT.
9 In the spinal cord, the first movement-related neurons to be activated are the Ia internuncials, which inhibit antagonistic motoneurons (Chapter 10).
10 α and γ motoneurons are supplied direct in the case of distal limb motoneurons, indirectly (via excitatory internuncials) in the case of axial and proximal limb muscles (Chapter 10). The pyramidal fibers to γMNs appear to originate in area 3a.
11 Renshaw cells allow versatility of action of the PT on motoneurons. A major function is to permit co-contraction of agonists and antagonists when required, by silencing Ia interneurons (Chapter 10).

Macrostimulation of the human area 4 gave rise to the belief that the PT neurons were organized in terms of movements. Microstimulation by intracortical electrodes (in monkeys) indicates that area 4 has a purely executive function; movement programs result from interplay between area 6, striatum, and cerebellum.

Most PT cells are constantly active at low firing rates. This accounts for tonic activation of inhibitory reticulospinal fibers to anterior horn cells, and tonic facilitation of flexor reflex internuncials (see later). Increased activity of PT cells to motoneurons is characterized by rapid summation.

A notable feature of corticomotoneuronal connections is *overlap* (Fig. 20-10). The spinal cell groups

supplying individual muscles are supplied by several cortical cell columns often several millimeters apart. Also, individual cell columns supply several cell groups by intraspinal branching of PT neurons. Single PT neurons to proximal arm motoneurons also supply proximal leg motoneurons. The reason is unknown. Overlap is much less for distal limb motoneurons.

There is positive feedback from muscles, joints, and skin to area 4, mostly via SI. Both actively contracting (agonist) and passively stretched (antagonist) muscle spindles provide feedback, especially from the hand. Contracting spindles operate a *long-loop stretch reflex* in response to obstruction of ongoing movements, increasing the discharge rate of the PT neurons operating the movement. The long-loop reflex is absent in paraplegic patients.

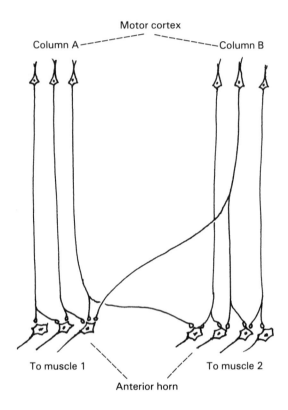

Fig. 20-10 Overlap in origin and termination of pyramidal tract neurons.

Proprioceptive feedback is particularly important for the execution of fine, skilled movement by the fingers. Otherwise, sensory deafferentation (by sensory nerve blocks) has little effect on motor performance, in the presence of ongoing visual supervision.

Note: There is controversy about the 'short latency' pathway from muscle spindles to the motor cortex. The dorsal column–lemniscal route to the thalamus (VPL) is accepted, but a direct projection from VPL to motor cortex seems doubtful. A relay from area 3a (which is specific for spindles) to area 4 is also unlikely, since 3a seems to project backward instead of forward (Fig. 20-6). A forward projection from area 2 is the strongest candidate at present; in addition to inputs from 3a, it may receive afferents from spindles as well as from joint capsules.

Sensory component

The chief targets are:
12 Striatum
13 Ventrobasal complex
14 Reticular formation
15 Dorsal column nuclei
16 Spinal posterior gray horn
17 Flexor reflex internuncials

12 The significance of the substantial input to striatum from PT and lamina III neurons of the sensory cortex is unknown. They are part of a comprehensive sensory input that includes lamina III inputs from visual and auditory association areas.

13 Collaterals from SI PT fibers synapse direct upon the dendrites of ventrobasal neurons projecting to SI (Fig. 20-11). They synapse distal to the lemniscal and spinothalamic inputs to these cells, and they facilitate sensory transmission during movement.

14 Collaterals are given to the nucleus ceruleus and nucleus raphe magnus, both of which inhibit nociceptive transmission in the posterior gray horn of the spinal cord (Chapter 15).

15 Fibers are distributed to excitatory and inhibitory internuncials in the dorsal column nuclei, but not directly to the principal cells. The function of these fibers is unclear. Excitatory effects could facilitate transmission from the hand since the rapidly and slowly adapting receptors of the finger pads (Chapter 5) give substantial direct contribution to these nuclei. However, the sensitivity of the hand does not seem to be increased during active exploration, since textured surfaces can be discriminated with equal accuracy whether they are actively palpated or are merely drawn across the stationary hand. Nevertheless, the identification of three-dimensional objects is much improved if they are actively explored rather than being passively enclosed by the hand. Proprioceptive information is added during active exploration and this may be integrated at SI level with collateral information arriving there from area 4.

16 In the substantia gelatinosa, PT fibers synapse upon inhibitory (?GABA) neurons which synapse in turn upon primary afferent neurons, to exert presynaptic inhibition. It is not known whether all primary afferents are subject to PT control in this way. The annulospiral afferents from neuromuscular spindles are so subject: injury to the PT removes a tonic inhibition and facilitates tendon reflexes (see 'Applied anatomy'). Tactile information from moving parts may also be suppressed at this level under certain conditions. Free voluntary movement of the hand (in tracking a spot of light) is accompanied by reduced sensitivity of the hand to touch, in direct proportion to the speed of movement.

17 PT fibers exert tonic facilitation of flexor reflex internuncials (see 'Applied anatomy').

APPLIED ANATOMY

Premotor cortex

Unilateral lesions of the premotor cortex (as revealed by CT scans) result in weakness of the shoulder and hip muscles on

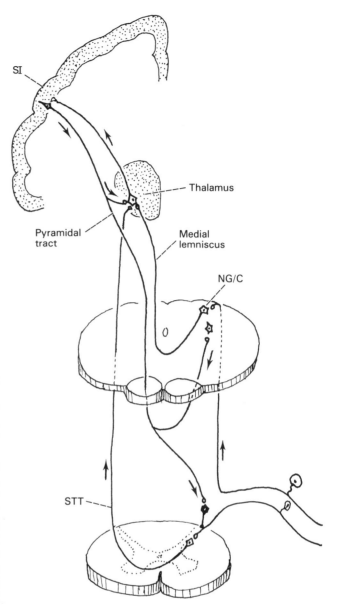

Fig. 20-11 Major sensory elements of the pyramidal tract. NG/C, nucleus gracilis or cuneatus; STT, spinothalamic tract.

the other side. In the shoulder, the weakness is in muscles normally used to raise the arm during routine activities of the hand. The hand itself is unimpaired. The limbs are not spastic, although muscle tone is slightly increased. Bilateral lesions of the premotor cortex are followed by faulty posture, which is shown by instability of stance and gait.

Supplementary motor area

Unilateral lesions result in severe impairment of spontaneous motor activity (mainly contralateral), of speech facility, and of bimanual co-ordination. Bilateral lesions result in long-lasting akinesia and mutism (loss of speech).

Comment The relevance of the effects of lesions of the premotor cortex and supplementary motor area (other than the effects on speech) to Parkinson's disease is obvious. The two areas receive major inputs from the basal ganglia via the ventral anterior nucleus of the thalamus. Although the mode of action of this nucleus on these areas in Parkinson's disease (and even in healthy people) is obscure, it seems likely that deranged input from it may have a bearing on the defective

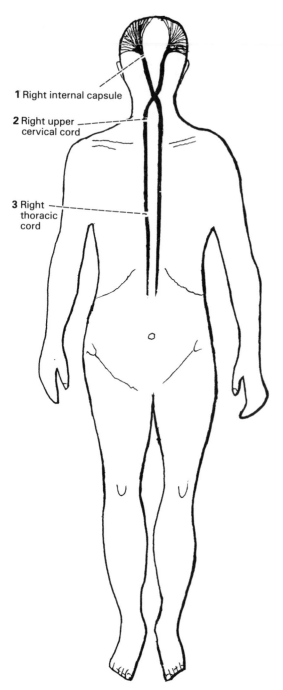

Fig. 20-12 Lesion 1 causes left hemiplegia. Lesion 2 causes right hemiplegia (face spared). Lesion 3 causes right crural (lower limb) monoplegia.

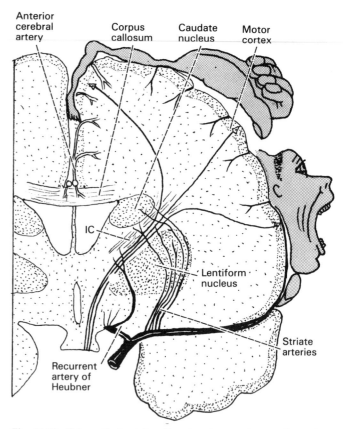

Fig. 20-13 Schematic frontal section showing arteries supplying the internal capsule (IC). (Homunculus adapted from Penfield and Rasmussen, 1950.)

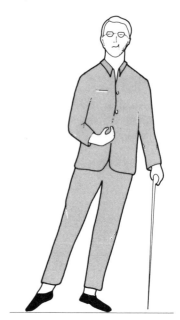

Fig. 20-14 Hemiplegic gait. The patient's right side is affected.

postural fixation typical of Parkinsonian patients, and upon their difficulty in initiating voluntary movements.

Pyramidal tract

A 'pyramidal syndrome' or 'upper motor neuron lesion' is characterized by weakness of movement, spasticity of affected muscles, and increased tendon reflexes. *PT lesions above the pyramidal decussation cause contralateral symptoms; lesions below it cause ipsilateral ones.*

Lesions *above the brainstem* involve corticobulbar as well as corticospinal fibers and result in supranuclear paralysis of cranial nerves (of variable extent; see below) in addition to contralateral hemiplegia (paralysis of upper and lower limb). Lesions *within the brainstem* often produce nuclear and supranuclear cranial nerve lesions (Chapter 12) as well as

contralateral hemiplegia. Lesions *below the brainstem* (i.e., in the spinal cord) produce ipsilateral paralysis of upper and lower limb if at cervical level, and ipsilateral paralysis of the lower limb (monoplegia) if at a thoracic or upper lumbar level (Fig. 20-12).

Possible causes of a pyramidal syndrome are numerous. The etiology may be congenital, inflammatory, traumatic, neoplastic, or degenerative. Much the commonest is a 'stroke', caused by thrombosis of the middle cerebral artery near its origin, resulting in ischemia of the internal capsule.

Less common (and more crippling) is hemorrhage from a striate artery (Fig. 20-13). Another frequent cause of hemi- or monoplegia is a plaque of demyelination associated with multiple sclerosis.

Bilateral PT disorders may be caused by spinal cord injury, whether through accident, prolapse of a cervical disc, or thrombosis of the anterior spinal artery or vein. A meningioma of the falx cerebri may compress the leg areas of the motor cortex on both sides, causing a *spastic paraplegia*.

After a thrombosis the patient initially has a flaccid hemiplegia (paralysis) without reflexes. Some return of movement may occur in trunk and limb girdle muscles within a day, with a Babinski sign (see Chapter 11). Within a week the limb muscles show resting tone (resistance to passive movement) and the tendon reflexes become hyperactive on the hemiplegic side.

Spasticity is the state of increased tone with heightened reflexes. Ankle clonus and wrist clonus (rhythmic flexion in response to sustained passive extension) may be elicited. The abdominal reflexes are absent on the hemiplegic side.

In the following weeks the patient may recover sufficient control over the limbs to be able to move about and perform simple tasks. The antigravity posture adopted by the lower limb may require an ankle brace to prevent the foot striking the ground during the swing phase of walking (Fig. 20-14). Delicate manual skills (such as buttoning an overcoat and tying shoelaces) never recover. Moderate wasting occurs in the distal parts of the affected limbs, owing to loss of anterior horn cells (up to 25%), perhaps from transneuronal degeneration.

Cranial nerves

Nerves III, IV and VI are not affected unless the lesion includes the projection from the frontal eye field, which descends in front of the PT. Supranuclear involvement of the cranial nerves may be hard to detect apart from a consistent lower facial weakness on the hemiplegic side. PT projects only contralaterally to the facial neurons supplying lip and cheek muscles (see Fig. 35-3). It projects bilaterally to facial neurons that normally operate in pairs – the frontalis (to raise the eyebrows) and orbicularis oculi (to close the eyes). The jaw, tongue, larynx, and pharynx usually operate in a paired manner and receive a bilateral supranuclear supply. However, the supply to jaw, tongue, and palate may be mainly contralateral, in which case the jaw deviates to the hemiplegic side when the mouth is opened (unopposed pull of normal genioglossus) and the uvula deviates to the normal side when the palate is elevated (unopposed pull of normal levator palati).

The sternomastoids are largely independent of each other, and each receives an *ipsilateral* supranuclear supply (turning the head to see what the same PT is doing with the opposite hand). The trapezius receives a *contralateral* supply, and there is weakness of elevation (shrugging) of the shoulder on the hemiplegic side.

What causes 'pyramidal signs'?

Spasticity and increased tendon reflexes

The *spasticity* of the pyramidal syndrome is of the clasp-knife variety, the initial resistance to passive flexion of the knee being followed by sudden collapse of resistance. In normal individuals rapid passive extension at a joint is accompanied by a small burst of α motoneuron activity produced by stretching of the muscle spindles. In spastic patients the EMG records show a large burst. This is not because fusimotor drive is elevated in the spastic muscles, but because α motoneurons are more responsive to the Ia fiber input. The heightened responsiveness could be due to (a) removal of tonic inhibitory drive by PT fibers from neurons exerting presynaptic inhibition on the central ends of Ia afferents, (b) removal of tonic Renshaw inhibition exerted by PT fibers, or (c) removal of tonic inhibition of the α motoneurons themselves by cortically driven reticulospinal fibers which bypass the medullary pyramids but which otherwise accompany the PT and would be damaged as well.

Some workers believe that the peculiar nature of clasp-knife rigidity can best be accounted for by a change in the viscoelastic properties of muscle, a change known as 'increased muscle stiffness'.

None of the above explanations adequately explains the fact that a 'pure' lesion of the medullary pyramid (very rare) is followed by a flaccid (atonic) hemiplegia.

Increased tendon reflexes may require a separate explanation because they are sometimes increased in the absence of significant spasticity. A clear answer is not available but the sprouting of Ia terminals to occupy sites vacated by the PT on α motoneurons or related excitatory internuncials may be significant. Such sprouting has been demonstrated following spinal cord injury, in which the tendon reflexes are notably exaggerated.

Lost abdominal reflexes

The abdominal reflex (twitch of abdominal muscles in response to stroking the skin) is a flexor reflex dependent upon tonic facilitation of excitatory interneurons by the PT.

Babinski sign (extensor plantar response). The normal response to stroking the sole is flexion of the toes (Chapter 11). In PT disease the great toe is dorsiflexed ('upgoing toe') and the other toes are fanned. Fanning results from simultaneous contraction of dorsiflexors and plantar flexors of the toes; the dorsiflexor wins in the great toe. Clearly there is a breakdown of reciprocal inhibition, which is replaced by reciprocal excitation.

The Babinski sign is absent in nearly 25% of individuals who have other evidence of PT disease. There is a high correlation of Babinski sign with PT injury to motoneurons at first sacral segmental level, which is shown by inability to wiggle the toes.

Readings

Allen, C.M.C., Hoare, R.D., Fowler, C.J. and Harrison, M.J.G. (1984) Clinico-anatomical correlations in uncomplicated stroke. *J. Neurol. Neurosurg. Psychiatry*, 47: 1251–1254.

Angel, R.W. and Malenka, R.C. (1982) Velocity-dependent suppression of cutaneous nerve sensitivity during movement. *Exp. Neurol.*, 77: 266–274.

Asanuma, H. (1981) Functional role of sensory inputs to the motor cortex. *Prog. Neurobiol.*, 16: 241–262.

Balagura, S. (1980) Undecussated innervation to the sternomastoid muscle: a reinstatement. *Ann. Neurol.*, 7: 84–95.

Benecke, R., Berthold, A. and Conrad, B. (1983) Denervation activity in the EMG of patients with upper motor neuron lesions: time course, local distribution and pathogenic aspects. *J. Neurol.*, 230: 143–151.

Brinkman, C. (1984) Supplementary motor area of the monkey's motor cortex: short- and long-term deficits after unilateral ablation and the effects of subsequent callosal section. *J. Neurosci.*, 4: 918–929.

Brown, W.F., Milner-Brown, H.S., Ball, M. and Girvin, J.P. (1978) Control of the motor cortex on spinal motoneurons in man. *Prog. Clin. Neurophysiol.*, 4: 246–262. Basel: Karger.

Burke, D. (1983) Critical examination of the case for or against fusimotor involvement in disorders of muscle and tone. In *Motor Control Mechanisms in Health and Disease* (Desmedt, J.E., ed.), pp. 133–150. New York: Raven Press.

Chokroverty, S., Rubino, F.A. and Haller, C. (1975) Pure motor hemiplegia due to pyramidal infarction. *Arch. Neurol.*, 32: 647–649.

Darian-Smith, I., Johnson, K.O. and Goodwin, A.W. (1979) Posterior parietal cortex: relations of unit activity to sensorimotor function. *Annu. Rev. Physiol.*, 41: 141–157.

Dietz, V. and Berger, W. (1983) Normal and impaired regulation of muscle stiffness in gait: a new hypothesis about muscle hypertonia. *Exp. Neurol.*, 79: 680–687.

Dimitrijevic, M.R., Nathan, P.W. and Sherwood, A.M. (1980) Clonus: the role of central mechanisms. *J. Neurol. Neurosurg. Psychiatry*, 43: 321–332.

Eklund, G., Hagbarth, K.-E., Hägglund, J.V. and Wallin, E.U. (1982) The 'late' reflex responses to muscle stretch: the 'resonance hypothesis' versus the long-loop hypothesis. *J. Physiol.*, 326: 79–90.

Felleman, D.J., Nelson, R.J., Sur, M. and Kaas, J.H. (1983) Representations of the body surface in areas 3b and 1 of postcentral parietal cortex of Cebus monkeys. *Brain Res.*, 268: 15–26.

Freund, H.-J. (1984) Premotor areas in man. *Trends Neurosci.*, /: 481–483.

Fromm, C. (1983) Contrasting properties of pyramidal tract neurons located in the precentral or postcentral areas and of corticorubral neurons in the behaving monkey. In *Motor Control Mechanisms in Health and Disease* (Desmedt, J.E., ed.), pp. 329–345. New York: Raven Press.

Hanaway, J. and Young, R.R. (1977) Localization of the pyramidal tract in the internal capsule of man. *J. Neurol. Sci., 34:* 63–70.

Jones, E.G. (1983) The nature of the afferent pathways conveying short-latency inputs to primate motor cortex. In *Motor Control Mechanisms in Health and Disease* (Desmedt, J.E., ed.), pp. 263–285. New York: Raven Press.

Juliano, S.L., Hand, P.J. and Whitsel, B.L. (1983) Patterns of metabolic activity in cyto-architectural area SII and surrounding cortical fields of the monkey. *J. Neurophysiol.*, 50: 961–980.

Kaas, J.H. (1983) What, if anything, is SI? Organization of first somatosensory area of cortex. *Physiol. Rev.*, 63: 206–231.

Lee, R.G., Murphy, J.T. and Tatton, W.G. (1983) Long latency myotatic reflexes in man: mechanisms, functional significance, and changes in patients with Parkinson's disease or hemiplegia. In *Motor Control Mechanisms in Health and Disease* (Desmedt, J.E., ed.), pp. 489–508. New York: Raven Press.

Meinck, H.M., Benecke, R., Küster, S. and Conrad, B. (1983) Cutaneomuscular (flexor) reflex organization in normal man and in patients with motor disorders. In *Motor Control Mechanisms in Health and Disease* (Desmedt, J.E., ed.), pp. 787–795. New York: Raven Press.

Morrison, J.H. and Magistretti, P.J. (1983) Monoamines and peptides in cerebral cortex. *Trends Neurosci.*, 6: 146–150.

Mountcastle, V.B. (1978) An organizing principle for cerebral function: the unit module and the distributed system. In *The Mindful Brain*, by Edelman, G.M. and Mountcastle, V.B. Cambridge, Massachusetts: MIT Press.

Murray, E.A. and Coulter, J.D. (1981) Organization of corticospinal neurons in the monkey. *J. Comp. Neurol.*, 195: 339–365.

Mykleburst, B.M., Gottlieb, G.L., Penn, R.D. and Agarwal, G.C. (1982) Reciprocal excitation of antagonistic muscles as a differentiating feature in spasticity. *Ann. Neurol.*, 12: 367–374.

Orgogozo, J.M. and Larsen, B. (1979) Activation of the supplementary motor area during voluntary movement in man suggests it works as a supramotor area. *Science*, 206: 847–850.

Penfield, W. and Jasper, H. (1954) *Epilepsy and the Functional Anatomy of the Human Brain*. Boston: Little Brown.

Penfield, W. and Rasmussen, G. (1950) *The Cerebral Cortex of Man: A Clinical Study of Localization of Function*. London: Macmillan.

Peters, A. and Jones, E.G. (1984) *The Cerebral Cortex, Vol. 1, Cellular Components*. New York: Plenum Press.

Phillips, C.G. (1979) The corticospinal pathway of primates. In *Integration in the Nervous System* (Asanuma, H. and Wilson, V.J., eds.), pp. 263–278. Tokyo: Igaku-Shoin.

Picard, C. and Olivier, A. (1983) Sensory cortical tongue representation in man. *J. Neurosurg.*, 59: 781–789.

Porter, R. (1981) Internal organization of the motor cortex for input-output arrangements. In *Handbook of Physiology, The Nervous System, Vol. 2, Motor Control* (Brooks, V.B., ed.), pp. 1063–1082. Bethesda: American Physiological Society.

Porter, R. (1982) The control of voluntary movement. In *Proprioception, Posture and Emotion* (Garlick, D., ed.), pp. 136–141. Sydney: University of New South Wales.

Powell, T.P.S. (1981) Certain aspects of the intrinsic organisation of the cerebral cortex. In *Brain Mechanisms and Perceptual Awareness* (Pompeiano, O. and Marsan, C.A., eds.), pp. 1–19. New York: Raven Press.

Roland, P.E., Skinhøj, E., Lassen, N.A. and Larsen, B. (1980) Different cortical areas in man in organization of voluntary movements in extrapersonal space. *J. Neurophysiol.*, 43: 137–150.

Sanes, J. and Evarts, E.V. (1983) Regulatory role of proprioceptive input in motor control of phasic or maintained voluntary contractions in man. In *Motor Control Mechanisms in Health and Disease* (Desmedt, J.E., ed.), pp. 47–59. New York: Raven Press.

Schwartz, A.S., Percy, A.J. and Azulay, A. (1975) Further analysis of active and passive touch in pattern discrimination. *Bull. Psychonom. Soc.*, 6: 7–9.

Sedgwick, E.M. (1982) Clinical neurophysiology in rehabilitation. In *Rehabilitation of the Neurological Patient*, by Illis, L.S., Sedgwick, E.M. and Glanville, H.J., pp. 85–122. Oxford: Blackwell.

Shanks, M.F. and Powell, T.P.S. (1980) An electron-microscopic study of the termination of thalamocortical fibers in areas 3b, 1 and 2 of the somatic sensory cortex in the monkey. *Brain Res.*, 218: 35–47.

Somogyi, P., Freund, T.F. and Cowey, A. (1982) The axo-axonic interneuron in the cerebral cortex of rat, cat and monkey. *Neuroscience*, 11: 2577–2607.

Strick, P.L. and Preston, J.B. (1978) Multiple representation in the primate motor cortex. *Brain Res.*, 154: 366–370.

Szentagothai, J. (1977) The neuron network of the cerebral cortex: a functional interpretation. *Proc. R. Soc. Lond. B.*, 201: 219–248.

Tanaka, R. (1983) Reciprocal Ia inhibitory pathway in normal man and in patients with motor disorders. In *Motor Control Mechanisms in Health and Disease* (Desmedt, J.E., ed.), pp. 433–443. New York: Raven Press.

Tanji, J. and Kurata, K. (1983) Functional organization of the supplementary motor area. In *Motor Control Mechanisms in Health and Disease* (Desmedt, J.E., ed.), pp. 421–431. New York: Raven Press.

Van Gijn, J. (1978) The Babinski sign and the pyramidal syndrome. *J. Neurol. Neurosurg. Psychiatry*, 41: 865–873.

Vogt, B.A. and Pandya, D.N. (1978) Corticocortical connections of the somatic sensory cortex (areas 3, 1 and 2) in the rhesus monkey. *J. Comp. Neurol.*, 177: 179–192.

Vogt, C. and Vogt, O. (1919) Allgemeinere Ergebnisse unserer Hirnforschung. *J. Psychol. Neurol., 25:* 279–461.

Wiesendanger, M. and Miles, T.S. (1982) Ascending pathway of low-threshold muscle afferents to the cerebral cortex and its possible role in motor control. *Physiol. Rev., 62:* 1234–1270.

Wise, E.P. and Evarts, E.V. (1981) The role of the cerebral cortex in movement. *Trends Neurosci., 4:* 297–300.

Young, J.L. and Mayer, R.F. (1982) Physiological alterations of motor units in hemiplegia. *J. Neurol. Sci., 54:* 401–412.

21
Limbic System: Limbic Cortex

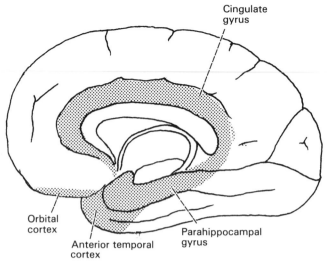

Fig. 21-2 Limbic cortex, medial view.

The limbic system, or visceral brain, is concerned with the affective (emotional) aspects of behavior, including the basic drives required for preservation of the individual and of the species. The principal executive arm of the limbic system is the hypothalamus.

The limbic system is prominent in primitive mammals and in amphibia. In these it is intimately concerned with defense and attack mechanisms and with procreation. Studies in higher mammals have revealed functions in laying down memory traces. It is richly interconnected with sensory association areas of the isocortex, on the one hand, and with the hypothalamus and reticular formation, on the other.

ANATOMY

The limbic system comprises the *limbic cortex (limbic lobe)* of the brain and related subcortical structures. 'Limbus' means a margin, and the term (coined by Broca in 1878) originally referred to the rim of cortex on the medial surface of the hemisphere, surrounding the corpus callosum and brain stem (Figs. 21-1, 21-2). The

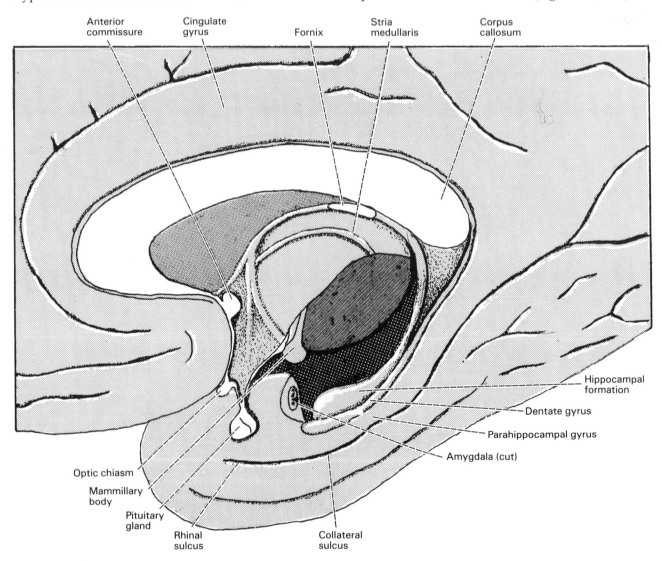

Fig. 21-1 Medial view of limbic cortex and related areas. Brain stem removed by a cut through the thalamus. (Adapted from Nauta and Haymaker, 1969.)

150

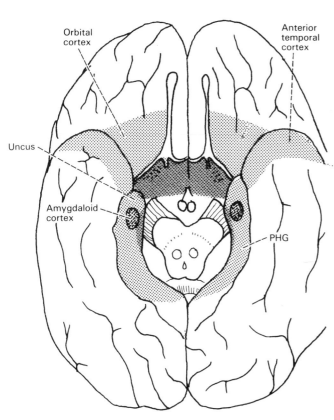

Fig. 21-3 Limbic cortex, from below. PHG, parahippocampal gyrus.

term has been extended to include the anterior temporal cortex, the posterior part of the orbital cortex of the frontal lobe (Fig. 21-3), and the insula. Apart from the insula, the limbic cortex now comprises a vertical limbus on each side surrounding the corpus callosum and a cerebral peduncle, and a horizontal limbus surrounding the midbrain.

The inner part of the horizontal limbus is three-layered allocortex. The remainder (called juxtallocortex) shows transitional features between allo- and isocortex.

The following areas of limbic cortex will now be described: parahippocampal gyrus, hippocampal formation, insula, and cingulate cortex.

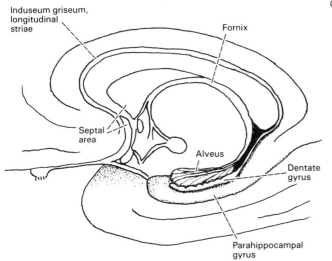

Fig. 21-4 Medial view showing structures on upper surface of parahippocampal gyrus.

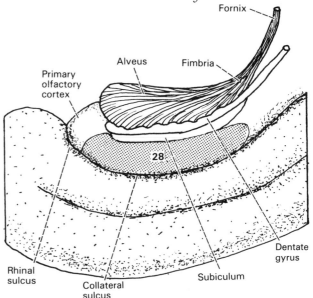

Fig. 21-5 Enlargement from Fig. 21-4 showing entorhinal cortex (area 28) and hippocampal formation. The hippocampus is covered by the alveus.

Parahippocampal gyrus

The parahippocampal gyrus (Figs. 21-4, 21-5) consists mostly of *entorhinal cortex* (area 28 of Brodmann). Area 28 is six-layered but the granular laminae tend to lie external to the pyramidal laminae rather than alternating with them. Anteriorly, it blends with the primary olfactory cortex at the *uncus*. Laterally, the gyrus merges with temporal isocortex in the floor of the rhinal sulcus in front and collateral sulcus behind. Medially, it blends with the subiculum.

The parahippocampal gyrus has two-way connections with all of the major cortical association areas (Fig. 21-6), and with the primary olfactory cortex and hippocampal formation.

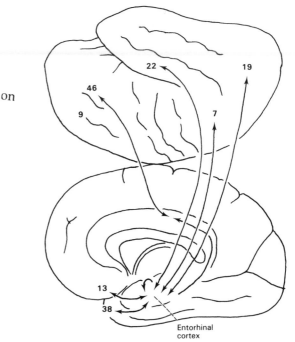

Fig. 21-6 Interconnections between entorhinal and association areas of right hemisphere. Numbers refer to Brodmann areas. (Adapted from Van Hoesen, 1982.)

151

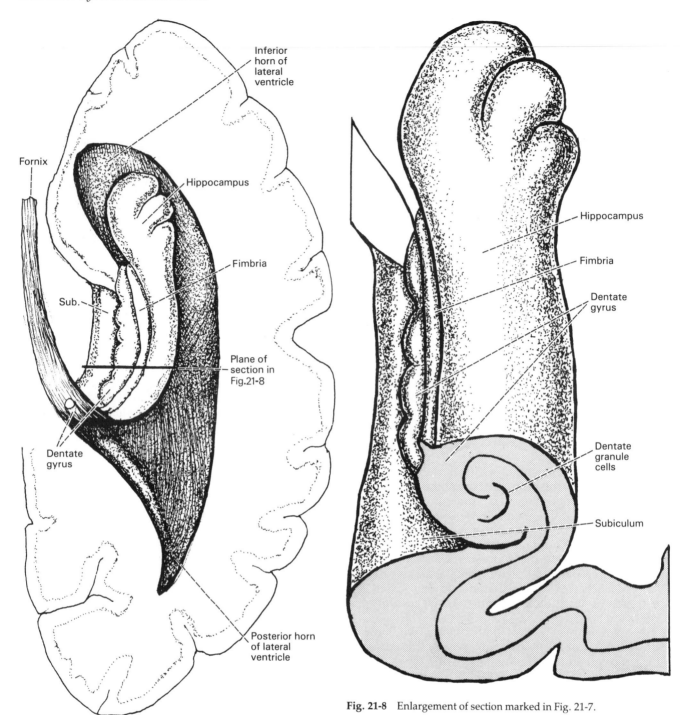

Fig. 21-7 Hippocampal formation and related structures, from above. Sub., subiculum.

Fig. 21-8 Enlargement of section marked in Fig. 21-7.

Interference with the parahippocampal gyrus, whether vascular or surgical, is known to be followed by an inability to retain new information acquired through any of the senses. This form of amnesia is very rare since the lesion must be bilateral. It has led to the view that information received in the sensory association areas is channeled to the parahippocampal gyrus, 'memorized' in the adjacent hippocampal formation, and returned to the association areas for long-term storage. However, although the parahippocampal gyrus is the largest output station of the hippocampal formation, the fornix is also large and lesions of the fornix pathway may result in amnesia for recent events.

Hippocampal formation

The hippocampal formation (Figs. 21-7, 21-8) comprises the subiculum, hippocampus, and dentate gyrus. It is composed of three-layered allocortex with prominent spiny principal cells – pyramidal cells in the subiculum and hippocampus, granule cells in the dentate gyrus.

The *subiculum* contains pyramidal and stellate cells. It merges with the *hippocampus*, which is also known as Ammon's horn (from an Egyptian deity with a ram's head). The hippocampus is a half-cylinder (C-shaped in section) of mainly pyramidal cells. It is conventionally divided into four CA (cornu ammonis) zones, of which CA1 and CA3 are the largest (Fig. 21-10).

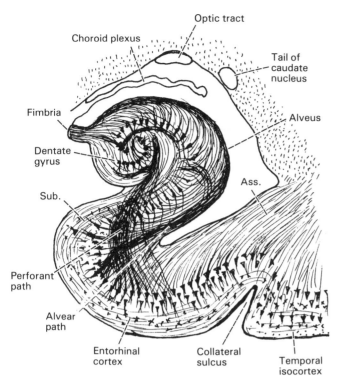

Fig. 21-9 Coronal section of temporal limbic cortex, bounded by the collateral sulcus. Ass., connections with association areas; Sub., subiculum.

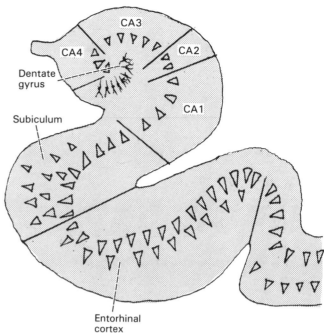

Fig. 21-10 Subdivisions of medial temporal cortex.

The *dentate gyrus* contains a half-cylinder of *granule cells* enclosing the CA4 zone.

Connections

Numbers 1–7 refer to Figs 21-11, 21-12.
1 The adjacent entorhinal cortex is richly interconnected with all of the sensory association areas.
2 From the lateral entorhinal cortex, the *perforant pathway* perforates the subiculum and synapses upon apical dendrites of dentate granule cells.
3 From the medial entorhinal cortex the *alvear pathway* contributes to a sheet of axons – the *alveus* – coating the surface of the hippocampus. The alvear pathway fibers synapse upon basal dendrites of CA1 pyramidal cells.
4 From the subiculum, some axons return into the entorhinal cortex and others traverse the alveus to enter the fornix (via the fimbria).
5 CA1 pyramidal-cell axons bifurcate to enter the subiculum and fornix.
6 CA3 pyramidal axons bifurcate to enter CA1 and fornix. Recurrent CA3 axons are called *Schaffer collaterals*. They synapse upon dendrites in CA1, on which they have a very powerful and prolonged excitatory effect (see later).
7 The axons of the dentate granule cells synapse upon the basal dendrites of CA3 pyramids, as well as on basket cells that inhibit other granule cells.

The hippocampal formation receives numerous afferents through the fornix, including (a) afferents from thalamus and hypothalamus and (b) monoaminergic fibers from basal forebrain and midbrain (Table 21-1).

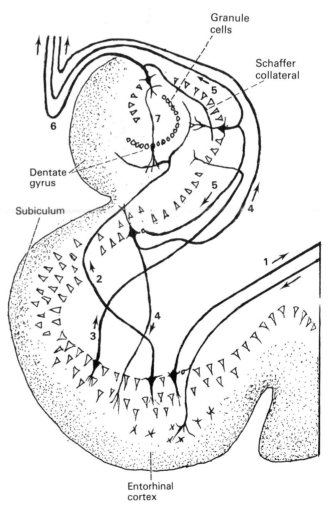

Fig. 21-11 Hippocampal connections (see text). 2 is perforant path, 3 is alvear path.

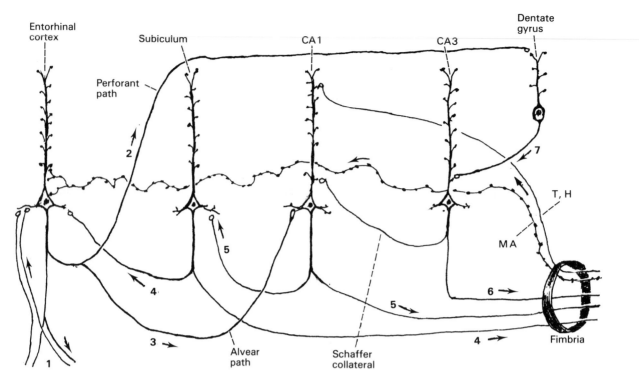

Fig. 21-12 Diagram of hippocampal connections (see text). MA, monoaminergic connections; T, H, thalamic and hypothalamic afferents.

Table 21-1 Monoamine neurons supplying the hippocampal formation via the fornix

Monoamines	Sources
Acetylcholine	Septal nucleus, substantia innominata
Dopamine	Ventral tegmental area
Norepinephrine	Nucleus ceruleus
Serotonin	Midbrain raphe nucleus

The monoamine content of the hippocampal formation has significant influence on memory functions in experimental animals.

Special qualities of hippocampal neurons

Hippocampal pyramidal cells are highly excitable. Repetitive stimulation leads to poststimulus facilitation which may last for hours or even weeks. This feature is shared by dentate granule cells.

The pyramidal cells show amazing anatomical *plasticity*. Stimulation of Schaffer collaterals for a few seconds causes a 50% increase in the number of Schaffer axospinous synapses on CA1 pyramidal cells within half an hour. If stimulation is prolonged the number of new synapses is reduced, indicating that the sprouting of new dendritic spines is temporary. Repeated training in rats (for example, learning to run a maze) is accompanied by an increase in RNA and protein synthesis in hippocampal pyramidal neurons. The metabolic changes are influenced by the monoaminergic neurons, which synapse directly upon the pyramidal somas.

Memory traces are not thought to be stored in the hippocampus, but to be dispersed to cortical association areas – probably via both entorhinal cortex and fornix. In the association areas, the spiny stellate cells, having an intimate synaptic relationship with cortical pyramidal cells, are prime candidates for imprinting memory traces. The mechanism of such imprinting is unknown.

Induseum griseum and longitudinal striae

The posterior end of the dentate gyrus arches over the splenium (posterior end) of the corpus callosum. Its gray and white matter become attenuated, forming the *induseum griseum* (gray) and *longitudinal striae* on the upper surface of the corpus callosum (Fig. 21-4); through them the dentate gyrus is linked to the septal area (Chapter 22).

Insula

The insular cortex is intermediate in structure between allocortex and isocortex. It is continuous with similar 'mesocortex' on the orbital surface of the frontal lobe and at the temporal pole. Stimulation of the anterior insula in patients produces hallucinations of taste and smell, and has a variety of autonomic effects. The posterior insula contains part of SII above and is interconnected with the primary auditory cortex below. It is also interconnected with the entorhinal cortex and amygdala.

The insula appears to be concerned with generating appropriate emotional and autonomic responses to stimuli reaching it from the external world.

The primary olfactory cortex is described in Chapter 27.

Cingulate cortex

The anterior cingulate cortex (ACC) receives a substantial number of inputs from the intralaminar thalamic nuclei, which are the chief targets of the spinoreticu-lothalamic tracts. Stimulation of the ACC does not cause pain but it does produce 'painful' responses: pupillary dilatation, cardiovascular changes, and shrill vocalization. The ACC is connected to the prefrontal cortex; section of this connection, or incision of the ACC (anterior cingulotomy) may relieve intractable pain. The pain itself is not diminished but its unpleasant, aversive quality is removed. This is also a feature of morphine treatment of pain, and it may be significant that the ACC contains abundant opiate receptors.

The posterior cingulate cortex is richly intercon-nected with the parietal association area, where tactile and visual information is integrated. The limbic connection may be responsible for the emotional 'tone' of tactile and visual sensations.

APPLIED ANATOMY

Disorders of mood and thought are believed to originate in the limbic system. These disorders include schizophrenia, depression, amnesia, anxiety states, and phobias. Only the first three will be discussed here.

Schizophrenia

Schizophrenia is prevalent throughout the world, with an incidence as high as 1% of the adult population in some countries. The disease has a variety of forms, but it is characterized by a blunting of emotional responses to everyday incidents ('blunting of affect'), withdrawal into a private world, and thought disorders, usually accompanied by paranoid delusions and auditory hallucinations.

At the biochemical level, schizophrenia is believed to be associated with overactivity of the mesolimbic dopaminergic (DA) system (Chapter 15), notably in the dominant hemisphere. This theory of origin arose from the fortuitous observation that drugs which block DA receptors in general, have a beneficial effect upon the symptoms of the disease. The chief side-effects of drugs in current use are the appearance of Parkinsonian effects (akinesia, rigidity, and tremor) because of concomitant blockade of DA receptors in the striatum (Chapter 18), and (in females) menstrual disorders and milk secretion because of suppression of the prolactin inhibitory factor (Chapter 16).

It is by no means clear that DA receptor malfunction is the root of the disorder. Increased DA activity is accepted, but it could conceivably be triggered by abnormal production of one or more peptide neuromodulators also found in the limbic system.

Depression

The depression syndrome consists of somatic complaints (pains and aches), anxiety and tension, guilt, and manifesta-tions of depressed mood. *Patients who may be dismissed in the mind as 'neurotics' should be suspected instead of being depressed.* Depression may be categorized as follows:

1 *Reactive* (about 65% of cases), occurring in response to bereavement, illness, and so on.
2 *Endogenous* (about 25%), a genetically determined inabil-ity to cope with the stresses of daily life. A sense of personal inadequacy and a suicidal tendency are characteristic.
3 *Manic-depressive* (about 10%), in which periods of depress-ion alternate with periods of elation and hyperactivity.

A current biochemical basis of explanation for depression is the *biogenic amine theory*. This theory originated in the observation that reserpine could cause deep depression in normal individuals. The effect was correlated with reser-pine's ability to reduce the concentrations of norepinephrine (noradrenaline) and serotonin (5-HT) in the limbic system and at other central receptor sites. It is now known that drugs which block the 'amine pump' (by which amines are normally retrieved from the synaptic cleft) have a significant antidepressant action, presumably by prolonging the availa-bility of amines for postsynaptic action. Inhibitors of monoamine oxidase (which normally degrades a significant amount of retrieved amine) may also be antidepressant.

Studies on the cerebrospinal fluid of depressed patients have shown that metabolites of norepinephrine in some patients, and of serotonin metabolites in others, are abnormally low.

Memory disorders

Bilateral injury of the hippocampal formation results in global learning disorder – so-called anterograde amnesia.

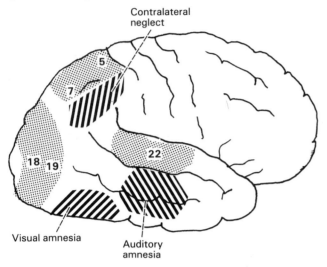

Fig. 21-13 Lesions (hatching) causing sensory–limbic disconnection.

Disconnection syndromes (Fig. 21-13)

Bilateral disconnection of the visual association cortex (areas 18, 19) from the entorhinal cortex results in failure to process newly acquired visual information through the memory pathway(s). Such specific disconnection is very rare and is produced by basilar artery insufficiency propagated into both posterior cerebral arteries. The critical zone is the white matter at the occipitotemporal junction. A patient with anterograde visual amnesia has no difficulty in finding his way in surroundings that are already familiar but he is at a loss in novel terrain; for instance, he cannot find his way around a strange hotel however long he stays there.

Conversations are processed by the dominant temporal cortex. Disconnection of the auditory association area (22) from the entorhinal cortex causes anterograde auditory amnesia: the patient is unable to memorize spoken words.

Disconnection of the parietal association cortex (areas 5, 7) from the entorhinal cortex causes the curious syndrome of *contralateral neglect*. Such a patient fails to recognize the contralateral side of the body as his own ('there is a stranger in my bed'), and he may have no capacity to deal with the contralateral sensory field as a whole: for example, if asked to draw a clock face he may put all the numbers on the ipsilateral half of the figure.

See also 'Cortical "watershed"' in Chapter 23.

Readings

Amaral, D.G. and Cowan, W.M. (1980) Subcortical afferents to the hippocampal formation in the monkey. *J. Comp. Neurol., 189:* 573–591.

Atrens, D. and Curthoys, I. (1982) *The Neurosciences and Behaviour,* 2nd ed. Sydney: Academic Press.

Braitenberg, V. and Schüz, A. (1983) Some anatomical comments on the hippocampus. In *Neurobiology of the Hippocampus* (Seifert, W., ed.), pp. 21–38. London & New York: Academic Press.

Breathnach, C.S. (1980) The limbic system, 1980. *J. Irish Med. Assoc., 73:* 331–339.

Carlton, P.L. and Menowitz, P. (1984) Dopamine and schizophrenia: an analysis of the theory. *Neurosci. Behav. Rev., 8:* 137–152.

Chronister, R.B. and DeFrance, J.F. (1979) Organization of projection neurons of the hippocampus. *Exp. Neurol., 66:* 501–523.

Gerstenbrand, F., Poewe, W., Aichner, F. and Sultuari, L. (1983) Klüver–Bucy syndrome in man: experience with posttraumatic cases. *Neurosci. Behav. Rev., 7:* 413–417.

Gold, P.E. and Zornetzer, S.F. (1983) The mnemon and its juices: neuromodulation of memory processes. *Behav. Neur. Biol., 38:* 151–189.

Halgren, E., Wilson, C.L., Squires, N.K., Engel, J., Walter, R.D. and Crandall, P.H. (1983) Dynamics of the hippocampal contribution to memory: stimulation and recording studies in humans. In *Neurobiology of the Hippocampus* (Seifert, W., ed.), pp. 529–572. London & New York: Academic Press.

Hollister, L. (1982) Antidepressants. In *Basic and Clinical Pharmacology* (Katzung, B.C., ed.), pp. 301–308. Los Altos: Lange.

Isaacson, R.L. (1982) *The Limbic System,* 2nd ed. New York & London: Plenum Press.

Klüver, H. and Bucy, P.C. (1938) An analysis of certain effects of bilateral temporal lobectomy in the rhesus monkey, with special reference to 'psychic blindness'. *J. Psychol., 5:* 33–54.

Krugilov, R.I. (1982) On the interaction of neurotransmitter systems in processes of learning and memory. In *Neuronal Plasticity and Memory Formation* (Marsan, C.A. and Matthies, H., eds.), pp. 339–351. New York: Raven Press.

Lee, K., Oliver, M., Schottler, F., Creager, R. and Lynch, G. (1979) Ultrastructural effects of repetitive synaptic stimulation in the hippocampal slice preparation. *Exp. Neurol., 65:* 478–480.

Leonard, B.E. (1982) Current status of the biogenic amine theory of depression. *Neurochem. Int., 4:* 339–350.

Leonard, B.E. (1984) Pharmacology of new antidepressants. *Prog. Neuro-Psychopharmacol. Biol. Psychiat., 8:* 97–108.

Livingston, K.E. and Escobar, A. (1971) Anatomical bias of the limbic system concept. *Arch. Neurol., 24:* 17–21.

Lopes de Silva, F.H. and Arnolds, D.E.A.T. (1978) Physiology of the hippocampus and related structures. *Annu. Rev. Physiol., 40:* 185–216.

Lynch, G.S. and Lee, K.S. (1982) Some capacities for structural growth and functional change in the neuronal circuitries of the adult hippocampus. In *The Neural Basis of Behavior* (Beckman, A.L., ed.), pp. 103–116. New York: SP Medical and Scientific Books.

Lynch, G., Halpin, S. and Baudry, M. (1983) Structural and biochemical effects of high frequency stimulation in the hippocampus. In *Neurobiology of the Hippocampus* (Seifert, W., ed.), pp. 253–264. London & New York: Academic Press.

Matthies, H. (1982) Plasticity in the nervous system – an approach to memory research. In *Neuronal Plasticity and Memory Formation* (Marsan, C.A. and Matthies, H., eds.), pp. 2–15. New York: Raven Press.

Meck, W.H., Church, R.M. and Olton, D.S. (1984) Hippocampus, time, and memory. *Behav. Neurosci., 98:* 3–22.

Mesulam, M.-M. and Mufson, E.J. (1982) Insula of the old world monkey. *J. Comp. Neurol., 212:* 1–52.

Nauta, W.J.H. and Domesick, V.B. (1982) Neural associations of the limbic system. In *The Neural Basis of Behavior,* pp. 175–206. New York: Spectrum.

Nauta, W.J.H. and Haymaker, W. (1969) Hypothalamic nuclei and fiber connections. In *The Hypothalamus* (Haymaker, W., Anderson, E. and Nauta, W.J.H., eds.), pp. 136–202. Springfield, Illinois: Thomas.

Paykiel, E.S. (ed.) (1982) *Handbook of Affective Disorders.* Edinburgh: Churchill-Livingstone.

Reynolds, G.P. (1983) Increased concentrations and lateral asymmetry of amygdala dopamine in schizophrenia. *Nature, 305:* 527–529.

Roberts, G.W., Ferrier, N., Lee, Y., Crow, T.J., Johnstone, E.C., Owens, D.G.C., Bacarese-Hamilton, A.J., McGregor, G., O'Shaughnessy, G., Polek, J.M. and Bloom, S.R. (1983) Peptides, the limbic lobe and schizophrenia. *Brain Res., 288:* 199–211.

Ross, E.D. (1982) Disorders of recent memory in humans. *Trends Neurosci., 5:* 170–173.

Shashoua, V.E. (1982) Molecular and cell biological aspects of learning: toward a theory of memory. *Adv. Cell Neurobiol., 3:* 97–141.

Squire, L.R. (1983) The hippocampus and the neuropsychology of memory. In *Neurobiology of the Hippocampus* (Seifert, W., ed.), pp. 491–511. London & New York: Academic Press.

Swanson, L.W. (1979) The hippocampus – new anatomical insights. *Trends Neurosci., 2:* 9–12.

Swanson, L.W. (1983) The hippocampus and the concept of the limbic system. In *Neurobiology of the Hippocampus* (Seifert, W., ed.), pp. 3–20. London & New York: Academic Press.

Thompson, R.F. (1983) Cellular processes of learning and memory in the mammalian CNS. *Annu. Rev. Neurosci., 6:* 447–491.

Van Hoesen, G.W. (1982) The parahippocampal gyrus: new observations regarding its cortical connections in the monkey. *Trends Neurosci., 5:* 345–350.

Walaas, I. (1983) The hippocampus. In *Chemical Neuroanatomy* (Emson, P.C., ed.), pp. 337–358. New York: Raven Press.

Zola-Morgan, S., Squire, L.R. and Mishkin, M. (1982) The neuroanatomy of amnesia: amygdala–hippocampus versus temporal stem. *Science, 218:* 1337–1339.

22

Limbic System: Subcortical Structures

The principal subcortical limbic structures are the fornix, the septal area, the habenular nucleus, the nucleus accumbens, and the amygdala. The majority of the hypothalamic nuclei may also be regarded as subcortical limbic components because they receive substantial inputs from all the structures listed except the habenular nucleus (Fig. 22-1).

FORNIX (Figs. 22-2, 22-3)

The *fornix* is a pathway linking the subiculum and hippocampus with the basal forebrain and brain stem. Each pillar of the fornix contains 1.2 million fibers – rather more than the pyramidal tract. The great majority are efferents from the hippocampal formation.

The fornix commences as the *fimbria*, which runs backward beside the dentate gyrus before rising up as the *posterior pillar* beneath the corpus callosum.

The two posterior pillars exchange fibers in the *posterior* or *hippocampal* commissure. The *body* of the fornix separates into two *anterior pillars*. Each anterior pillar divides above the anterior commissure. The *precommissural fornix* reaches the septal area. The *postcommissural fornix* sends half of its fibers to the

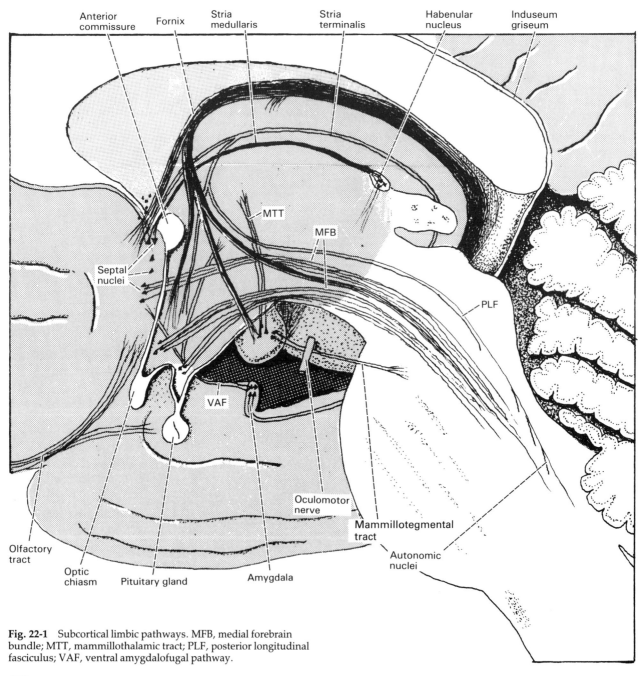

Fig. 22-1 Subcortical limbic pathways. MFB, medial forebrain bundle; MTT, mammillothalamic tract; PLF, posterior longitudinal fasciculus; VAF, ventral amygdalofugal pathway.

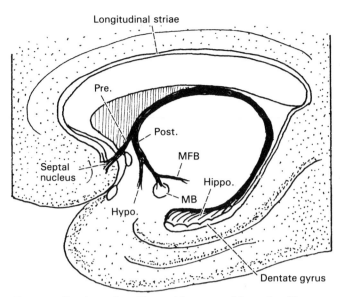

Fig. 22-2 Fornix, outline. Hippo., hippocampal formation; Hypo., hypothalamus; MB, mammillary body; MFB, medial forebrain bundle; Pre., Post., pre- and postcommissural fornix.

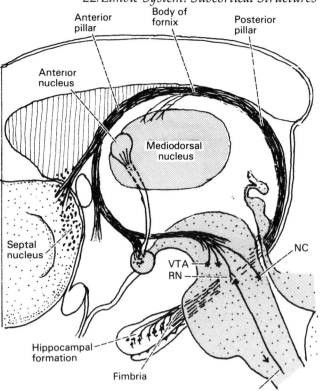

Fig. 22-3 Fornix, details. NC, nucleus ceruleus; RN, raphe nucleus; VTA, ventral tegmental area.

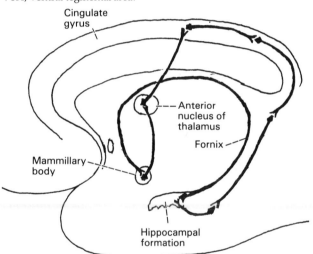

Fig. 22-4 Papez circuit.

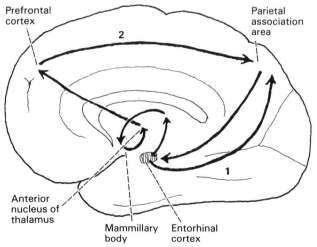

Fig. 22-5 1, direct, and 2, fornix route from entorhinal cortex to parietal association area.

mammillary body and anterior hypothalamus. The other half bypass the hypothalamus and reach the midbrain in the median forebrain bundle. Hippocampal efferents synapse in the reticular formation and periaqueductal gray matter. Afferents enter the *fornicohippocampal pathway* from monoaminergic neurons of midbrain (raphe nucleus and ventral tegmental area) and pons (nucleus ceruleus). The fornix also contains several kinds of peptidergic neurons – some afferent, some efferent.

From the mammillary body, the *mammillothalamic tract* enters the anterior thalamic nucleus, from which a large projection enters the posterior half of the cingulate gyrus. The cingulate is linked by polysynaptic connections with the entorhinal cortex. This completes the *Papez circuit* (hippocampal formation–mammillary body–anterior thalamus–cingulate cortex–entorhinal area–hippocampal formation: Fig. 22-4).

The mediodorsal nucleus of the thalamus receives fibers direct from the fornix and from the septal area. Lesions of the mediodorsal nucleus have been associated with dramatic *anterograde amnesia*, as severe as that associated with removal of the hippocampal formation. An alternate route for memory traces (separate from the entorhinal projections to association areas) seems to be one from the mediodorsal thalamus to the prefrontal cortex. The latter is richly interconnected with the sensory association areas.

Lesions of the fornix or mammillary bodies are *sometimes* accompanied by anterograde amnesia. *Korsakoff's psychosis* occurs in chronic alcoholics having vitamin B_1 deficiency. Anterograde amnesia, cerebellar ataxia, and polyneuropathy of peripheral nerves are characteristic. At autopsy (in untreated cases) the mammillary bodies are severely shrunken and there are hemorrhages in them and in the mediodorsal nucleus of the thalamus.

There are grounds for believing that the two routes to the isocortex from the hippocampus (Fig. 22-5) are concerned with subtly different aspects of memory imprinting.

SEPTAL NUCLEUS AND SEPTAL AREA (Fig. 22-6)

In the human brain, the medial and lateral septal nuclei are buried within the par019terminal gyrus, directly in front of the anterior commissure and lamina terminalis. A few cells extend into the septum pellucidum. The medial and lateral septal nuclei constitute the *septal nucleus*, and the *septal area* includes the septal nucleus and its extension into septum pellucidum.

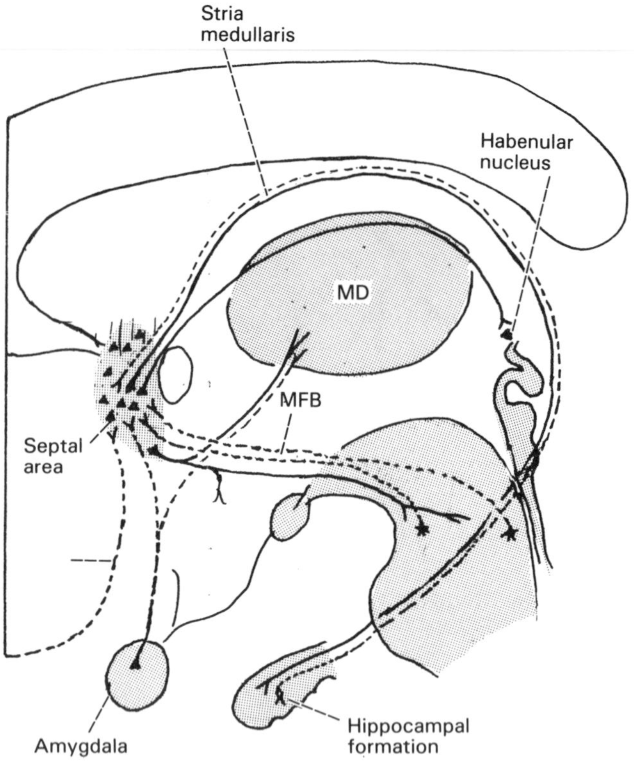

Connections

Afferents are received by the septal nucleus:
a from the hippocampal formation via the precommissural fornix;
b from the amygdala, mainly via the diagonal band of Broca;
c from the primary olfactory cortex via the medial olfactory stria;
d from brainstem monoamine neurons via the medial forebrain bundle (MFB).
Efferents run:
a to the mediodorsal thalamic nucleus;
b to the hippocampal formation via the fornix;
c to the habenular nucleus;
d to the lateral hypothalamus and midbrain tegmentum via the medial forebrain bundle.

Fig. 22-6 Afferent (dotted lines) and efferent connections of septal area. MD, mediodorsal nucleus; MFB, median forebrain bundle; Olf., olfactory tract.

Functions

1 The septal nucleus is responsible for the rhythmic slow wave activity (4–7 Hz), known as *theta rhythm*, found in groups of pyramidal cells in the hippocampus. The theta rhythm is abolished if the cholinergic septohippocampal pathway is put out of action. The biological significance of theta rhythm is not understood. It is found in other cortical areas besides the hippocampus. Theta rhythms are obvious in the EEG when the individual is performing routine motor tasks, and also during rapid-eye-movement sleep.
2 The septothalamic pathway is thought to be involved in the transfer of memory traces from the hippocampus to the prefrontal neocortex. However, there is no clear evidence that septal lesions produce memory defects in animals.
3 Through the medial forebrain bundle the septum exerts inhibitory effects on the lateral hypothalamus and reticular formation. Animals with septal lesions are hyperactive, and often show signs of 'septal rage'. Conversely, stimulation of the intact septum reduces or abolishes the rage produced by simultaneous stimulation of the lateral hypothalamus. The septal effects on rage may be due to stimulation of amygdalar fibers passing to or through the septal area.
4 Septal stimulation in humans may produce a euphoric state of mind – the sense of pleasure. Sometimes a sense of orgasm is felt. In animals, the septum is one of many 'reward areas' of the brain, on the evidence provided by self-stimulation experiments. Animals seem to find self-stimulation of the medial forebrain bundle even more pleasurable. They may self-stimulate in either of these areas (by pressing a lever activating an indwelling electrode) to the exclusion of all other activities, even to the point of death from starvation. Dopamine has been suggested as the transmitter substance required to achieve the sense of pleasure.

HABENULAR NUCLEUS (Figs. 22-1, 22-6)

The *habenular nucleus* lies above and in front of the pineal gland on each side. It receives septal fibers in the *stria medullaris thalami*. It communicates with its fellow through the *habenular commissure*. It gives rise to a cholinergic bundle (the *fasciculus retroflexus*) which enters the *interpeduncular nucleus* in the floor of the interpeduncular space of the midbrain. The interpeduncular nucleus projects into the reticular formation.

The significance of the habenular connections is unknown.

NUCLEUS ACCUMBENS

The nucleus accumbens septi (see Fig. 18-10) is regarded as a motor-effector nucleus of the limbic system. It belongs structurally to the basal ganglia, being structurally identical to the striatum.

AMYGDALA (Figs. 22-7, 22-8)

The amygdala (amygdaloid body, amygdaloid complex) lies above the inferior horn of the lateral ventricle. The subnuclei of the amygdala are in corticomedial and basolateral (including central) groups. The corticomedial group blends with the secondary olfactory cortex. The central nucleus gives rise to the two projection pathways to other brain centers:

1 The *stria terminalis* is a long strand of white matter which follows the curve of the caudate nucleus. Like the fornix, it splits into pre- and postcommissural fibers. The precommissural fibers terminate in the septal area. The postcommissural fibers enter the hypothalamus and medial forebrain bundle (MFB). The fibers entering the MFB supply all of the autonomic nuclei of the brain stem.

2 The *ventral amygdalofugal pathway* passes direct to the mediodorsal nucleus of the thalamus through the inferior thalamic peduncle. Its most anterior fibers enter the septal area (Fig. 22-1).

In cats and monkeys stimulation of the amygdala produces a full *defense reaction* with pupillary dilatation, snarling and aggressive gestures, piloerection, and increased respiratory rate and cardiac output. The effect is a duplicate of that produced by stimulating the 'rage center' in the lateral hypothalamus, and hypothalamic stimulation is ineffective if the amygdalas have been removed. The amygdala elicits the defense reaction through its input to the ventromedial nucleus, which controls the lateral hypothalamic 'rage' center.

In humans, stimulation of the amygdala most often produces a sense of *fear*, rarely a sense of anger. Bilateral amygdalectomy has been carried out on individuals subject to *rage attacks*, characterized by irritability, progressing over several hours to dangerous aggressiveness, and finally subsiding to a state of abject remorse. The operation has been successful in eliminating such attacks.

The amygdala has the highest concentration of opiate receptors in the entire brain. These receptors are likely to be activated, and the amygdalas 'switched on', in acutely stressful situations, in which endogenous opiates enter the bloodstream.

The largest inputs to the amygdala come from the superior, middle and inferior temporal gyri. The significance of these is unknown. The amygdala receives subcortical afferents from the majority of its target nuclei in the hypothalamus and brainstem; most travel in the stria terminalis, which is therefore a mixed, afferent–efferent pathway.

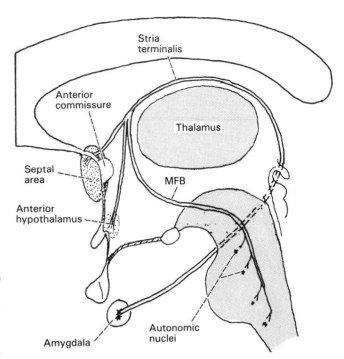

Fig. 22-7   Stria terminalis. MFB, median forebrain bundle.

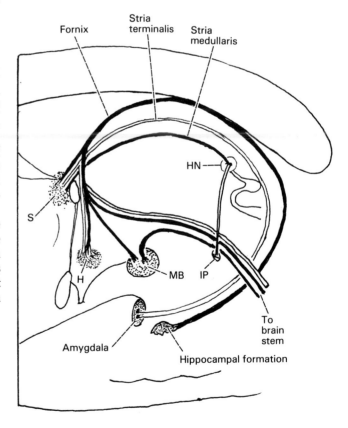

Fig. 22-8   Three limbic loops. H, hypothalamus; HN, habenular nucleus; IP, interpeduncular nucleus; MB, mammillary body; S, septal area.

Sex hormones and the amygdala

In rats, the amygdala is rich in estradiol receptors, and the stria terminalis exerts both excitatory and inhibitory effects on the secretion of gonadotropic hormones by the hypothalamus. In monkeys, a hormonal effect is presumed to underlie the hypersexuality that follows bilateral amygdalectomy. Such monkeys are hyperactive, constantly exploring their environment and putting objects in their mouths. They display no fear of natural enemies, and often attempt to copulate with other species. If they are returned to their natural habitat they are unable to conform to their own social group and are quickly driven out or killed.

Readings

Buchanan, S.L. and Powell, D.A. (1982) Cingulate cortex: its role in Pavlovian conditioning. *J. Comp. Physiol. Psychol., 96:* 755–774.

Krnjevic, K. and Ropert, N. (1981) Septo-hippocampal pathway modulates hippocampal activity by a cholinergic mechanism. *Can. J. Physiol. Pharmacol., 59:* 911–914.

Markowitsch, H.J. (1982) Thalamic mediodorsal nucleus and memory: a critical evaluation of studies in animals and man. *Neurosci., Behav. Rev., 6:* 147–165.

Mehler, W.R. (1980) Subcortical afferent connections of the amygdala in the monkey. *J. Comp. Neurol., 190:* 733–762.

Powell, E.W. and Leman, R.B. (1976) Connections of the nucleus accumbens. *Brain Res., 105:* 389–403.

Price, J.L. and Amaral, D.G. (1981) An autoradiographic study of the projections of the central nucleus of the monkey amygdala. *J. Neurosci., 1:* 1242–1259.

Roberts, G.W., Allen, Y., Crow, T.J. and Polak, J.M. (1983) Immunocytochemical localization of neuropeptides in the fornix of rat, monkey and man. *Brain Res., 263:* 151–155.

Shiosaka, S., Sakanaka, M., Inagaki, S., Senba, E., Hara, Y., Takatsuki, K., Takagi, H., Kawai, Y. and Tohyama, M. (1983) Putative transmitters in the amygdaloid complex with special reference to peptidergic pathways. In *Chemical Neuroanatomy* (Emson, P.C., ed.), pp. 359–390. New York: Raven Press.

Siegel, A. (1984) Anatomical and functional differentiation within the amygdala – behavioral state modulation. *Neurol. Neurobiol., 12:* 1–25.

Swanson, L.W. (1978) The anatomical organization of septo-hippocampal projections. In *Function of the Septo-Hippocampal System*, pp. 25–43. Amsterdam: Elsevier.

Vogt, B.A., Rosene, D.L. and Pandya, D.N. (1979) Thalamic and cortical afferents differentiate anterior from posterior cingulate cortex in the monkey. *Science, 204:* 205–207.

23
Blood Supply of the Hemispheres

The arterial blood supply to the brain is derived entirely from the internal carotid and vertebral arteries.

Each internal carotid artery enters the subarachnoid space by piercing the dural roof of the cavernous sinus. It gives off ophthalmic, posterior communicating and anterior choroidal branches before dividing into the anterior and middle cerebral arteries (Fig. 23-1).

The two vertebral arteries unite at the lower border of the pons to form the basilar artery. Together, the vertebral and basilar arteries supply the brain stem and

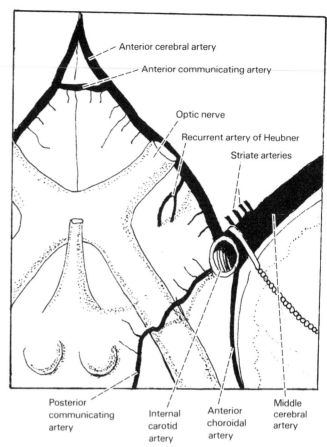

Fig. 23-2 Central branches from the circle of Willis. The internal carotid artery is pulled aside to show Heubner's artery.

cerebellum (Chapter 12). The basilar terminates by dividing into two posterior cerebral arteries, which complete the arterial circle of Willis (Fig. 23-2).

Each of the cerebral arteries gives rise to cortical and central branches.

CORTICAL ARTERIES (Figs. 23-3, 23-4, 23-5)

The cortical branches of the *anterior* cerebral artery supply the anterior two-thirds of the medial surface of the cerebral hemisphere, as well as a 2–3 cm strip of the adjoining orbital and lateral surfaces. The territory includes the supplementary motor area and the primary motor and sensory areas for the contralateral lower limb.

The cortical branches of the *middle* cerebral artery supply two-thirds of the lateral surface of the hemisphere, and the temporal pole. Important territories include the primary motor and sensory areas for the hand and face and (in the dominant hemisphere) Broca's and Wernicke's areas.

The cortical territories of the *posterior* cerebral artery include the primary and associative visual areas, and the hippocampus.

CENTRAL ARTERIES

Dozens of fine branches are given off by the constituent elements of the circle of Willis. They have been classified in various ways but are conveniently grouped into short and long branches. *Short* central

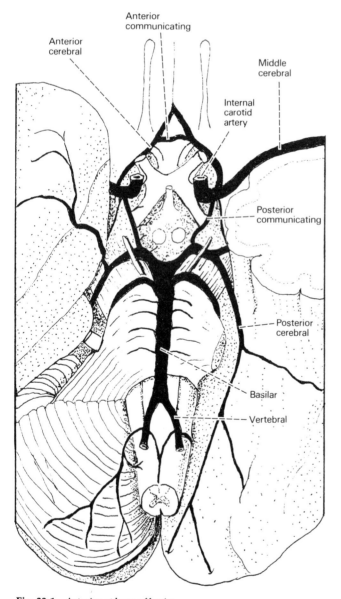

Fig. 23-1 Arteries at base of brain.

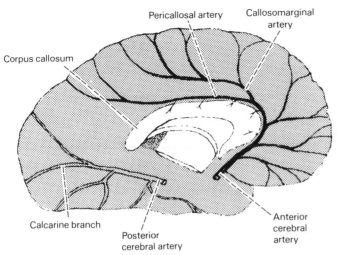

Fig. 23-3 Medial view of cerebrum, to show distribution of cortical branches of anterior and posterior cerebral arteries.

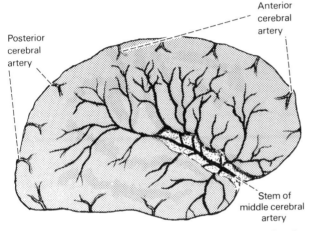

Fig. 23-4 Lateral view of cerebral hemisphere, showing distribution of cortical arteries. The lips of the lateral sulcus (opercula of the insula) have been pulled apart.

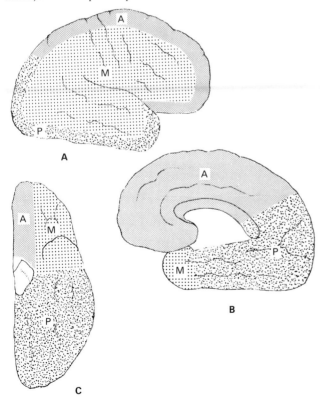

Fig. 23-5 A, lateral, B, medial, C, inferior surfaces of cerebral hemisphere, showing cortical territories of anterior (A), middle (M), and posterior (P) cerebral arteries.

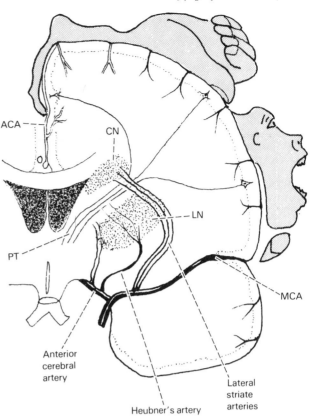

Fig. 23-6 Schematic coronal section to show distribution of anterior (ACA) and middle (MCA) cerebral artery. CN, caudate nucleus; LN, lentiform nucleus; PT, pyramidal tract.

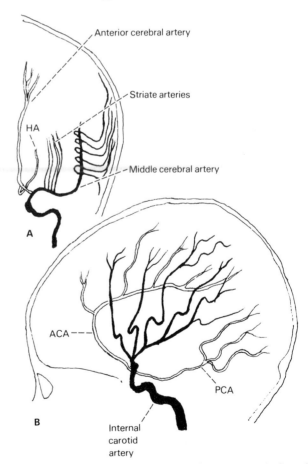

Fig. 23-7 Cerebral vessels as seen in carotid angiograms. A, frontal projection; B, lateral projection. Filling of the posterior cerebral artery (via the posterior communicating artery) is infrequent. ACA, PCA, anterior and posterior cerebral arteries; HA, artery of Heubner. (Adapted from Ascherl et al, 1980.)

branches arise from all of the elements, to supply the optic nerve, chiasm, and tract, and the hypothalamus. *Long* central branches arise from the three cerebral arteries and from the anterior choroidal. They penetrate deeply to supply the thalamus, internal capsule, and basal ganglia.

Striate arteries (Figs. 23-6, 23-7)

The long central branches of the anterior and middle cerebral are called the *striate arteries*; they create the foramina in the anterior perforated substance. *Medial striate arteries* come off the anterior and middle cerebral; they supply the anterior part of the thalamus, the basal ganglia, and the internal capsule. The largest of these is the *recurrent artery of Heubner*, from the anterior cerebral (Fig. 23-2). *Lateral striate arteries* come from the middle cerebral and anterior choroidal. They penetrate the lentiform nucleus at various levels and then pass across the internal capsule to end in the thalamus.

VENOUS DRAINAGE

The cerebral hemispheres are drained by superficial and deep cerebral veins. Like the intracranial venous sinuses, they are devoid of valves.

Superficial veins (Fig. 23-8)

The main superficial veins lie in the subarachnoid space overlying the hemispheres. The veins anastomose with one another, and pierce the arachnoid and dura prior to entering intracranial venous sinuses.

Superior superficial veins drain the frontal, parietal, and occipital cortices. They empty into the superior sagittal sinus. The more anterior ones enter the sinus more or less at right angles. The rest turn forward and enter against the direction of flow. The forward angulation is conferred during fetal life during the mainly backward expansion of the hemispheres.

A single, middle superficial vein occupies the lateral sulcus and drains the frontal, parietal, and temporal opercula. It empties into the cavernous or sphenoparietal sinus.

Inferior superficial veins drain the lateral and inferior surfaces of the temporal and occipital lobes. They empty into the transverse sinus.

Deep veins (Figs. 23-9, 23-10)

The deep cerebral veins commence in the walls and floor of the lateral ventricles. The *thalamostriate (terminal) vein* runs along the body and tail of the caudate nucleus. It drains the corpus striatum and the deep white matter of the frontal and parietal lobes. It unites with the *choroidal vein* (which drains the choroid plexus of the corresponding lateral ventricle) to form the *internal cerebral vein*. The internal cerebral veins of the two sides run backward in the tela choroidea of the transverse fissure of the brain and unite beneath the splenium of the corpus callosum, forming the *great cerebral vein* (of Galen).

The *deep middle cerebral vein* lies on the surface of the insula. It drains the insula, claustrum, and external capsule.

The *basal vein* (of Rosenthal) is formed in the subarachnoid space below the anterior perforated substance, by the union of the *anterior cerebral vein* (whose territory is similar to that of the anterior cerebral artery) and the deep middle cerebral vein. The basal vein runs around the crus cerebri and empties into the great cerebral vein.

The great cerebral vein is about 2 cm long. It curves below the splenium of the corpus callosum before piercing the arachnoid and dura to join the inferior sagittal sinus, thereby forming the straight sinus (Fig. 23-9). In addition to receiving the internal cerebral and basal veins, the great cerebral vein receives tributaries from the posterior part of the corpus callosum and from the adjacent parts of the cerebellum and midbrain.

Note: The anatomical details of the deep cerebral veins are important to neurosurgeons. They have only occasional relevance to general neurological practise.

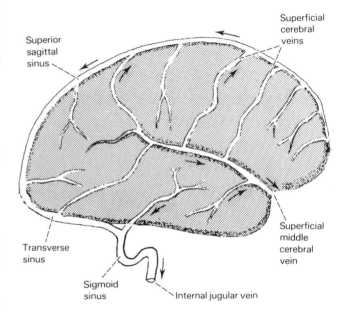

Fig. 23-8 Lateral view of cerebrum, to show superficial cerebral veins. Arrows indicate direction of blood flow.

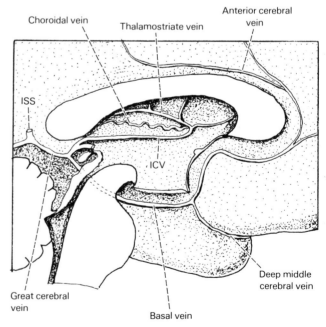

Fig. 23-9 Tributaries of the great cerebral vein, medial view. ICV, internal cerebral vein; ISS, inferior sagittal sinus.

APPLIED ANATOMY

Anastomotic and end arteries

In the circle of Willis, the blood in the three communicating arteries is normally static. Following occlusion of one of the three large arteries contributing to the circle, the other two compensate more or less completely, via the communicating arteries. With occlusion of one internal carotid, the other internal carotid may perfuse both anterior cerebral arteries. With occlusion of the basilar, each posterior cerebral artery may be perfused by the internal carotid of its own side.

Further anastomoses occur between cortical branches of the cerebral arteries, prior to penetration of the branches into the brain substance. Once the cortical and central branches have penetrated, they become end arteries, communicating only at capillary level.

In what follows, the term 'occlusion' embraces thrombosis, embolism, or hemorrhage of the affected arteries.

Anterior cerebral artery (ACA)

The effects of ACA occlusion depend upon whether the lesion is distal or proximal to the point of origin of Heubner's artery. If *distal*, the patient develops severe (flaccid) motor weakness, and sensory loss, in the contralateral leg. Mental confusion is usual because of 'decortication' of much of the frontal lobe. Bladder control is usually lost owing to interference with the bilateral pathway from the bladder area of the motor cortex to the pontine bladder control center (Chapter 40).

If the lesion is *proximal*, or if Heubner's artery is absent (it is missing in 3% of the population), the above picture will be complicated by the addition of contralateral spastic weakness of the arm, and contralateral facial weakness of upper motor neuron type.

Middle cerebral artery (MCA)

A typical 'stroke' is caused by occlusion of one of the *striate branches* of the MCA. The clinical picture is described in Chapter 20. Bilateral occlusion of one or more striate branches is liable to produce *pseudobulbar palsy*. In this condition, mastication, swallowing, and speech articulation are severely affected. These effects occur because cranial nerve nuclei V, VII, X and XII (except for the lower face element of VII) usually receive bilateral supply from the motor cortex.

The effects of occlusion of individual *cortical branches* of the MCA are described in Chapter 25. They include deficits in speech performance and comprehension.

Occlusion of the *stem* of the MCA devitalizes a large part of the cerebral hemisphere. Coma (often irreversible) is caused by the resultant cerebral edema (Chapter 24). Contralateral hemiplegia and hemianesthesia are severe and are usually permanent, as is hemianopsia (blindness of the opposite visual field, Chapter 29).

Posterior cerebral artery (PCA)

Occlusion of the *calcarine branch* produces contralateral hemianopsia. This effect is most commonly seen in adolescents suffering from migraine.

Occlusion of one of the *thalamic branches* devitalizes the posterior limb of the internal capsule. It is characterized by contralateral hemianopsia, together with contralateral hemianesthesia (the latter resulting from damage to fibers passing from thalamus to somesthetic cortex). A thalamic syndrome (Chapter 17) may be a distressing sequel.

Occlusion of the *stem* of the PCA causes contralateral hemianopsia and hemianesthesia, together with signs of severe cerebral edema.

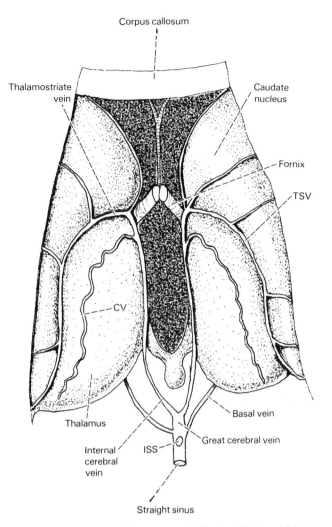

Fig. 23-10 Tributaries of the great cerebral vein. CV, choroidal vein; ISS, entry point of inferior sagittal sinus; TSV, thalamostriate vein.

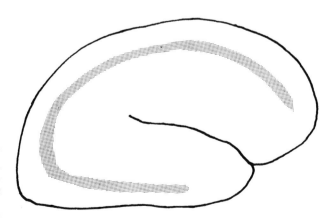

Fig. 23-11 The cortical 'watershed' (shaded) is the terminal cortical territory of the three cerebral arteries (compare with Fig. 23-4).

167

Occlusion of *branches to the midbrain* may cause a dorsal or ventral midbrain syndrome (Chapter 12).

Anterior choroidal artery

On its way to supplying the choroid plexus of the lateral ventricle, this artery passes alongside the optic tract. It supplies the tract, and gives central branches to the base of the internal capsule at this level. Occlusion of the main artery causes contralateral hemiplegia, hemianesthesia, and hemianopsia. The condition is distinguished from stem MCA occlusion by the absence of signs of cerebral edema.

Cortical 'watershed'

Cortical perfusion pressure is relatively weak along a semicircular strip between the main territories of the middle cerebral artery, on the one hand, and the anterior and posterior cerebrals, on the other (Fig. 23-11). Cerebral hypoxia (such as from severe hypotension or from carbon monoxide poisoning) may damage the underlying white matter anywhere along this strip, as well as the cortex. Fibers linking somesthetic or visual association areas with the entorhinal cortex may be interrupted, giving rise to a 'disconnection syndrome' (Chapter 21).

Some temporal branches of the PCA supply the entorhinal cortex and hippocampal formation. Unilateral occlusion of these branches does not seem to affect the memory functions (Chapter 21) of this area. A temporary bilateral occlusion may be caused by kinking of the *vertebral* arteries in an individual who has cervical spondylosis, with osteophytes encroaching on the foramina transversaria (through which the arteries run). If such an individual stares at an object directly overhead, he may stagger because of reduced perfusion in the labyrinthine arteries, and he may go blind for a few seconds from reduced perfusion of the occipital lobes. He may have no recollection of either event (or even of having looked up) because of reduced perfusion of the temporal lobes.

Subarachnoid hemorrhage (SAH)

SAH results from rupture of a localized 'berry' aneurysm on an artery in or near the circle of Willis.

The severity of the symptoms varies greatly, from mild headache (a small leak) to immediate coma (flooding of the subarachnoid space). Most commonly, the patient experiences sudden severe headache, and vomits because of raised intracranial pressure (Chapter 2). The patient becomes stuporous and shows neck rigidity because blood enters the posterior cranial fossa (Chapter 34). Focal signs may be present if cranial nerves are pressed upon or if the hemorrhage was initially intracerebral.

Subdural hematoma

Subdural hematomas may be acute, subacute, or chronic. In all cases there is rupture of one or more superficial cerebral veins in transit from the brain to an intracranial venous sinus.

Acute subdural hematoma may follow severe head injury, most often in children. Many of these cases result from child battering. It is always suspected if a child does not recover consciousness following head injury.

Subacute subdural hematomas may follow head injury at any age, after recovery of consciousness for up to three weeks. Signs of raised intracranial pressure appear. About half of these cases develop a hemiparesis which may be contralateral or ipsilateral following uncal herniation (Chapter 2).

Chronic subdural hematoma is the commonest of the three forms. It nearly always occurs in people over 40. In these older people, moderate shrinkage of the brain puts tension on the transit veins, which become increasingly brittle with advancing age. Head injury may be mild or even absent. The overall incidence of trauma is unknown, because a significant number of these patients are alcoholics with impaired blood clotting. Presenting symptoms are variable and include personality changes, headaches, and epileptic seizures.

Readings

Ascher, G.F., Ganti, S.R. and Hilal, S.K. (1980) Cerebral angiography. In *The Science and Practice of Clinical Medicine, Vol. 5, Neurology* (Rosenberg, R.N., ed.), pp. 643–644. New York: Grune & Stratton.

Bannister, R. (ed.) (1978) Disorders of the cerebral circulation. In *Brain's Clinical Neurology*, 5th ed., pp. 253–282. Oxford: Oxford University Press.

Capra, N.F. (1984) Anatomy of the cerebral venous system. In *Cerebral Venous System and its Disorders* (Kapp, J.P. and Schmidek, H.H., eds.), pp. 1–36. New York: Grune & Stratton.

Carpenter, M.B. (1978) Blood supply of the central nervous system. In *Core Text of Neuroanatomy*, pp. 317–340. Baltimore: Williams & Wilkins.

Gomes, F., Dujovny, M., Umansky, F., Ausman, J.-I., Diaz, F.G., Ray, W.J. and Mirchandani, H.G. (1984) Microsurgical anatomy of the recurrent artery of Heubner. *J. Neurosurg., 60*: 130–139.

Patten, J. (1978) The cerebral hemispheres. 2: vascular diseases. In *Neurological Differential Diagnosis*, pp. 86–98. London: Harold Starke; New York: Springer-Verlag.

Weisberg, L.A., Strub, R.L. and Garcia, C.A. (1983) Stroke. In *Essentials of Clinical Neurology*, pp. 147–166. Baltimore: University Park Press.

Blood–Brain Barrier and the Cerebrospinal Fluid

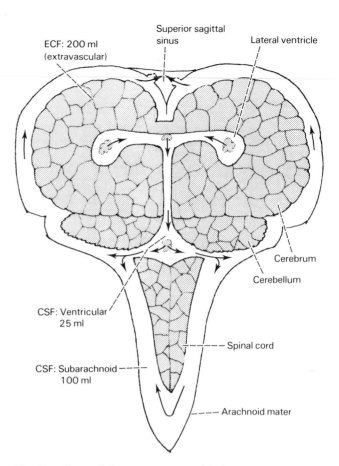

Fig. 24-1 Extracellular compartments of the brain. Arrows indicate circulation of cerebrospinal fluid (CSF). ECF, extracellular fluid.

The nervous system is isolated from the blood by a barrier system that provides a stable and optimal environment for the parenchymal cells (neurons and neuroglia). The environment consists of the *brain extracellular fluid* (ECF) (in the present context, 'brain' includes spinal cord). The term 'brain ECF' does not include the cerebrospinal fluid in the ventricles and subarachnoid space (Fig. 24-1), although the ECF and CSF are chemically similar.

The brain ECF accounts for 15–18% of total brain volume. In electron micrographs prepared by standard methods the apparent extracellular space is minute, owing to the tissue swelling that occurs within seconds after death.

SOURCES OF BRAIN ECF

Source	Percentage
Choroid plexus	50–60
Brain capillaries	30–40
Metabolic water	<10>

The blood–brain barrier (BBB) has two components (Fig. 24-2). One barrier is between the choroidal capillaries and the CSF. The other barrier is between the brain capillaries and the ECF.

THE BLOOD–CSF BARRIER (Fig. 24-3)

The choroid plexuses secrete about 500 ml CSF per day into the ventricles. CSF passes from the lateral ventricles into the third (through the foramen of Monro), from the third to the fourth (through the aqueduct), and from the fourth into the subarachnoid space through the median and lateral apertures. The CSF circulates around the brain and spinal cord before entering the superior sagittal sinus by way of the arachnoid granulations. The subarachnoid space is sealed off by the arachnoid mater, whose cells are bonded by tight junctions. On the other hand, no seals exist between the CSF and the brain parenchyma: the pia–glial and ependyma–glial membranes (Chapter 2) are freely permeable. The net flow through these membranes is outward: ventricular CSF diffuses into brain ECF, and brain ECF diffuses into the subarachnoid space.

The blood–CSF barrier resides in specialized ependymal epithelium overlying the choroidal capillaries.

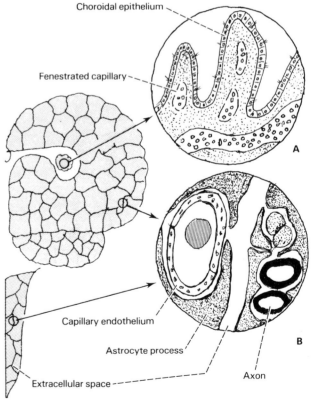

Fig. 24-2 The two elements of the blood–brain barrier. A, choroidal epithelium; B, capillary endothelium of the CNS.

This *choroidal epithelium* differs from the general ependymal epithelium in three ways:

1 Cilia are scarce and surface microvilli are numerous.

2 The cells are bonded by tight junctions. The tight junctions are pericellular belts of membrane fusion and they are the actual site of the blood–CSF barrier. If a high-molecular-weight tracer (e.g. lanthanum) is injected into the circulation (in animals), it passes freely through the fenestrated choroidal capillaries but it is arrested at the level of the tight junctions.

3 Histochemically, the choroidal epithelium contains numerous enzymes specifically involved in ion transport. Na^+-K^+-ATPase within the microvilli provides a pump driving sodium into the CSF and potassium into the plasma. Sodium transport is optimized by movement of bicarbonate ions in the same direction. This is provided for by the presence of carbonic anhydrase enzyme, which hydrates intracellular carbon dioxide.

The convoluted choroid plexuses expose a large epithelial surface to the ventricles – about 200 cm² in all, equivalent in area to the palms of two hands. About 25% of plasma water leaves the capillary bed between its arterial and venous ends. This very large movement of water is assisted by movement of sodium. The flow of CSF through the ventricles in experimental animals is arrested if the Na^+-K^+-ATPase is specifically inhibited (by ouabain). Hydrostatic pressure appears to be insignificant in water transfer.

Energy-dependent carrier systems operate within the choroidal epithelial cells: they transport many chemicals from plasma to CSF, including monosaccharides, amino acids, and other organic acids and bases.

THE BLOOD–ECF BARRIER

The blood–ECF barrier resides in the *capillary endothelium of the brain*. Brain capillaries differ from those of other tissues in four important ways (Fig. 24-4):

1 The cells are bonded by tight junctions, which are impermeable to large molecules.

2 Pinocytic vesicles are rare, and fenestrations are absent. Pinocytotic vesicles and fenestrations are important thoroughfares for macromolecules in other tissue capillaries.

3 The cells have specific enzymes regulating transport both into and out of the CSF. The cells are highly active metabolically, containing ten times more mitochondria than the capillaries of skeletal muscle. The transport systems are the same as those of the choroidal epithelium.

4 The cells are not contractile. In non-nervous tissues, capillary endothelium contains filaments resembling the actomyosin of smooth muscle. The filaments contract in response to a surge of histamine, causing the endothelial cells to separate and render the local capillary bed permeable to blood plasma. The absence of filaments from brain capillaries protects the brain from allergic and other systemic disorders in which histamine is released into the circulation.

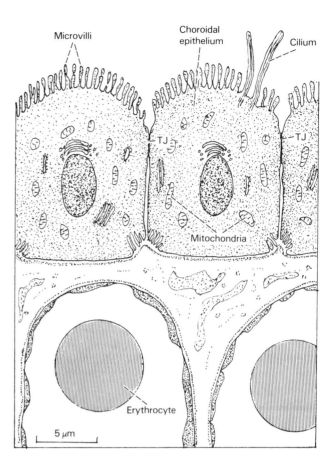

Fig. 24-3 Ultrastructure of the choroid plexus. TJ. tight junction.

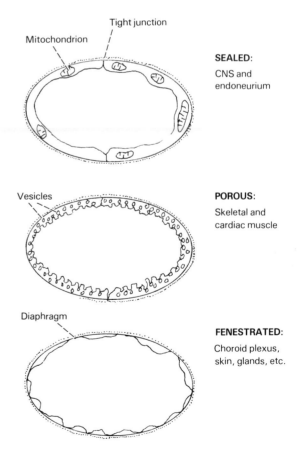

Fig. 24-4 The three types of tissue capillary.

(The occasional pericytes around brain capillaries may respond to local release of norepinephrine from neurons within the brain. Blood flow is reduced when these neurons are active.)

The area of the brain capillary bed is enormous: 150 cm^2/g of brain weight. In a 1500 g brain the area is 100000 cm^2 – 5000 times greater than that of the choroidal epithelium. The huge capillary area accounts for the brain's consuming 20% of basal oxygen intake even though brain weight is only 2% of total body weight.

METABOLIC WATER

Brain metabolism generates water and electrolytes, which diffuse through the pia–glial membrane into the subarachnoid space. This 'sink' movement of ECF is essential because the brain is virtually devoid of the lymphatics which remove metabolic water in other tissues. *Metabolic water is the only element of the CSF which does not pass through a blood–brain barrier.*

CONTROL SYSTEMS IN THE BBB

To reach the brain ECF from the blood, solutes must penetrate the choroidal epithelium or the brain capillary endothelium. Immediate access is provided to molecules soluble both in water (plasma) and in membrane lipid. Other molecules must be manipulated across by carrier proteins.

The BBB and glucose

Glucose is actively transported by a specific carrier protein. CSF glucose concentration is only two-thirds that of the blood's because of constant glucose consumption by brain cells. The ECF glucose level is more stable than the blood's because the transport system becomes saturated when blood glucose rises and is hyperactive when it falls. Stability of ECF glucose is essential for normal neuronal function. In severe *hyperglycemia*, with perhaps a threefold increase in blood glucose, ketone bodies and lactic acid accumulate in the brain ECF and depress neuronal activity (diabetic coma). In severe *hypoglycemia* the CNS becomes overactive. The patient exhibits mental confusion and sweating, with a rapid pulse. Hypoglycemia may finally silence brain neurons if their main source of nutrition becomes exhausted (insulin coma).

The BBB and potassium

The molarity of K$^+$ in the brain ECF and CSF is maintained at about 3 mmol/l, whereas in other extracellular fluids it ranges from 4 to 5.5 mmol/l. Active transport systems in the choroidal epithelium and CNS capillaries operate in both directions. The transport systems from the blood quickly become saturated as blood K$^+$ levels rise, and normal CSF values obtain even when the blood K$^+$ is doubled. Conversely, if excess K$^+$ is instilled into the ventricular system (in animals), it is quickly cleared by active transport *into* the blood. The rigorous control of brain K$^+$ concentration allows the neurons to generate high electrical potentials without interference from K$^+$ fluctuations generated in other body systems.

The BBB and neurotransmitters

The BBB is impermeable to circulating epinephrine, nor-epinephrine, acetylcholine, and dopamine. If it were not, their effects would be disastrous. Epinephrine, in particular,

floods the circulation in response to physical or emotional stress, and it would profoundly alter brain function should it reach the brain ECF.

As well as blocking access of transmitters from the outside, the barrier conserves transmitters from the inside. Transmitters liberated by brain cells are (in general terms) taken up by the synaptic boutons from which they were liberated, and are used again. Considerable economy is provided by the capillary bed being closed to them. However, an appreciable loss does occur into the CSF along with the metabolic water that provides 10% of CSF volume. For this reason, fluctuations of CNS transmitter output can be detected by analysis of the CSF, and sometimes even of the blood (into which the CSF escapes).

THE PERIVASCULAR SPACES (Fig. 24-5)

The perivascular spaces (of Virchow–Robin) are extensions of the subarachnoid space around the vessels penetrating the brain surface. The spaces taper progressively, but they are continuous with the pericapillary spaces. Although they are *inward* extensions in the anatomical sense, the flow of ECF is *outward*, into the subarachnoid space. The perivascular spaces are involved in autoregulation of brain arterioles.

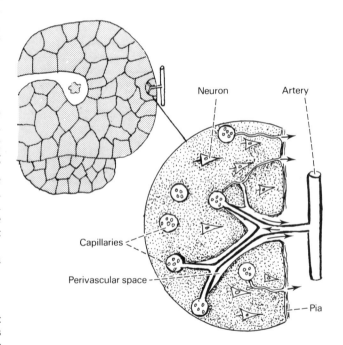

Fig. 24-5 Movement of fluid into and out of the cerebral cortex (arrows).

Autoregulation

Autoregulation is defined as a tissue's capacity to regulate its own blood supply. The H$^+$ ion concentration in the perivascular space is the chief *external* source of autoregulation of cerebral blood vessels. A rising H$^+$ (usually following hypercapnia – excess plasma CO$_2$) travels along the perivascular space from the capillary bed, and it inhibits vascular muscle, perhaps by reducing ionized calcium levels. On the other hand, hypocapnia causes vasoconstriction.

The chief *internal* source of autoregulation is the adjustment of arterial muscle tone in response to intraluminal pressure changes (Fig. 24-6). Cerebral blood flow remains at 60–70 ml/100 g/min during systemic blood pressure changes ranging from 80 to 180 mmHg (11–24 kPa). This is achieved by a direct, *myogenic* response to distension produced by rising intraluminal pressure.

Neuroregulation

Still in its infancy is the concept of cerebral vascular control by central neurons. Potential candidates for this function include norepinephrine, cholecystokinin, vasoactive intestinal polypeptide, serotonin, substance P, and neuropeptide Y.

CIRCUMVENTRICULAR ORGANS (Fig. 24-7)

Patches of brain tissue close to the third and fourth ventricles have fenestrated capillaries. These patches comprise the median eminence, neurohypophysis, subfornical organ, OVLT (organum vasculosum of the lamina terminalis), pineal gland, and area postrema. In the median eminence and neurohypophysis the fenestrations permit hypothalamic neurosecretions to enter the capillary beds. The subfornical organ, OVLT, and area postrema are *chemoreceptor zones*, from which neural responses are triggered by alterations in the composition of the blood plasma. The area postrema is the *chemoreceptor trigger zone*, which activates the underlying *vomiting center* (Chapter 36). The trigger zone may be excited by toxins or drugs which are unable to cross the BBB.

BLOOD–NERVE BARRIER

Peripheral nerve fibers have the same protection as those in the CNS. The endoneurial capillaries are sealed by tight junctions (Chapter 3).

SUMMARY OF BBB FUNCTIONS

1 To modulate the entry of metabolic substrates, notably glucose.
2 To pump ions – notably K^+ – into and out of the blood.
3 To restrict entry of macromolecules and of polar compounds (i.e., water-soluble but lipid-insoluble). The entry of lipid-soluble compounds is relatively unrestricted and does not require carrier systems in the BBB.
4 To block the entry of transmitters from the blood – notably epinephrine – and to conserve its own transmitters.
5 To block the entry of toxins, either because the toxins are bound to plasma albumin or because their solubilities are inappropriate.

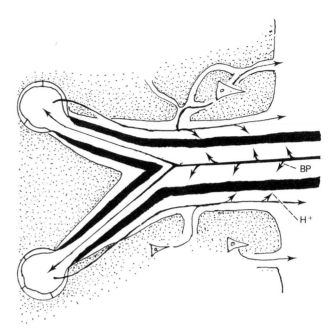

Fig. 24-6 Autoregulation: smooth muscle inhibition by H^+ ions (arrows in perivascular space); myogenic response to rising blood pressure (BP, arrows in arterial lumen).

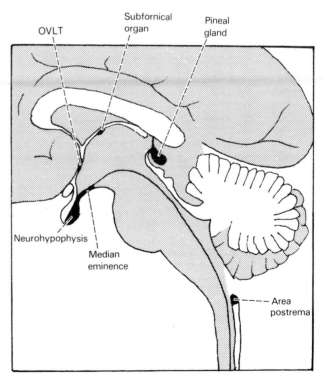

Fig. 24-7 Circumventricular organs. OVLT, organum vasculosum of lamina terminalis.

SUMMARY OF CSF FUNCTIONS

1 To provide protection for the brain. The CSF 'water-jacket' acts as a shock-absorber in the event of a blow to the head or spine, or a heavy fall. The entire CNS is suspended in CSF by webs of pia–arachnoid attached to the dura mater. The total amount of CSF can be reduced (by increased expulsion) to accommodate venous blood when the head is down, or during straining. A hemorrhage or tumor within the cranium can also be accommodated in this way – within limits.
2 To remove the products of brain metabolism (carbon dioxide, lactate, and so on).
3 To provide a stable chemical environment for the cells of the CNS. This function is executed by the BBB.
4 To participate in autoregulation of cerebral arterioles.

APPLIED ANATOMY

Kernicterus is a condition of neonates in which the brain (especially the striatum) shows a yellow discoloration. It occurs in *hemolytic disease of the newborn*, which arises from Rhesus incompatibility between the parents. The yellow stain is bilirubin derived from red cell hemolysis. It was long thought that kernicterus was caused by immaturity of the BBB. In fact, mature tight junctions are already present at the 12th week of gestation. The fault lies in the *liver*: bilirubin is normally conjugated to plasma proteins, and the conjugate is unable to pass the BBB. The neonatal liver is inefficient in this respect, and free bilirubin predominates in hemolytic disease.

The neonatal BBB *is* immature in one respect. The cerebral capillaries have pinocytotic vesicles capable of carrying large molecules from blood to ECF. Thus, the albumin level in the CSF is about 100 mg/dl at birth and dwindles to the adult values of 20–40 mg during the first postnatal year.

Cerebral edema
The normal autoregulatory mechanisms may be overpowered by severe hypercapnia or by severe hypertension. In either case the blood flow in the capillary bed may be large enough to disrupt the tight junctions between the endothelial cells. In experimental animals, either condition may also cause the capillaries to display pinocytotic activity. The end result is an increase in the ECF, or *brain edema*, which in turn alters the electrical activity of neurons.

Examples
1 Patients with severely *reduced alveolar ventilation* in the lungs (as in pulmonary or heart disease, or after surgery) may suffer from progressive mental confusion and drowsiness, leading to coma and death.
2 Patients suffering from arterial hypertension are liable to attacks of *hypertensive encephalopathy*. The attacks follow a rise in blood pressure to more than 170 mmHg (22.6 kPa), which the myogenic response may not withstand. In these cases the edema causes severe headache, visual disturbances and vomiting, sometimes progressing to convulsions and coma.
3 *Injury* to the brain is always followed by cerebral edema. The injury may be caused by a blow on the head or by a spontaneous vascular lesion, such as cerebral hemorrhage or thrombosis. The edema is caused in part by the osmotic effect of cellular necrosis (death) and in part by free blood in the extracellular space. Liberation of serotonin causes capillary pinocytosis, with aggravation of the edema.

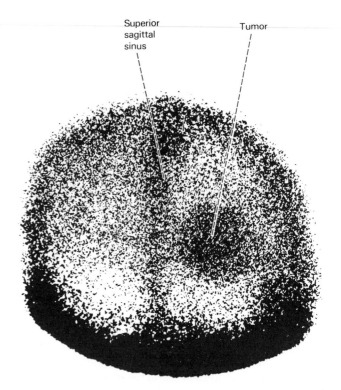

Fig. 24-8 Anteroposterior radiograph showing a glioma penetrated by technetium-99m following intravenous injection. A lateral view showed the tumor to be located in the frontal lobe. (From film kindly supplied by Dr J.P. Murray.)

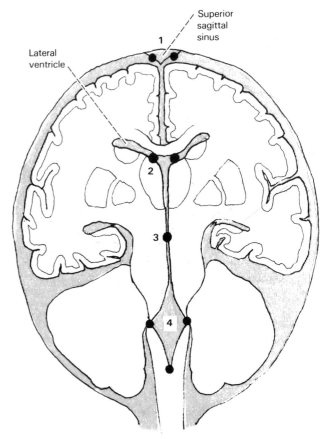

Fig. 24-9 Potential sites of obstruction to CSF circulation. 1, arachnoid granulations; 2, interventricular foramen; 3, aqueduct; 4, exit foramina of fourth ventricle.

Infections

Infections of the brain (encephalitis) or of the meninges (meningitis) are accompanied by breakdown of the BBB. The breakdown may be caused by large-scale emigration of leukocytes through brain capillary walls from the blood. The breakdown can be exploited clinically by the use of powerful non-lipid-soluble antibiotics, notably penicillin and chlortetracycline, in treatment.

Brain tumors

Astrocytomas are the commonest brain tumors, and they are accompanied by local breakdown of the BBB. The astrocyte foot processes withdraw from their usual intimacy with the capillary bed, whereupon the capillaries become fenestrated. Astrocytes may have a normal function of inducing brain capillaries to become specialized. When astrocytes are replaced by tumor cells from other regions, for example by a secondary cancer from the breast or lung, the capillaries growing into the tumor are fenestrated. The breakdown of the BBB in astrocytomas and metastatic cancers is detectable clinically. Radioactive tracers too large to penetrate the normal BBB (such as ^{32}P-tagged albumin, or technetium) will enter these tumors, where they can be detected radiologically (Fig. 24-8).

Pathology of CSF circulation

Hydrocephalus (Gr., water in the head) signifies accumulation of CSF within the skull. In the great majority of cases the condition is caused by obstruction to CSF circulation (Fig. 24-9). If the obstruction is within the ventricular system the hydrocephalus is called *internal*. If the obstruction is at the level of the arachnoid granulations it is called *communicating*.

A major cause of hydrocephalus is the *Arnold–Chiari malformation*, in which the vermis of the cerebellum is extruded into the vertebral canal in prenatal life. The fourth ventricle is also displaced, and an internal hydrocephalus results from blockage of the exit foramina to the subarachnoid space. In untreated cases the child's head may become as large as a football and the cerebral hemispheres may become paper-thin. The condition is nearly always associated with *spina bifida* (Chapter 11). Early treatment is essential to prevent severe brain damage: the obstruction can be bypassed by passing a catheter from a lateral ventricle into the internal jugular vein.

The posterior cranial fossae are abnormally small in Arnold–Chiari cases, and experimental evidence suggests that the small posterior fossae may be the cause, rather than the result, of cerebellar herniation. In the *Dandy–Walker syndrome* (rare) the posterior fossae are abnormally small, but the hydrocephalus in this condition is caused by failure of normal development of the ventricular exit foramina.

In later life the fourth ventricular foramina may be obstructed by a tumor in the posterior cranial fossa or by an ill-advised lumbar puncture (Chapter 2).

The *aqueduct* may be narrowed by congenital stenosis (rare) or by being deformed by an uncal hernia. It is occasionally blocked by a cyst within the third ventricle. An *interventricular foramen* is rarely obstructed.

The arachnoid granulations often suffer from moderate obstruction in patients suffering from cerebral meningitis or hemorrhage into the subarachnoid space.

Drugs and the BBB

Three factors determine the rate and extent to which drugs enter the brain from the blood stream.

Lipid solubility
Since the brain capillaries are not fenestrated, some degree of lipid solubility is required to permit a drug to pass through

the outer and inner plasma membranes of the cerebral capillaries. Rapidly acting general anesthetics (thiopental [thiopentone], halothane, cyclopropane, nitrous oxide, etc.) are intensely lipid-soluble. So too are caffeine, nicotine, steroids, and of course most of the psychoactive drugs. Alcohol is only moderately lipid-soluble; this accounts for its relatively slow action and for the fact that fat and thin people are almost equally susceptible to its central effects.

The antibiotics are weakly lipid-soluble and require high doses to be effective in the CNS. Penicillin is ineffective (unless capillary structure has been altered by disease) because penicillin is completely ionized at plasma pH (see later).

Plasma protein binding
Only the *free* drug can penetrate the BBB. Many drugs are partly bound to plasma albumin, and their effectiveness in the CNS is inversely proportional to their degree of protein binding.

Ionization
The drug must be in the non-ionized form at plasma pH (7.4) in order to penetrate the blood–brain barrier.

Computed X-ray tomography

Iodine is radio-opaque. Some iodinated compounds can be safely injected intravenously. They reach the brain capillary bed and in CT scans the contrast between gray and white matter is enhanced (the gray matter has four times as many capillaries). The opacity of tumors is also enhanced because of their capillary support.

Readings

Adams, P. (1984) Perivascular nerve fibres and the cerebral circulation. *Trends Neurosci., 7:* 135–138.

Alksne, J.F., Smith, R.W., Marshall, L.F. and Ignelzi, R.J. (1980) Acute brain injury. In *Neurology* (Rosenberg, R.N., ed.), pp. 370–381. New York & London: Grune & Stratton.

Astrup. J. (1982) Energy-requiring cell functions in the ischemic brain. *J. Neurosurg., 56:* 482–497.

Bradbury, M.W.B. (1984) The structure and function of the blood–brain barrier. *Fed. Proc., 43:* 186–190.

Cervos-Navarro, J., Artigas, J. and Mesulja, B.J. (1983) Morphofunctional aspects of the normal and pathological blood-brain barrier. *Acta Neuropathol. [Suppl.] (Berl.), 7:* 1–19.

Davson, H. (1984) Formation and drainage of the cerebrospinal fluid. In *Hydrocephalus* (Shapiro, K., Marmarou, A. and Portnoy, H., eds.), pp. 3–40. New York: Raven Press.

Eisenberg, H.M. (1983) New ways of looking at the blood–brain barrier. In *Concepts in Pediatric Neurosurgery*, Vol. 2 (Eisenberg, H.M. and Suddith, R.L., eds.), pp. 127–136. New York: Plenum Press.

Gaab, M.R. and Koos, W.Th. (1984) Hydrocephalus in infancy and childhood: diagnosis and indication for operation. *Neuropediatrics, 15:* 173–179.

Goldstein, G.W. and Betz, A.L. (1983) Recent advances in understanding brain capillary function. *Ann. Neurol., 14:* 389–395.

Groothuis, D.R. and Vick, N.A. (1982) Brain tumors and the blood–brain barrier. *Trends Neurosci., 5:* 232–235.

Hauw, J.J. and Lefauconnier, J.M. (1983) Blood–brain barrier. 1. Morphological data. *Rev. Neurol., 11:* 611–624.

Hirano, A. (1983) Morphological aspects of brain edema. In *Adv. Cell Neurobiol., 4:* 224–247.

Jennett, B., Teasdale, G., Fry, J., Braakman, R., Minderhoud, J., Heiden, J. and Kurze, T. (1980) Treatment for severe head injury. *J. Neurol. Neurosurg. Psychiatry, 43:* 289–295.

Klatzo, I. (1983) Disturbances of the blood–brain barrier in cerebrovascular disorders. *Acta Neuropathol. [Suppl.] (Berl.), 8:* 81–88.

Krentzberg, G.W. and Toth, L. (1983) Enzyme cytochemistry of the cerebral microvessel wall. *Acta Neuropathol. [Suppl.] (Berl.), 7:* 35–41.

Kuschinsky, W. and Wahl, M. (1978) Local chemical and neurogenic regulation of cerebral vascular resistance. *Physiol. Rev., 58:* 656–688.

Lefauconnier, J.M. and Hauw, J.J. (1984) La barrière hémato-encéphalique. *Rev. Neurol. (Paris), 140:* 3–13; 89–109.

Masuzawa, T. and Sato, F. (1983) The enzyme histochemistry of the choroid plexus. *Brain, 106:* 55–99.

Meisenberg, G. and Simmons, W.H. (1983) Peptides and the blood–brain barrier. *Life Sciences, 32:* 2611–2623.

Oldendorf, W.H. (1982) Some clinical aspects of the blood–brain barrier. *Hospital Practice*, February 1982, pp. 143–164.

Pollay, M. (1984) Research into human hydrocephalus: a review. In *Hydrocephalus* (Shapiro, K., Marmarou, A. and Portnoy, H., eds.), pp. 301–314. New York: Raven Press.

Porliskock, J.T. and Levine, J.E. (1984) Cerebrospinal fluid absorption. In *Cerebral Venous System and its Disorders* (Kapp, J.P. and Schmidek, H.H., eds.), pp. 251–274. New York: Grune & Stratton.

Raichle, M.E. (1983) Neurogenic control of blood–brain barrier permeability. *Acta Neuropathol. [Suppl.] (Berl.), 7:* 75–79.

Weindl, A. (1983) The blood–brain barrier and its role in the control of circulating hormone effects on the brain. In *Central Cardiovascular Control* (Ganten, D. and Pfaff, D., eds.), pp. 151–186. Berlin: Springer-Verlag.

25

Hemispheric Asymmetries

There is abundant evidence that the left and right hemispheres often have distinct modes of processing sensory information. Clinically the most important difference resides in the left hemisphere dominance for speech in 95% of males and 80% of females. Because of this faculty, the left is termed the dominant hemisphere, and the right the minor hemisphere. It is now apparent that the right hemisphere has information-processing capabilities quite different from those of the left, but perhaps equally important. These often subtle differences are grouped under the heading of *cognitive style*.

Some general information about cognitive style is presented first (for details see textbooks of psychology). Control of speech and related matters will be considered later.

TESTS OF COGNITIVE STYLE

Hemispheric dominance for particular information-processing functions has been investigated by presenting information to both hemispheres simultaneously. Three methods have been used:
1 Dichotic listening: two different sounds are presented to the left and right ears through a headset.
2 Dichhaptic touch: two different objects are palpated simultaneously.
3 Tachistoscopic vision: two different images are flashed in the left and right visual fields.

Results show that the left hemisphere is superior in processing information that is suceptible to *sequential analysis* (in other words, where one detail can be dealt with after another). Latent in this finding is the inference that such information is susceptible to *verbal* analysis; that is, it can be described in words. The right hemisphere is *holistic*, having the ability to perceive spatial relationships. This ability is particularly evident in the analysis of shapes that cannot be described in words. The right hemisphere is also more aware of the emotional content of visual images.

An example of the distinction is provided by *facial recognition* tests. Presentation of photographs for 0.1 milliseconds in the right or left visual hemifield demonstrates that the left hemisphere is superior for processing differences that can be verbalized (such as the presence of a moustache), whereas the right hemisphere is superior for subtle differences in facial contours.

The right hemisphere's superiority for spatial relationships appears to be a function of the *superior parietal lobule*, which lies between the sensory association cortex (area 5) and the visual association cortex,

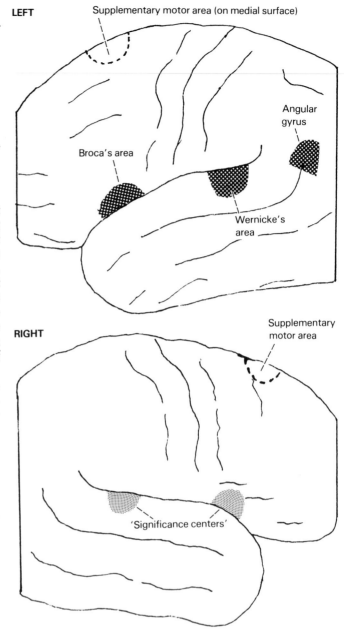

Fig. 25-1 Speech centers. The 'significance centers' are concerned with the meaning of what is expressed or heard.

and integrates information from both. *Contralateral sensory neglect* is usually more pronounced in lesions of the right superior parietal lobule than in lesions of the left one. After a lesion of the right superior parietal lobule the patient may pay no attention to the left visual field and may deny that his left limbs are his own (he may even report 'a stranger in bed with him').

Dichotic listening tests show that the right hemisphere attends to music of all kinds, including song, whereas the left is superior for word sounds (strictly, it is superior for consonants: vowels are 'musical').

The right hemisphere's emotional function is expressed during spontaneous smiling. Smiling may originate in the limbic system in response to appropriate sensory inputs, but it is evidently mediated by the basal ganglia en route to the facial nerve (Chapter 20). A spontaneous smile is usually observed first (or only) on the left side of the face.

THE SPEECH CENTERS (Fig. 25-1)

Although left hemisphere dominance for speech is universally known, it has become apparent that the right hemisphere is significant in appreciating the emotional tone of spoken words, and in imparting appropriate tone and emphases to verbal replies.

Five brain areas are functionally concerned with speech: Broca's area, Wernicke's area, the angular and supramarginal gyri, and the supplementary motor area. 'Siding' of the speech centers can be determined by the Wada test during carotid angiography: amobarbital sodium (amylobarbitone sodium) is injected into each internal carotid artery during the perfusion while the patient counts aloud. The amytal briefly interrupts speech on the dominant side. Positron emission tomography (PET) is a noninvasive method which is equally reliable: it detects the greater increase in blood flow in the dominant speech areas.

Broca's area

Broca's area (44) is the *motor speech center*. It occupies the left inferior frontal gyrus directly in front of the area of motor cortex controlling the brain stem nuclei serving speech. A lesion confined to Broca's area results in *expressive aphasia*: the patient knows what he wants to say but has great difficulty in saying it. Speech is slow and labored, and characteristically 'telegraphic' in style: important nouns and verbs are spoken (often incompletely) but prepositions and conjunctions are omitted. Broca's area receives auditory word information from Wernicke's area, and it projects to the motor cortex.

Wernicke's area

Wernicke's area (posterior part of area 22) is the *sensory speech center*. Lesions here produce severe disturbances of speech content. Fluency is quite normal, but three kinds of abnormality occur in the use of nouns:
1   Circumlocution. Instead of 'I use a knife', 'I use the thing you cut with'.
2   Verbal paraphrasia (the use of words of allied meaning). Instead of 'I cut with a knife', 'I cut with a fork'.
3   Phonemic paraphrasia (the use of made-up words having appropriate sounds. Instead of 'knife and fork', 'bife and dork'.

Table 25-1 Comparison of Broca's and Wernicke's aphasia

	Aphasia	
	Broca's	*Wernicke's*
Articulation	Slurred	Normal
Speed	Halting	Rapid
Comprehension	Good	Poor
Awareness	Yes	No

The patient is unaware of his errors (Table 25-1). Wernicke's area receives inputs from the auditory association area (area 21 and remainder of area 22) and from the angular gyrus. It projects to Broca's area via the arcuate fasciculus, and to the premotor cortex.

Angular gyrus

The *left angular gyrus* is the *visual–auditory conversion area*. It is area 39, which caps the superior temporal

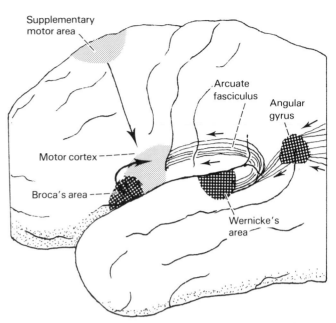

Fig. 25-2   The left angular gyrus receives from the visual association cortex and projects to Wernicke's area. Wernicke's area projects to Broca's area. Broca's area projects to the face area of the motor cortex. The supplementary motor area is also thought to project to the face area.

sulcus. It receives from the visual association cortex on its own side and from its partner opposite through the corpus callosum. It projects to Wernicke's area (Fig. 25-2).

The left angular gyrus is essential for the conversion of the written word to its auditory equivalent (from graphemes to phonemes). A lesion here causes written words to become meaningless hieroglyphics (*alexia*). This is because we need to 'hear' the written word while reading. Most dyslexic people have an impairment of function within the angular gyrus. Significant improvement in reading ability can be achieved by simultaneous presentation of word sounds during reading (in effect, bypassing the angular gyrus).

Reading aloud

The anatomic pathway for reading aloud is as follows (commissural connections between the two angular gyri have been omitted) (Fig. 25-3).
1   Retinogeniculate tracts.
2   Geniculocalcarine tracts.
3   Transfer to visual association cortex.
4   Transfer from right to left hemisphere via splenium of corpus callosum.
5   Composite visual picture passed to angular gyrus for auditory transformation.
6   Transfer from angular gyrus to Wernicke's area, for comprehension.
7   Transfer to Broca's area via arcuate fasciculus.
8   Transfer to motor cortex.

See also Fig. 25-4.

Angular gyrus syndrome

A lesion (usually vascular) involving the angular gyrus on the dominant side is typically accompanied by

179

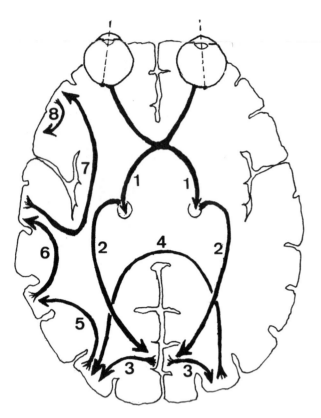

Fig. 25-3 Minimal pathway for reading aloud. For identification of numbers see text.

alexia together with Gerstmann's syndrome: agraphia (inability to write), acalculia (inability to do simple sums), difficulty in distinguishing right from left, and 'finger agnosia' (inability to tell how many of the examiner's fingers are held up for inspection (a variant of acalculia).) Patients with angular gyrus syndrome may be thought to have Alzheimer's disease – a relatively common degenerative disease of the cerebral cortex.

Supramarginal gyrus (Fig. 25-5)

The supramarginal gyrus surrounds the upturned posterior end of the lateral sulcus. Lesions here which include the *underlying white matter* may result in conductive aphasia and facial apraxia.

Conductive aphasia

The term derives from interrupted conduction in the arcuate fasciculus, deep to the gyrus (Fig. 25-2). The symptoms are those of Wernicke's aphasia, with the additional inability to repeat even the simplest phrases spoken by the examiner.

Facial apraxia

Apraxia denotes the inability to perform a given movement on request, in the presence of otherwise normal cerebration and motor power. Facial apraxia is attributed to interruption of long association fibers passing from the visual and auditory association areas to the premotor cortex, for relay to the lower end of area 4. If the visual connections alone are lost, the

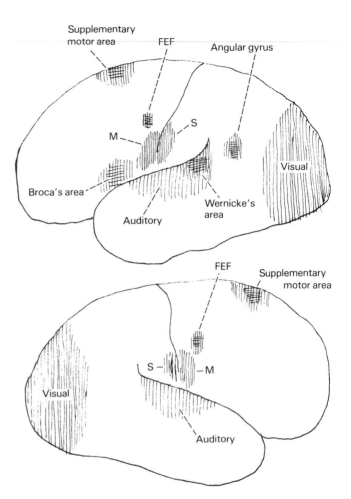

Fig. 25-4 Areas of increased cortical blood flow during reading aloud. FEF, frontal eye field; M, motor cortex for lips, tongue, jaw, and larynx; S, sensory cortex receiving from lips, tongue, jaw, and larynx.

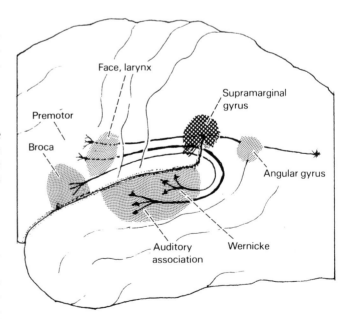

Fig. 25-5 Three sets of long association fibers underlie the supramarginal gyrus.

patient cannot mimic facial movements carried out by the examiner (pursing the lips, squeezing the eyes shut, and so on), but he can respond to a spoken request for such movements. If the auditory connections are also lost, the spoken request is ineffective. Upper limb apraxia may be added if the lesion is more extensive.

Facial apraxia also occurs in association with Broca's aphasia in the presence of anterior lesions large enough to affect the premotor cortex.

Facial apraxia is bilateral, indicating that the contralateral hemisphere is normally activated through the corpus callosum.

The significance of the *cortex* of the supramarginal gyrus is unknown. It is likely to be significant since it is comparable with the angular gyrus in its degree of enlargement in the human brain. Both are rudimentary in apes (which have minimal speech) and in monkeys (which have none). Together they constitute the *inferior parietal lobule.*

Supplementary motor area

Although the SMA shows bilateral increase in blood flow during speech, its contribution to the speech function is enigmatic. It may be involved in integrating pyramidal tract output from the face area of the motor cortex on the two sides: the two SMAs are cross-connected through the corpus callosum (see Chapter 20).

Notes

Broca's and Wernicke's areas are larger on the left side in 70–80% of brains. This asymmetry is already present before birth, suggesting very early hemispheric specialization for language. However, language function can be taken over by the contralateral hemisphere following brain injury in early childhood. Interhemispheric transfer ability is lost after the age of six.

Electrical stimulation of the exposed cortex in conscious subjects arrests ongoing language tests. It has shown that language functions are not restricted to Broca's and Wernicke's areas, but extend along the whole length of the cortex bordering the lateral sulcus, except for the foot of the sensorimotor cortex.

Speech centers in sinistrals

The 3% of people having the speech centers in the right hemisphere are made up of sinistrals (left-handers) and ambidextrals. Sinistrals constitute 9% of the population, and their speech centers are on the left side in 6% or 7% of the 9%. However, sinistrals recover better than dextrals from aphasia, regardless of the side of the aphasia-producing lesion in the particular case. Dextrals having a sinistral in their immediate family (parent, sibling or offspring) also recover better. We may infer that some degree of bilateral speech control exists in sinistrals.

The right hemisphere contribution

Although the left hemisphere is dominant in the majority, the right hemisphere does make a significant contribution. At the physical level, there is some increase in blood flow during speech, in areas matching those of the left side. Speech may also be interrupted by electrical stimulation of the exposed right cortex, in several areas bordering the Sylvian fissure.

Lesions of the right hemisphere are now believed to affect speech just as often as lesions of the left hemisphere. However, right hemisphere disturbance is much more subtle. On the motor side, there is loss of the inflections and emphases which are part of normal speech: the patient speaks in a dull monotone, and risks being treated for depression for this reason. On the sensory side, the patient is unable to say, for example, whether the clinician is speaking in an angry or soothing tone. This failure includes inability to distinguish happy from sad facial expressions. To detect this, the clinician has to act out various facial expressions and ask the patient (his reading ability is unaffected) to select the mime from a written list of facial demeanors.

Right hemisphere speech impairments are known as *aprosōdias.*

Absence of complementarity

Statistically, the left hemisphere is usually dominant for linguistic functions, and the right hemisphere for spatial functions. However, for an individual we cannot assume that attribution of linguistic ability to one hemisphere implies attribution of spatial ability to the other hemisphere. For example, about 20% of males having left-hemisphere dominance for speech have left-hemisphere dominance for spatial tasks as well. For females, the figure rises to about 30%.

Blood supply (Fig. 25-6)

The middle cerebral artery supplies all of the cortical areas involved in speech. The great majority of aphasias are caused by thrombosis within the territory of the left MCA. Main artery thrombosis in the stem of the lateral sulcus gives rise to *global aphasia* (a combination of Broca's and Wernicke's) together with left-sided apraxia.

Accurate diagnosis of aphasias and apraxias requires considerable clinical experience. Altered consciousness, confusion, and cognitive (thinking) disorders may give misleading information.

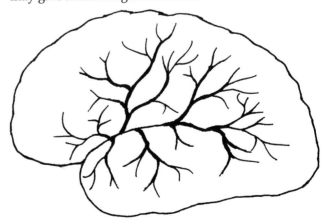

Fig. 25-6 Cortical branches of the middle cerebral artery.

181

CORPUS CALLOSUM

The corpus callosum interconnects matching areas of the two cerebral hemispheres. It contains 300 million fibers and is by far the largest fiber tract in the brain.

Callosal axons arise from pyramidal neurons in laminae II, III, V, and VI. They terminate in all laminae but mainly in the matching ones. Groups of callosal fibers tend to alternate with thalamocortical fibers in most parts of the cortex.

In the *primary* sensory areas (visual, auditory, and somesthetic) callosal interconnections are restricted to the respective representations of the midline region. In area 17, the interconnections have an obvious function in cortical activity from the *vertical meridian* of the binocular visual field. When any object is fixated, its cortical representation is split into two halves. For example, when the eyes see the word 'cortex', 'cor' is inverted and reversed onto the macular part of area 17 on the right, and 'tex' is similarly represented on the left. The two halves of the word are 'brought together' by callosal fibers. Cortical neurons in the vertical meridian are all binocular because of callosal interconnections.

In the somesthetic cortex, callosal interconnections are restricted to the trunk and head regions. They serve to integrate sensations received from the anterior and posterior midline.

In the auditory cortex, the corpus callosum converts monaural neurons into binaural neurons in the cortex receiving from the anterior and posterior midline regions of the left and right auditory fields.

Secondary sensory areas (visual, somesthetic, and auditory association areas) are very freely interconnected by callosal fibers. A composite copy of sensory information is sent to the contralateral association area, and is sent to the entorhinal cortex for processing into memory. It is a matter of ordinary experience that learned motor tasks based on sensory experience on the right side can be carried out later on the left side. However, if the corpus callosum has been sectioned the left side must be trained independently.

Callosal interruption (Fig. 25-7)

The splenium of the corpus callosum is supplied by the posterior cerebral artery, the remainder by the anterior cerebral.

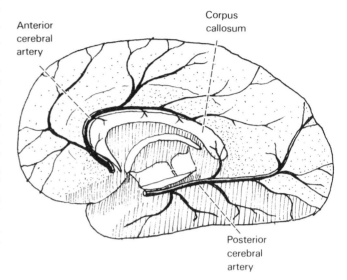

Fig. 25-7 Arterial supply of corpus callosum.

If the artery to the *splenium* undergoes thrombosis (rare), interhemispheric transfer from the right visual association cortex to the left becomes impossible. Such a patient would have no difficulty in reading material in the right half of the visual field, but material in the left half would be meaningless.

If the *trunk* of the corpus callosum is interrupted, familiar objects held in the left hand (with eyes closed) cannot be named, although the patient can indicate by gestures that he has identified them. The condition, called 'tactile aphasia', is the result of interrupted transfer of composite tactile information from the right superior parietal lobule to the left; the left is linked to Broca's area.

Readings

Benson, D.F., Cummings, J.L. and Tsai, S.Y. (1982) Angular gyrus syndrome simulating Alzheimer's disease. *Arch. Neurol., 39:* 616–620.

Berlucchi, G. (1981) Recent advances in the analysis of the neural substrates of interhemispheric communication. In *Brain Mechanisms and Perceptual Awareness* (Pompeiano, O. and Marsan, C.A., eds.), pp. 133–152. New York: Raven Press.

Bhatnager, S. and Andy, O.J. (1981) Language in the non-dominant right hemisphere. *Arch. Neurol., 40:* 728–731.

Bryden, M.P., Hécaen, H. and DeAgostini, M. (1983) Patterns of cerebral organization. *Brain and Language, 20:* 249–262.

Damasio, A.R. and Geschwind, N. (1984) The neural basis of language. *Annu. Rev. Neurosci., 7:* 127–147.

Gazzaniga, M.S. and Smylie, C.S. (1983) Facial recognition and brain asymmetries: clues to underlying mechanisms. *Ann. Neurol., 13:* 536–540.

Geschwind, N. (1966) Disconnection syndromes in animals and man. *Brain, 88:* 237–294.

Geschwind, N. (1972) Language and the brain. *Sci. Am., 226:* 76–83.

Geschwind, N. (1974) The anatomical basis of hemispheric differentiation. In *Hemisphere Functions in the Human Brain* (Dimond, S.G. and Baumont, J.G., eds.), pp. 7–24. New York: Wiley.

Joanette, Y., Lecours, A.R., Lepage, Y. and Lamoureux, M. (1982) Language in right-handers with right-hemisphere lesions: a preliminary study including anatomical, genetic, and social factors. *Brain and Language, 20:* 217–248.

Lynn, R.B., Buchanan, D.C., Fenichel, G.M. and Freemon, F.R. (1980) Agenesis of the corpus callosum. *Arch. Neurol., 37:* 444–445.

Lyons, J. (1981) Language and speech. *Philos. Trans. R. Soc. Lond. B, 295:* 215–222.

Marlsen-Wilson, W.D. and Tyler, L.K. (1981) Central processes in speech understanding. *Philos. Trans. R. Soc. Lond. B, 295:* 317–332.

McGlone, J. (1984) Speech comprehension after unilateral injection of sodium amytal. *Brain and Language, 22:* 150–157.

Naeser, M.A. (1982) Language behavior in stroke patients. Cortical v. subcortical lesion sites in CT scans. *Trends Neurosci., 5:* 53–59.

Phillips, C.G., Zeki, S. and Barlow, H.B. (1984) Localization of function in the cerebral cortex. *Brain, 107:* 327–361.

Ross, E.D. (1981) The aprosodias: functional–anatomic organization of the affective components of language in the right hemisphere. *Arch. Neurol., 38:* 561–569.

Ross, E.D., Harney, J.H., de Lacoste-Utamsing, C. and Purdy, P.D. (1981) How the brain integrates affective and propositional language into a unified behavioral function. *Arch. Neurol., 38:* 745–748.

Weintraub, S., Mesulam, M.-M. and Kramer, L. (1981) Disturbances in prosody. *Arch. Neurol., 38:* 742–744.

Willanger, R., Danielsen, V.T. and Ankerhus, J. (1981) Visual neglect in right-sided apoplectic lesions. *Acta Neurol. Scand., 64:* 327–336.

26
Plasticity and Recovery of Function

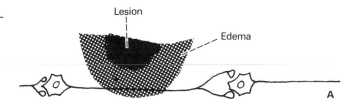

Fig. 26-1 Recovery of synaptic effectiveness. A, edema blocking conduction. B, conduction resumes when edema subsides.

In view of the general inability of the CNS to regenerate, the recuperative power of the brain is remarkable. Provided the patient survives the initial insult to the brain, significant functional recovery is often observed.

NEURAL SHOCK

Severe injuries to the CNS are followed by widespread inhibition of function which may last for several days. This is the state known as 'neural shock'. Its mechanism is uncertain, but it seems to be initiated by neurons in the area of the lesion. In animals, a lesion of the cerebral cortex is followed by depressed neuronal function in the matching part of the contralateral hemisphere as well – but not if the corpus callosum has been cut. Some of the effects may be produced by extensive vasoconstriction around the site of injury, others by hypothalamic responses to stress.

Only when neural shock wears off can a baseline be drawn for the assessment of functional recovery from a lesion.

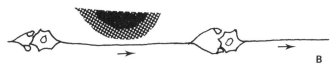

Fig. 26-2 Synaptic hypereffectiveness. A, transmitter passes from cell body to all terminals. B, reduction of axonal territory may cause transmitter to accumulate in the surviving boutons.

SPECIFIC RECOVERY MECHANISMS

Many different mechanisms have been shown to account for functional improvement in the weeks following vascular or traumatic injury to the nervous system:
1 Recovery of synaptic effectiveness
2 Synaptic hypereffectiveness
3 Denervation supersensitivity
4 Persistence of hyperinnervation
5 Recruitment of silent synapses
6 Sprouting–regenerative and collateral
7 Vicarious function
8 Behavioral substitution

In most situations more than one mechanism is likely to be involved.

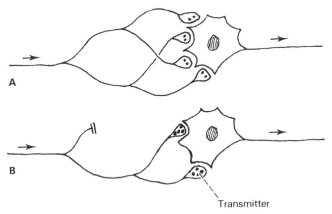

Fig. 26-3 Denervation supersensitivity. A, target cell innervated by two axons. B, depleted innervation results in supersensitivity to reduced supply of neurotransmitters.

Recovery of synaptic effectiveness (Fig. 26-1)

Following a vascular accident or brain surgery, many synapses are ineffective merely because parent fibers close to the lesion are compressed by edema. Considerable recovery of motor, sensory, and cognitive function takes place within one to two weeks as the edema subsides.

Example. Temporary homonymous hemianopsia following hemorrhage into the internal capsule (Chapter 29).

Synaptic hypereffectiveness (Fig. 26-2)

If some branches of a neuron are severed, all of the transmitter substance synthesized in the perikaryon travels to the intact nerve endings, and provides them with an extra load.

Example from the peripheral nervous system. In partially denervated skeletal muscle, the surviving motor end plates show a pronounced increase in acetylcholine, giving increased synaptic effectiveness.

Denervation supersensitivity (Fig. 26-3)

Removal of synaptic boutons is followed by the appearance of additional specific receptors in the

184

postsynaptic membrane. The new receptors respond to transmitter released by neighboring boutons.

Example. The supersensitivity of striatal neurons to dopamine, following loss of nigrostriatal neurons in Parkinson's disease (Chapter 18).

Persistence of hyperinnervation (Fig. 26-4)

In all mammals, the young nervous system contains a superabundance of neurons. The most effective and appropriate neurons survive and the remainer die off. However, interference with normal competitive interaction may cause neurons that would normally die off to persist and become functional.

Example. In monkeys, the left-eye, right-eye ocular dominance columns are segregated by the end of the sixth postnatal week. Prior to this there is overlap of geniculocalcarine inputs from the two eyes into each dominance column. If one eye is closed before the end of the third week the dominance columns from the normal eye become twice as wide by six weeks, and those from the inactive eye become only half as wide. The effect is not due to the growth of new fibers, but to the persistence of fibers which would otherwise die off.

This observation provides a rationale for the treatment of *amblyopia* in children. In amblyopia one eye dominates the other at an early age (one to two years). A mild squint is often responsible, the image from the misdirected eye being suppressed. The usual treatment is to cover the dominant eye in order to promote full development of dominance columns from the other eye. The dominant eye should be uncovered at intervals to ensure balanced development of the columns.

Recruitment of silent synapses (Fig. 26-5)

Many parts of the nervous system are supplied with synapses which appear to be inactive under physiological conditions. These 'silent synapses' are unmasked by removal of normally functioning inputs.

Examples from the pyramidal tract

a In Chapter 20 it was noted that 10% of pyramidal tract fibers enter the lateral corticospinal tract on the same side (that is, without entering the pyramidal decussation). These are very fine fibers and they evidently terminate in the anterior gray horn on both sides of the cord. They seem to be inactive unless the crossed CST is injured. If the lateral CST is severed on one side during a cordotomy operation for intractable pain, the patient has a severe motor weakness in the leg on that side but recovers almost completely within two weeks. If a second, equally extensive cordotomy is then carried out on the other side, *both* legs become permanently paralyzed. Evidently the fibers crossing lower down become functional in the interval between the two operations but are severed on the second occasion (Fig. 26-5).

b Completely uncrossed lateral corticospinal tract

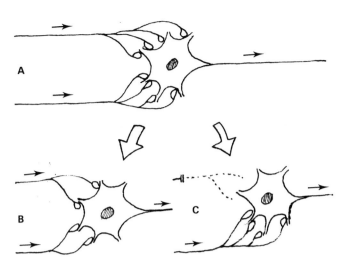

Fig. 26-4 Persistent hyperinnervation. A, usual arrangement in perinatal period. B, normal adult neuron, with reduced innervation. C, partial denervation in childhood may allow additional boutons to persist through lack of competition for space on target neurons.

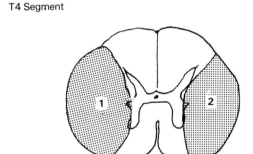

T4 Segment

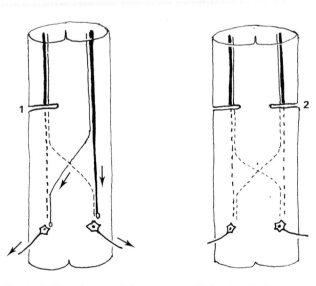

Fig. 26-5 Recruitment of silent synapses. Following the first cordotomy (1), function is restored by corticospinal fibers crossing lower down. The second cordotomy (2) causes complete paralysis because all the fibers crossing lower down have been cut.

fibers may be responsible for recovery of voluntary movement following pyramidal tract injury. Virtually an entire cerebral hemisphere is occasionally removed in adults because of an advanced glioma. These patients show a similar pattern of recovery to that after stroke: early return of flexion and adduction of the arm, and of extension and adduction of the thigh, but poor recovery of the hand.

c   The spoken command, 'make a fist with your left hand' is interpreted in Wernicke's area, forwarded to the left premotor cortex, transferred to the right premotor cortex and from here to the motor cortex (Fig. 26-6). If the corpus callosum has been cut, the patient can nevertheless make a left fist on command (uncrossed pyramidal tract fibers may be responsible), but he cannot perform fine movements. Fine movements of the left hand are carried out normally if the patient merely *sees* the movements being performed by the examiner; the signals are carried from left visual field to right visual cortex without traversing the corpus callosum.

d   In monkeys, destruction of the entire 'hand' area of the motor cortex makes the contralateral hand almost useless for manipulating test objects. However, normal skill is largely regained after a few weeks. If the motor cortex is again exposed, the cortex adjacent to the lesioned area now produces hand movements when stimulated. Destruction of the new area of 'hand' cortex causes a severe and permanent paralysis of the hand.

Sprouting

Sprouting is the new growth of axonal branches following injury. Two types of sprouting may occur: regenerative, and collateral.

Regenerative sprouting (Fig. 26-7)

In this case axons have been severed along with their target neurons. The *injured* axons may respond by issuing short (100 µm or less) side sprouts which form new synapses on other neurons in the area.

Example.   When the spinal cord is transected, the corticospinal and other tracts fail to bridge the gap, but they form numerous fresh synapses on neurons proximal to it.

Collateral sprouting (Fig. 26-8)

Neurons that have been denervated attract side sprouts from nearby, *uninjured* axons. In the CNS this is called *reactive synaptogenesis*.

Examples from the cerebellum.   (a) The dendritic trees of Purkinje cells receive climbing fibers from the inferior olivary nucleus. If the olive is partly destroyed, many of the degenerated climbing fiber synapses are replaced by collateral sprouts from uninjured climbing fibers nearby.

(b) Parallel fibers also synapse on Purkinje dendrites, and they too can be replaced by sprouts from other parallel fibers, following a lesion of the granule

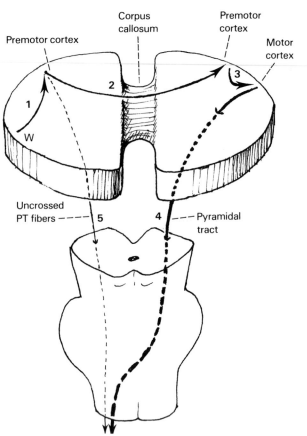

Fig. 26-6   1–4, normal pathway for left-sided response to a spoken command. 5, ipsilateral PT fibers appear to be active if either 2 or 4 is interrupted. W, Wernicke's area.

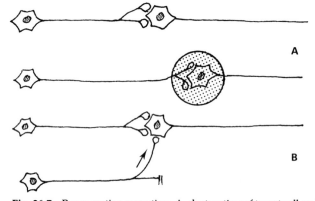

Fig. 26-7   Regenerative sprouting. A, destruction of target cell and afferent terminals. B, sprouting (arrow) of the injured axon into a different target cell.

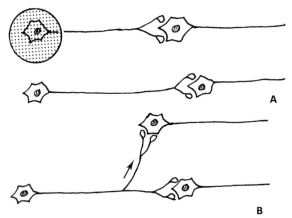

Figure 26-8   Collateral sprouting. A, lesion causes depletion of afferents to one target cell. B, uninjured neuron sprouts (arrow) to supply the deafferented cell.

cell layer. However, parallel fibers will not replace climbing fiber synapses, or vice versa.

Examples from the peripheral nervous system. In the PNS, collateral sprouting occurs following partial denervation of muscle or skin. The sprouts enter vacated Schwann sheaths, follow them, and form functional nerve endings.

Combinations of recruitment of silent synapses and sprouting

Under experimental conditions it can be shown that activity of previously ineffective synapses (immediate effect) can be followed by reactive synaptogenesis (late effect) in the same pathway.

Examples from the dorsal column–lemniscal pathway

a Under physiological conditions the nucleus gracilis responds to stimulation of the hind limb and nucleus cuneatus to stimulation of the trunk and forelimb. In cats, if the fasciculus gracilis is inactivated by cooling it, some cells in the nucleus gracilis respond for the first time to stimulation of the trunk. The response occurs within a few minutes and cannot be caused by collateral sprouting; moreover, it disappears when the fasciculus gracilis warms up. On the other hand, if fasciculus gracilis is destroyed collateral sprouting occurs slowly and gives a permanent trunk representation in the nucleus.
b The same immediate and late effects are observed in the ventroposterior nucleus of thalamus, and in the somesthetic cortex, following interruption of the posterior columns.
c In monkeys, the areas serving each digit can be mapped on the somesthetic cortex by taking cortical records while the digits are being stimulated. If the median nerve is cut, the cortical areas serving the lateral three digits (supplied by the median) fall silent for a few hours, then respond to stimulation of the medial two digits for the first time. This initial response seems to result from activation of silent synapses. If the median is not allowed to regenerate, the thalamocortical fibers serving the medial two digits extend their territory into the area previously receiving from the lateral digits.

Vicarious function

Theoretically, if one pathway were put out of action, its function could be served (vicariously) by another. This concept has been invoked to account for recovery of function in the limbs following injury to central motor or sensory pathways.

That any pathway can assume an additional function de novo is doubtful. In the sensory pathways, *parallel processing* of information is the rule. Thus, the posterior columns have a major function in conscious proprioception and the spinothalamic tract has a minor one. The spinocerebellar tracts have a major function in unconscious proprioception and the posterior columns have a minor one (via relays from the gracile and cuneate nuclei to the cerebellum). In the motor

system, the corticospinal tract has a major role in initiating voluntary movements, particularly those of a skilled nature; the corticoreticulospinal pathways have a role in the more automatic and unskilled voluntary movements. Interruption of a major sensory or motor pathway may permit a minor one to be used to the full rather than endowing it with novel functions.

Behavioral substitution

Special stratagems may be used to bypass a neurological deficit. A patient with homonymous hemianopsia can read normally by merely turning the head so that the intact half-field spans the page. Various tricks are devised by patients to circumvent muscle paralysis: for example, when the deltoid is paralyzed, they can abduct the arm by rotating the scapula.

ADAPTIVE AND NON-ADAPTIVE RESPONSES

Anatomical and/or functional responses to injury are called *adaptive* if they are beneficial. The great majority of responses are adaptive to some degree. The term 'plastic' has the same connotation; thus, the CNS is said to show remarkable 'plasticity' in response to injury.

Changes that are not beneficial are called *non-adaptive.*

Examples of non-adaptive responses

1 When the spinal cord is injured, the fibers of severed descending pathways form fresh synapses in the gray matter immediately above the lesion. They are functionally inert, and may even deter such fibers from continued regenerative activity.
2 When the spinal cord is transected, primary afferent fibers below the lesion extend their territory by taking up synaptic sites vacated by severed descending tracts. They acquire exaggerated central effects, often producing severe flexor reflex spasms in the lower limbs in response to stimulation of the skin, for instance when pulling on a pair of trousers.
3 In the PNS, skin grafts may sweat excessively, even in cool conditions. The sweating reflects inadequate reinnervation of sweat glands by sympathetic fibers. The glands are showing denervation supersensitivity, responding to minute amounts of circulating acetylcholine. (Sympathetic fibers to sweat glands are cholinergic; see Chapter 6.)

Readings

Bach-y-Rita, P. (1983) Rehabilitation versus passive recovery of motor control following central nervous system lesions. In *Motor Control Mechanisms in Health and Disease* (Desmedt, J.E., ed.), pp. 1085–1092. New York: Raven Press.
Björklund, A. and Steveni, U. (1971) Growth of central catecholamine neurons with smooth muscle grafts in the rat mesencephalon. *Brain Res.*, 31: 1–20.
Braddick, O.J. and Atkinson, J. (1983) Some recent findings on the development of human binocularity: a review. *Behav. Brain Res.*, 10: 141–150.

Brown, M.C. (1984) Sprouting of motor nerves in adult muscle: a recapitulation of ontogeny. *Trends Neurosci., 7:* 10–14.

Brown, M.C. and Ironton, R. (1977) Motor neurone sprouting induced by prolonged tetrodotoxin block of nerve action potentials. *Nature, 265:* 459–461.

Chen, S. and Hillman, D.E. (1982) Plasticity of the parallel-fiber–Purkinje cell synapse by spine takeover and new synapse formation in the adult rat. *Brain Res., 240:* 205–222.

Cotman, C.W., Matthews, D.A., Taylor, D. and Lynch, G.S. (1973) Synaptic rearrangement in the dentate gyrus: histochemical evidence of adjustments after lesions in immature and adult rats. *Proc. Natl Acad. Sci. USA, 70:* 3473–3477.

Cotman, C.W., Nieto-Sampedro, M. and Harris, E.W. (1981) Synapse replacement in the nervous system of adult vertebrates. *Physiol. Rev., 61:* 684–784.

Edds, M.V. (1953) Collateral nerve regeneration. *Or. Rev. Biol., 28:* 260–276.

Finger, S. and Stein, D.G. (1982) Behavioral recovery and development. In *Brain Damage and Recovery*, by Finger and Stein, pp. 135–152. New York: Academic Press.

FitzGerald, M.J.T., Martin, F. and Paletta, F.X. (1967) Innervation of skin grafts. *Surg. Gynecol. Obstet., 124:* 808–812.

Goldberger, M.E. and Murray, M. (1974) Restitution of function and collateral sprouting in the cat spinal cord: the deafferented animal. *J. Comp. Neurol., 158:* 37–54.

Goldman-Rakic, P.S. (1981) Development and plasticity of primate frontal association cortex. In *The Organization of the Cerebral Cortex* (Schmidt, F.O., Worden, F.G., Adelman, G. and Dennis, S.G., eds.), pp. 69–97. Oxford: Oxford University Press.

Hopkins, W.G., Brown, M.C. and Keyens, R.J. (1981) Nerve growth from nodes of Ranvier in inactive muscle. *Brain Res., 222:* 125–128.

Illis, L.S., Sedgwick, E.M. and Glanville, H.J. (1982) Plasticity in the adult nervous system. In *Rehabilitation of the Neurological Patient* (by Illis, L.S., Sedgwick, E.M. and Glanville, H.J.), pp. 44–77. Oxford: Blackwell Scientific.

LeVay, S., Wiesel, T.N. and Hubel, D.H. (1980) The development of ocular dominance columns in normal and visually deprived monkeys. *J. Comp. Neurol., 191:* 1–51.

Le Vere, T.E. (1980) Recovery after brain damage: a theory of the behavioral deficit. *Physiol. Psychol., 8:* 297–308.

McMahon, S.B. and Wall, P.D. (1983) Plasticity in the nucleus gracilis of the rat. *Exp. Neurol., 80:* 195–207.

Merrill, E.G. and Wall, P.D. (1978) Plasticity of connection in the adult nervous system. In *Neuronal Plasticity* (Cotman, C.W., ed.), pp. 97–112. New York: Raven Press.

Nathan, P.W. and Smith, M.C. (1973) Effects of two unilateral cordotomies on the motility of the lower limb. *Brain, 96:* 471–494.

Pockett, S. and Slack, J.R. (1982) Pruning of axonal trees results in increased efficacy of surviving nerve terminals. *Brain Res., 243:* 350–353.

Prendergast, J., Murray, M. and Goldberger, M.E. (1981) Sprouting and reflex recovery after spinal nerve lesions in cats. *Exp. Neurol., 73:* 732–749.

Purves, D. and Njå, A. (1978) Trophic maintenance of synaptic connections in autonomic ganglia. In *Neuronal Plasticity* (Gotman, C.W., ed.), pp. 27–48. New York: Raven Press.

Raisman, G. (1969) Neuronal plasticity in the septal nuclei of the adult brain. *Brain Res., 14:* 25–48.

Reis, D.J., Ross, R.A., Gilad, G. and Joh, T.H. (1978) Reaction of central catecholaminergic neurons to injury: model system for studying the neurobiology of central regeneration and sprouting. In *Neuronal Plasticity* (Gotman, C.W., ed.), pp. 197–276. New York: Raven Press.

Sherman, S.M. and Spear, P.D. (1982) Organization of visual pathways in normal and visually deprived cats. *Physiol. Rev., 62:* 738–855.

Swindale, N.V. (1982) The development of columnar systems in the mammalian visual cortex. *Trends Neurosci., 6:* 235–241.

Tieman, S.B. and Hirsch, H.V.B. (1982) Exposure to lines of only one orientation modifies dendritic morphology of cells in the visual cortex of the cat. *J. Comp. Neurol., 211:* 353–362.

Tsukahara, N. (1980) Synaptic plasticity in the mammalian central nervous system. *Annu. Rev. Neurosci., 4:* 351–379.

Veraa, R.P. and Grafstein, B. (1981) Cellular mechanisms for recovery from nervous system injury: a conference report. *Exp. Neurol., 71:* 6–75.

Weddell, G., Guttmann, L. and Guttmann, E. (1941) The local extension of nerve fibers into denervated areas of skin. *J. Neurol. Psychiat., 4:* 206–225.

VI

SMELL AND TASTE, VISION, AND HEARING

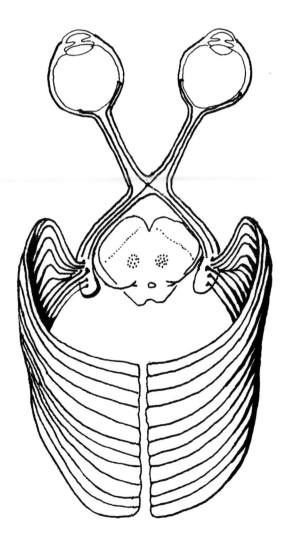

27
Smell and Taste

SMELL

The olfactory system is unique in four respects:
1 The peripheral (primary) olfactory neurons lie at the body surface, in the epithelium lining the roof of the nose.
2 The axons of the primary olfactory neurons enter the allocortex of the olfactory bulb directly. In all other sensory systems second-order neurons intervene between primary afferents and cerebral cortex.
3 The primary olfactory neurons undergo continuous turnover, being replaced from stem cells in the olfactory epithelium. No other neuron in the nervous system is replaced from stem cells.
4 Although the left and right olfactory pathways are cross-connected through the anterior commissure, the pathway to the highest cortical centers (in the orbitofrontal cortex) is ipsilateral. All other sensory pathways have a mainly (auditory) or entirely crossed cortical representation.

Olfactory epithelium (Figs. 27-1, 27-2)

The olfactory epithelium lines the upper one-fifth of the lateral and septal walls of the nasal cavity. This epithelium contains three cell types:

Bipolar olfactory neurons. The dendrite of each neuron reaches the epithelial surface and forms a *dendritic bulb*, from which cilia radiate into the covering film of watery mucus. The axon of each neuron is extremely fine (0.1–0.3 μm). It ascends through the cribriform plate of the ethmoid bone and the meninges, pierces the overlying olfactory bulb, and terminates in an olfactory glomerulus. The bipolar neurons have a limited life span.

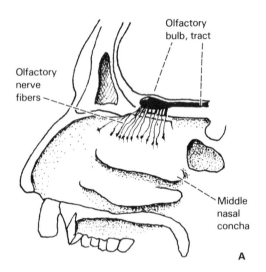

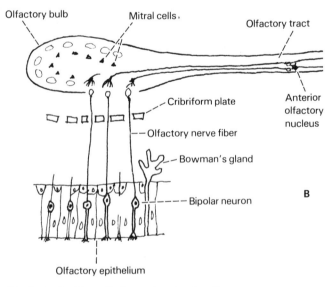

Fig. 27-1 A, side wall of nose showing the olfactory nerve ascending to the olfactory bulb. B, the fibers arise in the olfactory epithelium.

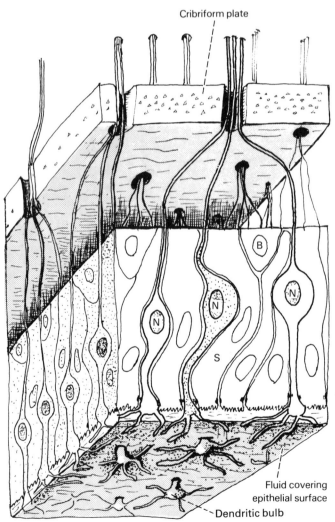

Fig. 27-2 Bipolar neurons (N), supporting cells (S) and basal cells (B) in olfactory epithelium, viewed from below.

Sustentacular (supporting) cells are interposed among the bipolars; their free surfaces bear microvilli.

Basal cells lie between the other two types. Their function is to form fresh bipolar neurons. If the olfactory nerve fibers are severed above the cribriform plate in a monkey the bipolar neurons degenerate and are completely replaced from basal cells within 30 days.

Olfactory bulb (Fig. 27-3)

The olfactory bulb has a shell of three-layered allocortex. The principal cortical neuron is the *mitral cell*, whose dendrites enter several olfactory glomeruli and receive the axons of some 1000 bipolar neurons. Mitral-cell axons form the bulk of the olfactory tract.

Inhibitory neurons

Two types of inhibitory internuncials are found in the olfactory bulb. Both types exert lateral (surround) inhibition on other mitral cells outside the immediate zone of excitation.

1 The (GABAergic) *periglomerular cell* receives excitatory synapses from bipolar neurons. Its axon enters another glomerulus, where it forms inhibitory axodendritic synapses.
2 The (dopaminergic) *granule cell* is remarkable in having no axon. Its processes are spiny dendrites which make dendrodendritic synapses with mitral cells.

The level of activity of both cell types can be raised by centrifugal fibers from the contralateral anterior olfactory nucleus (see later).

Olfactory tract (Fig. 27-4)

Mitral-cell axons proceed centrally along the olfactory tract. Collaterals are given off to the *anterior olfactory nucleus* (AON), which is made up of scattered multipolar neurons within the tract. The AON sends axons through the anterior commissure to excite inhibitory neurons in the contralateral bulb.

The olfactory tract divides into lateral, intermediate, and medial *olfactory striae*. The lateral stria (the

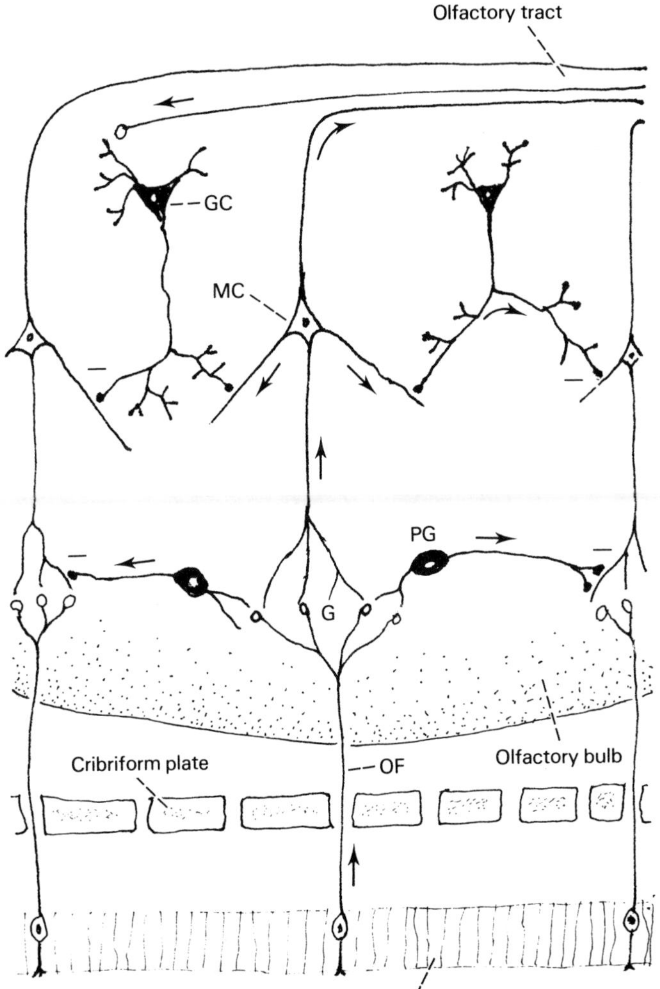

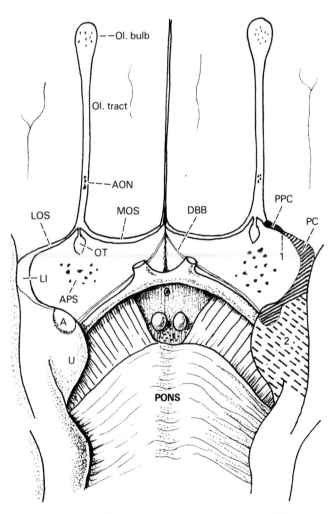

Fig. 27-3 In a glomerulus (G) active olfactory fibers (OF) excite on-line mitral cells (MC) and inhibit off-line mitral cells via periglomerular cells (PG). Off-line mitral cells are also inhibited by granule cells (GC) via dendrodendritic synapses. Granule cells can be activated from central sources.

Fig. 27-4 Central olfactory connections. A, amygdala; AON, anterior olfactory nucleus; APS, anterior perforated substance; DBB, diagonal band of Broca; LI, limen insulae; LOS, lateral olfactory stria; MOS, medial olfactory stria; PC, pyriform cortex; OT, olfactory tubercle; PPC, prepyriform cortex; U, uncus; 1, 2, primary and secondary olfactory cortex.

191

largest) gives collaterals to the *prepyriform cortex* – a thin sleeve of investing allocortex – and terminates in the *pyriform cortex*. The pyriform cortex includes the cortex of the most medial part of the insula (limen insulae) and the cortical amygdala. The amygdalar projection to the anterior hypothalamus accounts for parasympathetic responses (tachycardia and gastric contractions) to unpleasant odors.

The intermediate olfactory stria terminates in the *olfactory tubercle*, an area of allocortex rostral to the anterior perforated substance.

The medial olfactory stria enters the septal area.

Primary, secondary, and tertiary olfactory cortex

The *primary olfactory cortex* comprises the prepyriform and pyriform cortex. The *secondary olfactory cortex* occupies the anterior end of the entorhinal cortex. It includes the uncus. An unusual form of epilepsy (uncinate epilepsy) has its focus in the uncus. Prior to the convulsive seizure, the patient experiences an 'olfactory aura' characterized by an unpleasant sense of smell.

The *tertiary olfactory cortex* occupies the posterior part of the orbitofrontal cortex (Fig. 27-5). Its lateral part receives association fibers from the primary and secondary cortex. Its medial part receives from the mediodorsal nucleus of the thalamus, which receives from the primary olfactory cortex.

Descending connections enter the medial forebrain bundle from the olfactory tubercle, cortical amygdala, and septal area. They terminate in the pontine reticular formation and account for the arousal effect of olfactory stimulation (Chapter 14).

Functional anatomy

The human brain can distinguish about 3000 different odors. Although the olfactory bipolar neurons are morphologically uniform, the specific receptor proteins, embedded in the ciliary plasma membranes, differ from cell to cell. Odoriferous substances must be volatile in order to enter the nasal air and water-soluble in order to penetrate the fluid film bathing the cilia. All of the bipolars display 'background' electrical activity, and the olfactory bulb appears to be designed to facilitate central transmission from the more active bipolars. Contralateral excitation of inhibitory internuncials (via the anterior commissure) gives ipsilateral enhancement, to indicate the source of olfactory stimulation.

Microelectrode studies (in monkeys) indicate that odor discrimination improves slightly as one progresses from olfactory bulb to primary and secondary olfactory cortex, and shows marked improvement in the lateral part of the orbitofrontal cortex. However, the medial orbitofrontal cortex does not appear to participate in odor discrimination, and its function is still unknown.

TASTE

The gustatory system is structurally more advanced than the olfactory system. It resembles the visual,

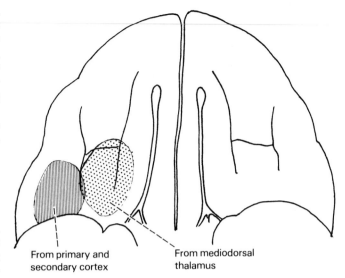

From primary and secondary cortex

From mediodorsal thalamus

Fig. 27-5 Tertiary olfactory cortex, in a monkey.

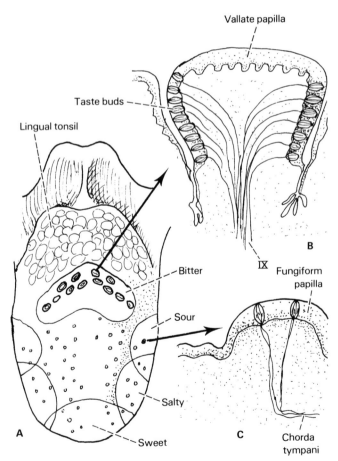

Fig. 27-6 A, dorsal surface of tongue, showing distribution of the four primary taste sensations. B, vallate papilla. C, fungiform papilla. IX, glossopharyngeal nerve.

auditory, and vestibular systems in having a receptor cell separated from the primary afferent neuron by a synapse, in having a second-order neuron in the brain stem, and in relaying to the neocortex via the thalamus. Surprisingly, the primary neurons of the taste pathway are unipolar, whereas those for the other four special senses are bipolar.

Taste buds

The taste buds of the tongue occupy the vallate, fungiform, and foliate papillae (Fig. 27-6). Some buds are also scattered in the epithelium lining the hard and soft palate, the epiglottis, and the upper end of the esophagus.

The four basic taste sensations are *sweet, sour, salty,* and *bitter*. Note that the flavor of a foodstuff (the 'taste' of chocolate, coffee, etc.) is detected by primary olfactory neurons, stimulated by volatile substances carried in the air from oropharynx to nasal cavities. It is commonplace to find that the sense of 'taste' (in reality, olfaction) is dulled during a head cold.

Structure (Fig. 27-7)

Each taste bud contains about 50 cells and is innervated by about 50 nerve fibers. Four cell types can be distinguished: parietal, sustentacular, basal, and gustatory. Autoradiographic studies using tritiated thymidine (a DNA label) have shown that the cells of a bud undergo continuous turnover: the parietal cells give rise to the sustentacular and basal cells, and the basal cells mature to become gustatory cells. The mature gustatory cells survive for only seven to ten days, being replaced from basal cells. The total number of taste buds declines throughout life at a rate of about 1% per year.

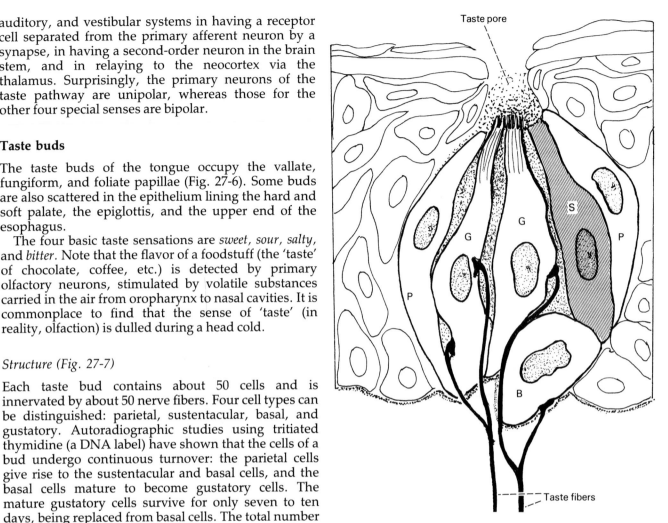

Fig. 27-7 The cells of a taste bud. B, basal cell; G, gustatory cell; P, parietal cell; S, supporting cell.

The sustentacular and gustatory cells extend the full length of the bud, and both display surface microvilli which occupy a taste *pit* beneath the taste *pore*. The necks of these cells contain contractile filaments which enable the cells to retract under strong stimulation, particularly by acids.

The sustentacular cells are dark, with a high content of rough endoplasmic reticulum and free ribosomes. Their secretion contains protein and mucopolysaccharides. The gustatory cells have fewer organelles, but lysosomes are numerous and are presumably responsible for autolysis of these cells. Each gustatory cell synapses upon one or more nerve endings. It is assumed that dissolved molecules bind with specific receptor proteins in the plasma membrane of gustatory microvilli, and that the receptors activate ion channels. Gustatory innervation is characterized by overlap:

1 The individual parent axons, which are unmyelinated, supply several gustatory cells in several taste buds.

2 About a dozen separate parent fibers contribute to the innervation of each bud.

3 The individual gustatory cell is not taste-specific: it responds maximally to one taste quality and gives smaller responses to the other three. Every gustatory cell therefore has receptors for all four qualities, with a preponderance of one type. But why?

Taste pathways

Taste buds in the anterior two-thirds of the tongue are supplied with taste fibers by the chorda tympani nerve. The vallate papillae are supplied by the glossopharyngeal. The epiglottis is supplied by the vagus, and the palate by the greater petrosal. The taste somas mainly occupy the geniculate ganglion, and their central processes synapse in the rostral end of the nucleus solitarius (see Chapter 36). Second-order neurons travel mainly contralaterally, in company with the medial lemniscus. They terminate in the ventroposteromedial nucleus of thalamus, where they are relayed to the cortical center for taste, located behind the face/tongue area of the somesthetic cortex.

APPLIED ANATOMY

Anosmia is the absence of the sense of smell. Bilateral anosmia (rare) is usually congenital. Unilateral anosmia may follow fracture of the anterior cranial fossa; it may be accompanied by *rhinorrhea*, a persistent leakage of cerebrospinal fluid. Unilateral anosmia is sometimes detected in patients having a meningioma in the floor of the anterior cranial fossa. The sense of smell can easily be tested by having the patient sniff a strong odor (such as coffee or peppermint) through one nostril, then through the other.

Readings

Altner, H. (1981) Physiology of taste. In *Fundamentals of Sensory Physiology*, 2nd ed. (Schmidt, R.F., ed.), pp. 218–227. New York, Heidelberg & Berlin: Springer-Verlag.

Arvidson, K., Cottler-Fox, M. and Friberg, U. (1981) Taste buds of the fungiform papillae in Cynomolgus monkey. *J. Anat., 133:* 271–280.

Erickson, R.P. (1984) The foundation of the four primary positions in taste. *Neurosci. Behav. Rev., 8:* 105–127.

Graziadei, P.P.C. (1973) Cell dynamics in the olfactory mucosa. *Tissue and Cell, 5:* 113–131.

Harding, J., Graziadei, P.P.C., Graziadei, G.A.M. and Margolis, F.L. (1977) Denervation in the primary olfactory pathway of mice. IV. Biochemical and morphological evidence for neuronal replacement following nerve section. *Brain Res., 132:* 11–28.

Henkin, R.I., Graziadei, P.P.C. and Bradley, G.F. (1969) The molecular basis of taste and its disorders. *Ann. Int. Med., 71:* 791–821.

Mattern, C.F.T. and Paran, V. (1974) Evidence of a contractile mechanism in the taste bud of the mouse fungiform papilla. *Exp. Neurol., 44:* 461–469.

Moran, D.T., Rowley, J.C., Jafek, B.W. and Lovell, M.A. (1982) The fine structure of the olfactory mucosa in man. *J. Neurocytol., 11:* 721–746.

Shepherd, G.M. (1978) Microcircuits in the nervous system. *Sci. Am., 238:* 93–103.

Takagi, S.F. (1979) Brain mechanism of olfaction. In *Integrative Control Functions of the Brain*, Vol. 2, pp. 51–66. Tokyo: Kodansha; Amsterdam: Elsevier.

Tamarin, A. (1975) *Illustrated Syllabus of Selected Topics in Oral Histology and Embryology*. Seattle: University of Washington Press.

Yamamoto, T. (1982) Neural mechanisms of taste function. *Front. Oral Physiol., 4:* 102–130.

Zalewski, A.A. (1974) Neuronal and tissue specifications involved in taste bud formation. *Ann. N.Y. Acad. Sci., 228:* 344–349.

28
Vision: Retina

Despite its peripheral location, the retina is part of the central nervous system. It is an outgrowth of the diencephalon. The stalk of white matter attaching the retina to the brain becomes the optic nerve.

Structurally, the nervous layer of the retina contains (a) photoreceptors, which are highly modified neurons with no exact homologue elsewhere in the sensory system, (b) bipolar neurons homologous with the primary afferent neurons of peripheral nerves, and (c) multipolar ganglion cells homologous with relay neurons of the posterior gray horn of the spinal cord. The ganglion cells are therefore second-order sensory neurons, and they duly project to the thalamus, half of their number crossing the midline en route.

Substantial processing of visual information takes place in the retina; this processing includes spatial and color coding, and contrast detection.

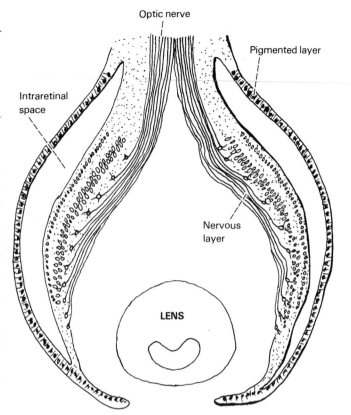

Fig. 28-1 Embryonic retina.

GENERAL FEATURES

Embryology (Fig. 28-1)

The retina is formed by an outgrowth from the diencephalon known as the optic vesicle. The vesicle is invaginated by the lens and becomes the two-layered optic cup. The outer, *pigmented (melanin) layer* becomes the pigment layer of the mature retina. The inner, *nervous layer* gives rise to the neurons of the mature retina. A potential intraretinal space persists between the two layers throughout life. In *retinal detachment*, the nervous layer lifts away, being anchored to the pigment layer only around the optic nerve head behind, and at the anterior edge of the retina (*ora serrata*) in front.

Inversion of the retina

The retina of all vertebrates is inverted. Light must pass through the entire thickness of the nervous layer to reach the photoreceptors. However, at the fovea centralis (the point of maximum visual acuity, in the line of the visual axis) the superficial layers lean away so that light strikes the photoreceptors directly (Fig. 28-2).

Reversal of the image (Fig. 28-3)

Objects in the upper half of the field of vision come into focus on the lower half of the retina, and *vice versa*. Images are also reversed in the horizontal plane.

Visual fields and retinal fields

In Fig. 28-4 the eyes are shown focused on an object directly in front. A second object (arrow) is introduced into the *left visual field*. Light reflected from this object

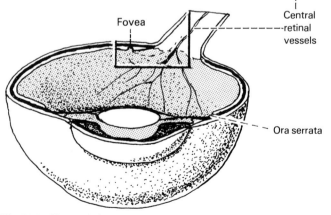

Fig. 28-2 Horizontal section of eyeball, with enlargement above.

196

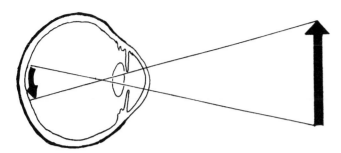

Fig. 28-3 Vertical or horizontal section of eyeball, showing reversal of the image on the retina.

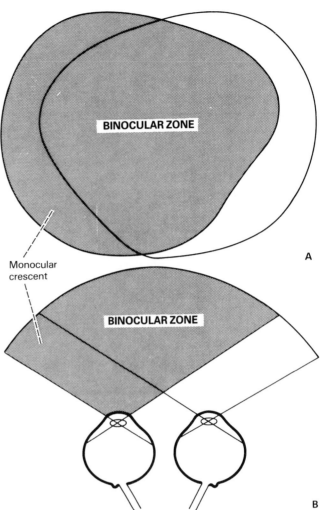

A

B

Fig. 28-5 A, frontal view, showing binocular zone and monocular crescent. B, horizontal section of binocular zone and monocular crescent.

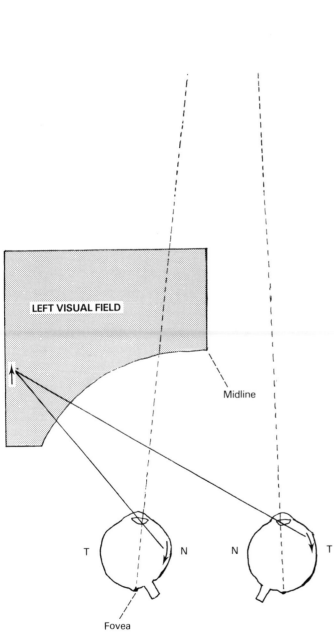

Fig. 28-4 An object in the left hemifield images on the left nasal (N) and right temporal (T) hemiretina.

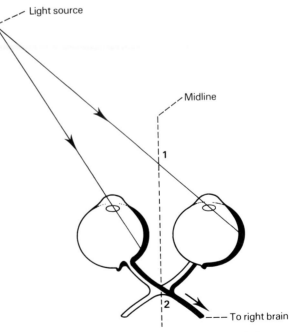

Fig. 28-6 Light crosses the midline in space (1) to reach the contralateral temporal hemiretina. Light reaching the ipsilateral nasal hemiretina is coded in nerve impulses which cross in the optic chiasm (2).

falls on the inner or *nasal field (nasal hemiretina)* of the left eye, and on the outer, *temporal field* of the right eye. The nasal and temporal hemiretinas meet in the center of the foveal centralis.

Light from the middle two-thirds of the field of vision registers on both retinas. This is the *binocular zone* (Fig. 28-5). The outer one-sixth of the field of vision on each side is the *monocular zone* or *crescent.*

An object in the left visual field registers in the right visual cortex. The image on the left nasal hemiretina is processed by neurons that cross the midline in the optic chiasm (Fig. 28-6). The image on the right temporal hemiretina *has already crossed the midline in space.* It is processed without further crossing. This is why nerve fibers from the nasal hemiretinas cross in the chiasm and fibers from the temporal hemiretinas do not.

The fovea centralis is only 0.5 mm in diameter, and the two halves of each project to opposite hemispheres (i.e., fibers from the nasal hemifoveas cross in the chiasm).

STRUCTURE OF THE RETINA

Radial neurons (Fig. 28-7)

The nervous layer of the retina includes three types of neurons radially disposed in tandem: photoreceptor, bipolar, and ganglion. Each of the three types of neurons can be subdivided into two classes.

Photoreceptor neurons

The *photoreceptor neurons* are either rod or cone neurons. The *rods* function only in dim light, being extremely sensitive to low illumination. They are absent from the fovea and increase in number peripherally. They are insensitive to color.

Cone neurons respond to bright illumination. They are concerned with visual detail and with color vision.

Each rod or cone has an outer and an inner *segment* with a narrow *connecting piece.* The outer segment is composed of hundreds of membranous discs produced by infolding of the plasma membrane. Infolding is a continuous process: new discs are added just above the connecting piece and old membrane is shed (after three weeks' passage through the outer segment) into the pigmented layer, where it is digested by phagosomes. The visual pigment molecules are synthesized in the inner segment and are passed through the connecting piece to be incorporated in the membranous discs.

An astonishing feature of both kinds of photoreceptor is that they are inactivated by light. In darkness, they continuously leak Na^+ ions and have a low negative potential (-30 mV). This is insufficient to generate action potentials, but enough to cause leakage of transmitter substance on to the bipolar neurons. Neurotransmission is arrested by light. *The photoreceptors are the only sensory receptors in the body to be inactivated by their specific stimulus.*

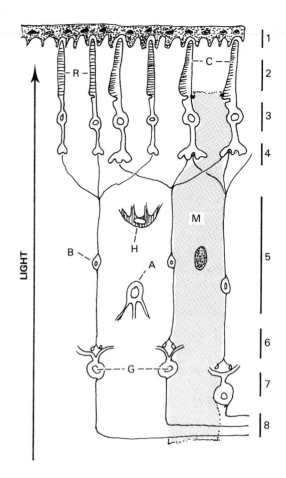

Fig. 28-7 Layers of the retina:
1 Pigmented layer
2 Layer of rods (R) and cones (C)
3 Outer nuclear layer (nuclei of rods and cones)
4 Outer synapse layer
5 Inner nuclear layer contains nuclei of amacrine cells (A), bipolar cells (B), horizontal cells (H), and Müller's cells (M). Müller's cells are neuroglial
6 Inner synapse layer
7 Ganglion cell (G) layer
8 Nerve fiber layer

Bipolar neurons

The *bipolar neurons* are either depolarizing or hyperpolarizing. *These terms are used with reference to their response to light* – in other words, to the arrest of transmission by photoreceptors. *Depolarizing* neurons are also called *invaginating* because they invaginate the bases of the photoreceptors (Fig. 28-8). The synaptic vesicles here run along active zones known as *synaptic bars (ribbons)* to reach the presynaptic membrane. The invaginating bipolars are inhibited by the transmitter during darkness. Conversely, they are released from inhibition by light: their negative electrotonus is increased sufficiently to permit them to release transmitter substance (again from synaptic bars) onto ganglion cells.

Hyperpolarizing bipolars are inactivated by light. They are also called *flat* bipolars because they do not invaginate the photoreceptors. Although they receive the same transmitter as the invaginating bipolars, their *receptors* are different, and induce biochemical changes causing hyperpolarization.

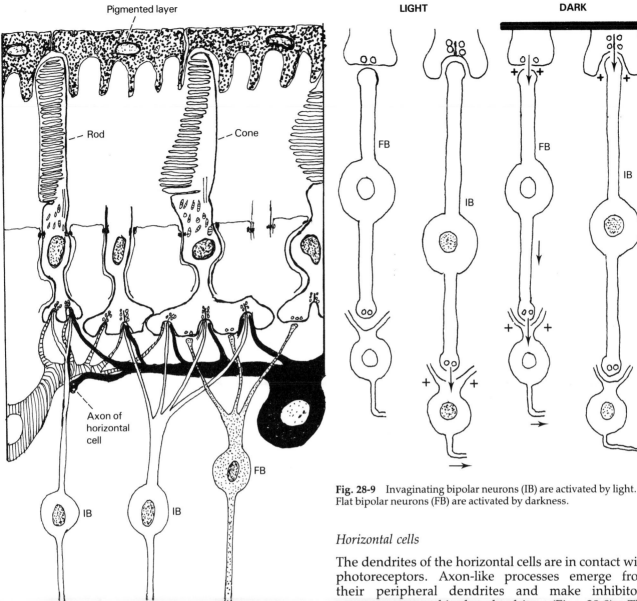

Fig. 28-8 Invaginating bipolars (IB) receive ribbon synapses from photoreceptor neurons. Flat bipolars (FB) receive conventional, 'flat' synapses. Horizontal cells (black and shaded) receive from the ribbon synapses and form inhibitory axodendritic synapses upon bipolar cell dendrites.

Fig. 28-9 Invaginating bipolar neurons (IB) are activated by light. Flat bipolar neurons (FB) are activated by darkness.

Ganglion neurons

The principal *ganglion neurons* are either 'on' type or 'off' type, in accordance with their bipolar connections (Fig. 28-9). 'On' cells are driven by depolarizing bipolars when their photoreceptors are illuminated. 'Off' cells are driven by hyperpolarizing bipolars when their photoreceptors are in the shade (as when receiving the image of black print on a page).

Tangential neurons

Tangential neurons are of two kinds – horizontal and amacrine.

Horizontal cells

The dendrites of the horizontal cells are in contact with photoreceptors. Axon-like processes emerge from their peripheral dendrites and make inhibitory synapses upon bipolar dendrites (Fig. 28-8). The function of the horizontal cells is to inhibit bipolar cells of like kind outside the immediate zone of excitation. The excited cells are said to be 'on line', the inhibited ones 'off line'. This mechanism serves to heighten contrast by inactivating bipolars (and hence ganglion cells) outside the area of the stimulus.

Amacrine cells

The amacrine cells resemble the granule cells of the olfactory bulb in having no definable axons. However, they do form synapses of conventional type upon ganglion cell dendrites. They enter into reciprocal synapses with bipolar neurons (Fig. 28-10).

Amacrines are the least understood cell type in the retina. Some ten different transmitter substances (some excitatory, others inhibitory) have been identified in different amacrine cells. The amacrines and the ganglion cells are the only neurons in the retina that give rise to action potentials. The amacrines may be at least as important as horizontal cells in generating 'off-line' inhibition of ganglion cells.

199

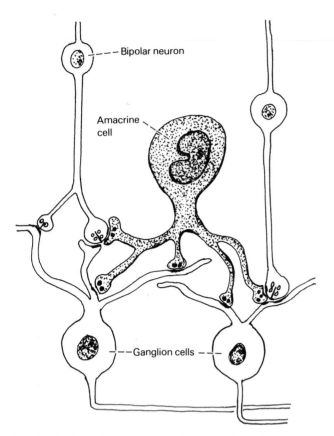

Fig. 28-10 Amacrine cell dendrites forming reciprocal synapses with bipolar neurons and conventional synapses upon ganglion cell dendrites.

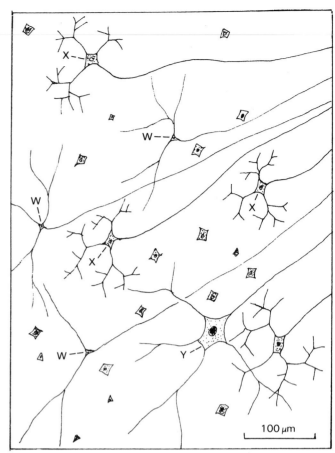

Fig. 28-11 W, X and Y cells in a surface view of the retina. Most are represented only by their cell bodies.

FUNCTIONAL ASPECTS

W, X and Y ganglion cells (Fig. 28-11)

The majority of the ganglion cells are called X, or 'sustained' cells. They give a sustained 'on' or 'off' response to a spot of light on the overlying photoreceptors. X cells of 'on' type are deeper (nearer to the vitreous) than X cells of 'off' type. X cells analyze fixated objects in terms of their shapes and colors.

Y cells are relatively scarce. They are called 'transient' because they give only momentary responses ('on' or 'off') when a spot of light appears, and again when it is switched off. Y cells respond well to rapidly moving stimuli, as do some of the amacrine cells that synapse upon them. The Y cells have large axons that project to the superior colliculus as well as to the thalamus. Their probable function is (a) to signal to the visual cortex the entry of fast-moving objects into the visual field, and (b) to switch the gaze (saccade, Chapter 32) in order to 'foveate' moving objects for analysis by X cells.

W cells are intermediate in number between X and Y cells. They have very small somas and project fine axons to the thalamus and superior colliculus. W cells provide the afferent limb of the pupillary light reflex (Chapter 31).

Coding for color

There are three biochemical types of cone. One is maximally sensitive (inhibited) to green light, one to

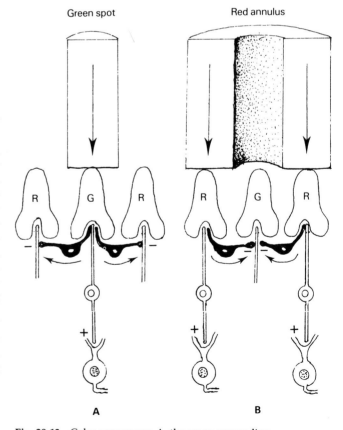

Fig. 28-12 Color opponency. A, the green-responding photoreceptor (G) is on-line and the red receptors (R) are off-line. B, when the red receptors are on-line the green receptor is off-line.

red light, and one to blue. Each is connected to 'on' or 'off' ganglion cells by invaginating or flat bipolar cells, respectively.

1 Invaginating bipolars attached *exclusively* to *green* cones cause their ganglion cells to be 'on' only for a spot of green light on the overlying retina (i.e., on-line). The same ganglion cells are inhibited by the complementary color – *red* – when the red is presented as a ring surrounding the spot originally lit by green (Fig. 28-12). The ganglion cell is off-line for the red annulus, and it is inhibited by red-responsive horizontal cells.

2 'On' type ganglion cells which are on-line for a *red* spot are off-line for a *green* annulus.

3 'On' type ganglion cells which are on-line for a *blue* spot are off-line for a complementary annulus of *yellow* light, derived from green and red cones acting together.

Sets of 'off' ganglion cells operate in a reverse manner, being inactivated by a green, red or blue spot and activated by an annulus of complementary color.

Black and white

White light is a mixture of green, red and blue. In bright conditions it is encoded by green, red, and blue cones, *all connected to common on-line ganglion cells*. The same cells are inhibited by a dark, off-line annulus. Both 'on' and 'off' type ganglion cells are involved in black-and-white vision just as in color vision.

In dim light only the rods are active, and colored objects appear in varying shades of gray. The rods are subject to the same rules as cones, showing center–surround antagonism between white and black, and being connected to 'on' and 'off' ganglion cells.

Visual acuity

The macula lutea ('yellow spot') measures 1.5 mm in diameter. The yellow pigment is carotene, contained in the photoreceptors. The macula is bowl-shaped, with a further, V-shaped depression in its central 0.5 mm. The latter is the *fovea centralis*. It is the point of acutest vision and contains 20–25 000 cones and no rods. The *foveola* is the exact center of the fovea. It contains 2000 very slender cones, each linked by one bipolar neuron to one ganglion cell. Visual acuity is maximal at this spot, which subtends an arc of only 0.5°. Acuity diminishes progressively toward the margins of the macula.

APPLIED ANATOMY

In *color blindness*, one or more of the three pigments required for normal color vision is reduced or absent. Color blindness due to retinal disease is rare but inherited color blindness is common. The genes for green and red cone pigments are carried by the X chromosome. The gene for blue is autosomal. Since males have only one X chromosome, blindness for green or red is much commoner in males (8%) than in females (0.25%). Green deficiency is three times commoner than red deficiency. Blindness for blue is extremely rare in both sexes. (For examples of red and green color blindness, see paintings by Cézanne or Paul Henry.)

Readings

Brecha, N. (1983) Retinal neurotransmitters: histochemical and biochemical studies. In *Chemical Neuroanatomy* (Ernson, P.C., ed.), pp. 85–130. New York: Raven Press.

Daw, N.W. (1984) The psychology and physiology of colour vision. *Trends Neurosci.*, 7: 330–335.

Dowling, J.E. (1975) The vertebrate retina. In *The Nervous System* (Tower, D.B., ed.), Vol. 1, *The Basic Neurosciences* (Brady, R.O., ed.), pp. 91–100. New York: Raven Press.

Fain, G.L., Ishida, A.T. and Callery, S. (1983) Mechanisms of synaptic transmission in the retina. *Vision Res.*, 23: 1239–1249.

Friedlander, M.J. and Sherman, S.M. (1981) Morphology of physiologically identified neurons. *Trends Neurosci.*, 5: 211–214.

Frisen, L. (1980) The neurology of visual acuity. *Brain*, 103: 639–670.

Kaneko, A. (1983) Retinal bipolar cells: their function and morphology. *Trends Neurosci.*, 5: 219–222.

Nelson, R., Famiglietti, E.V. and Kolb, H. (1978) Intracellular staining reveals different levels of stratification for on- and off-center ganglion cells in cat retina. *J. Neurophysiol.*, 41: 472–483.

Peichl, L. and Wässle, H. (1981) Morphological identification of on- and off-centre brisk transient (Y) cells in the cat retina. *Proc. R. Soc. Lond. B*, 212: 139–156.

Saito, H.-A. (1983) Morphology of physiologically identified X-, Y- and W-type retinal ganglion cells of the cat. *J. Comp. Neurol.*, 221: 279–288.

Wässle, H., Boycott, B.B. and Illing, R.-B. (1981) Morphology and mosaic of on- and off-beta (X) cells in the cat retina and some functional considerations. *Proc. R. Soc. Lond. B*, 212: 177–195.

29

Visual Pathways and Visual Cortex

The pathway from retina to visual cortex contains first-, second- and third-order sensory neurons. The somas of the first- and second-order neurons occupy the retina. The somas of the third-order neurons occupy the lateral geniculate nucleus.

First-order neurons

The bipolar neurons in the retina are homologous with the bipolar neurons of other special senses and with the unipolar neurons of the peripheral sensory nerves. In the eye, they link the photoreceptor cells to the retinal ganglion cells.

Second-order neurons

The ganglion cells of the retina are homologous with the projection cells of the posterior gray horn of the spinal cord. Their axons give rise to the optic nerves and optic tracts. The optic nerve differs from a true peripheral nerve in the following ways:
1 Embryologically, the retina is an outgrowth from the forebrain, and the optic nerve is forebrain white matter.
2 Histologically, the optic nerve contains oligodendrocytes, astrocytes, and microglia whereas true peripheral nerves contain Schwann cells and fibroblasts. Being identical to white matter in all respects, the optic nerve does not regenerate after injury.
3 Grossly, the optic nerve is invested with pia, arachnoid and dura mater, like all other parts of the CNS.

OPTIC NERVE AND TRACT

Each optic nerve contains about one million axons, which acquire myelin as they penetrate the sclera. Fibers from the macula enter the center of the nerve; they are surrounded by fibers from the four retinal quadrants (Fig. 29-1).

At the optic chiasm, fibers from the nasal hemiretina enter the contralateral optic tract; those from the temporal hemiretina enter the ipsilateral tract. The ratio of crossed to uncrossed fibers is 53 : 47, there being rather more ganglion cells in the nasal hemiretina.

The optic tract undergoes a 90° inward twist, carrying fibers from the upper retina to its medial side and those from the lower retina to its lateral side. The tract winds around the midbrain and divides into a medial and a lateral root. The medial root (10%) enters the midbrain via the superior brachium. The lateral

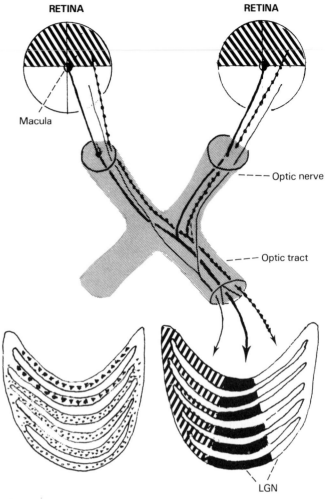

Fig. 29-1 Projection from retina to lateral geniculate nucleus (LGN).

root (90%) enters the lateral geniculate nucleus of the thalamus.

Medial root of optic tract

Medial root fibers enter the superior colliculus and the pretectal nucleus.

Superior colliculus: function

From the superior colliculus, the tectoreticular, tectobulbar, and tectospinal tracts serve to turn the eyes, head and trunk toward the source of a visual stimulus. The tectoreticular fibers synapse in gaze centers controlling conjugate movements of the eyes (Chapter 32). Tectobulbar fibers activate the sternomastoid to rotate the head. Tectospinal fibers descend in the anterior funiculus of the cord and excite motoneurons to axial muscles for rotation of the trunk. The afferent limb of the *visual turning reflex* is provided by fast-conducting Y ganglion cells in the retina, which are highly responsive to moving objects.

A poorly understood pathway runs from the superior colliculus to the visual association cortex via the pulvinar of the thalamus. This pathway has been invoked to account for the phenomenon known as 'blindsight'. A patient whose occipital lobe has been removed may be able to point toward a bright spot in the contralateral visual field, although he can 'see' nothing there. A visual perceptive function for the

202

superior colliculus would not be surprising on phylogenetic grounds, since it is the sole source of visual perception in reptiles. A simpler explanation of 'blindsight' after surgery may be that the anterior tip of the primary visual cortex (containing some monocular crescent cells, Fig. 29-5) was not removed.

Pretectal nucleus: function

The prectectal nucleus contains the internuncial neurons for the light reflex (Chapter 31), which is of major clinical importance. Other medial root fibers descend to the inferior olivary nucleus, to influence vestibulo-ocular reflexes (Chapter 33).

Lateral root of optic tract

The lateral root terminates in the lateral geniculate nucleus of the thalamus. The fibers enter the principal (dorsal) nucleus of the lateral geniculate in line with their positions within the optic tract.

LATERAL GENICULATE NUCLEUS (LGN)

Laminar arrangement

Six well-defined cellular laminae are present in the LGN. Crossed retinotectal fibers terminate in laminae I (deepest), IV and VI. Uncrossed fibers end in laminae II, III and V.

The principal cells in each lamina (third-order neurons) project to the primary visual cortex. In addition to the optic tract, they receive corticogeniculate fibers from the primary visual cortex, which are presumed to facilitate transmission by the principal cells.

Electrical records show little transformation in the LGN of impulses received from the optic tract. All of the principal cells are center-surround (either 'on' or 'off'), and all project to the primary visual cortex.

Laminae I and II are *magnocellular*. Three quarters of the cells are X-type, broad-spectrum (black-and-white). One quarter are Y-type, responding best to movement.

Laminae III–VI are *parvocellular*, and consist of X-type, color-opponent cells.

Geniculocalcarine tract

The geniculocalcarine tract, or *optic radiation*, is of major clinical importance because of its frequent entrapment in lesions of the posterior half of the cerebral hemisphere. It travels from the lateral geniculate nucleus to the primary visual cortex (area 17), located in the walls of the calcarine sulcus.

The anatomy of the tract is shown in Figs. 29-2, 29-3, and 29-4. Fibers destined for the lower half of area 17 begin in the lateral part of LGN and sweep forward into the temporal lobe (Meyer's loop) before turning back to join those traveling to the upper half. The tract passes through the retrolentiform part of the internal capsule and continues in the white matter underlying the parietotemporal junction. It runs outside the posterior horn of the lateral ventricle before turning medially to enter the occipital cortex.

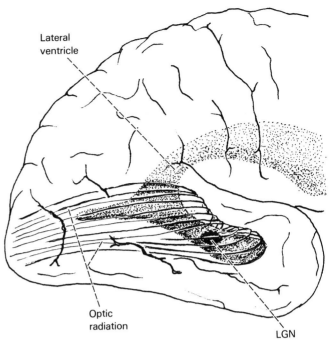

Fig. 29-2 Optic radiation seen through the brain surface. LGN, lateral geniculate nucleus.

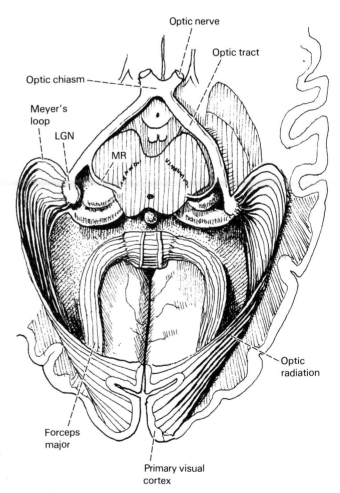

Fig. 29-3 Visual pathways, from below. LGN, lateral geniculate nucleus; MR, medial root of optic tract.

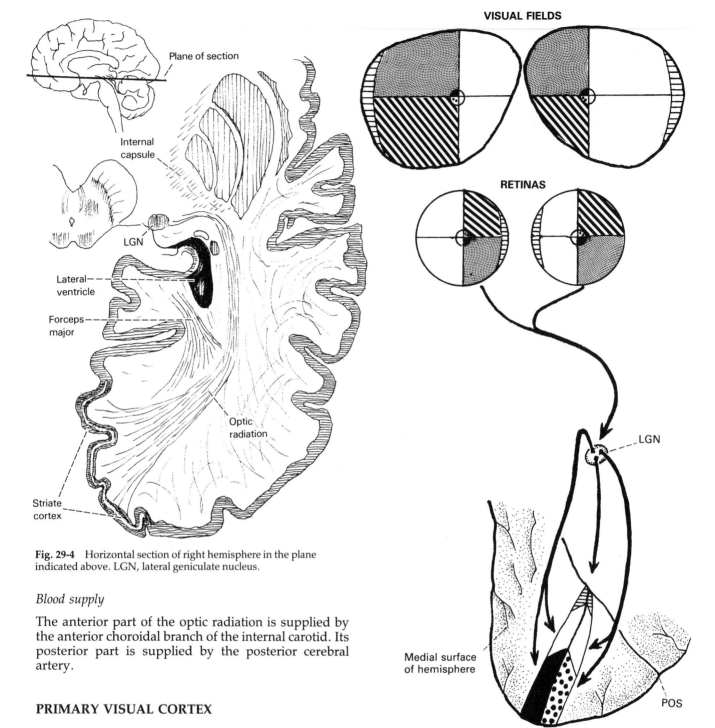

Fig. 29-4 Horizontal section of right hemisphere in the plane indicated above. LGN, lateral geniculate nucleus.

Blood supply

The anterior part of the optic radiation is supplied by the anterior choroidal branch of the internal carotid. Its posterior part is supplied by the posterior cerebral artery.

PRIMARY VISUAL CORTEX

The primary visual cortex is called the *calcarine cortex* because it occupies the walls of the calcarine sulcus, which is 10 mm deep. It extends 10 mm onto the medial surface above and below the sulcus, and 10 mm onto the occipital pole of the brain, giving a total area of 25 cm². It is easily identified in the freshly cut brain by a narrow strip of white matter – the *visual stria* (stria of Gennari) – within the gray matter.

Retinotopic map (Fig. 29-5)

The contralateral visual field is represented upside down, the plane of the sulcus representing the horizontal meridian. The retinal representation is posteroanterior, with the macula at the back of area 17

Fig. 29-5 Representation of left visual fields in right calcarine cortex. LGN, lateral geniculate nucleus; POS, parieto-occipital sulcus.

and the monocular crescent at the front end. The macular cortex is about 150 mm² in area; this is a huge magnification of the 0.2 mm² of the combined half foveas, and a reflection of the extensive visual processing required of the macular cortex.

Structure

The striate cortex is the thinnest part (2 mm) of the cerebral cortex. It is highly granular, containing an abundance of stellate cells in lamina IV. These stellate cells are split into inner and outer groups by the visual stria, which is mainly composed of geniculostriate axons. The great majority of the axons synapse in the two groups of stellate cells.

The general structure and connectivity resembles that of the somesthetic cortex. Pyramidal cells of laminae II and III project to the visual association cortex (areas 18 and 19). Lamina V projects to the superior colliculus and lamina VI to the lateral geniculate nucleus.

Ocular dominance columns

In the monkey, if radiolabeled proline is injected into the vitreous humor of one eye it is taken up by retinal neurons and sent to the LGN by rapid orthograde transport. The principal cells of LGN pick up the label at retinogeniculate synapses and send it to area 17. The label can be identified by autoradiography: it is distributed in vertical stripes, alternating with un-labeled stripes of equal width. The same effect can be obtained by shining a light in one eye while injecting labeled deoxyglucose intravenously. Cortical cells with increased metabolism (in response to the light) take up large amounts of deoxyglucose from the capillary bed.

In humans the *ocular dominance columns* are hard to detect histologically but are about 1 mm wide. They represent alternating left-eye, right-eye inputs from the LGN (Fig. 29-6). The geniculocalcarine projections are so ordered that matching points from the two retinas are registered side by side in contiguous columns. This arrangement is ideal for binocular vision, since cortical neurons at the edge of a column can readily receive from both eyes simultaneously.

Electrical responses

Electrical records taken from individual cortical cells (in animals) while the eyes are looking at various shapes and colors projected onto a screen fall into four categories. The cells concerned are called 'concentric', 'simple', 'complex', and 'hypercomplex'. 'Concentric' and 'simple' cells are found in lamina IV, the other two in higher and lower laminae and in visual association cortex. All four categories are divided into *contrast cells*, which respond only to black or white, and *color-opponent cells*, whose opponency is of the same spectral nature as in the retina and LGN.

'Concentric' cells have the same features as those of the retina and LGN. The centers and surrounds are mutually antagonistic. All are monocular, being driven from one eye only. All are stellate cells at the bottom of lamina IV.

'Simple' cells respond to slits of light and shade (or of opponent colors) rather than to spots. They respond well whether the slit is stationary or moving, but each responds only to a particular *orientation* (tilt) of the slit. The character of simple cells is explained on the grounds that they receive from 'concentric' cells of suitable orientation (Fig. 29-7). They are mostly monocular, nearly always stellate, and are at the top of lamina IV.

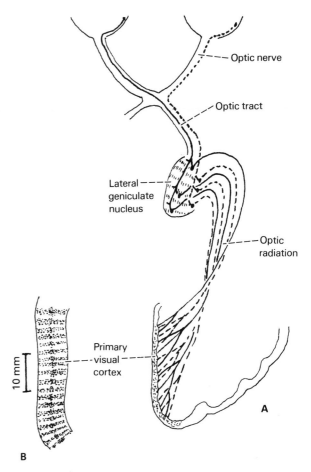

Fig. 29-6 Ocular dominance columns. A, diagram to show alternating inputs to area 17 from left and right eyes. B, radiolabeling following ³H proline injection into one eye.

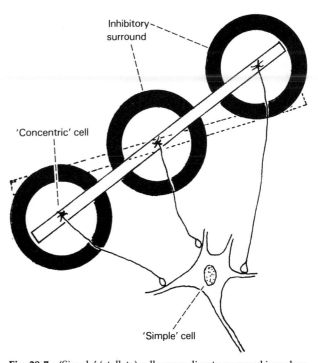

Fig. 29-7 'Simple' (stellate) cell responding to summed impulses from three 'concentric' (stellate) cells responding to a bar of light in the 'on' position for each. Changing the orientation of the bar (dotted outline) puts it in the 'off' position for two of the cells; the 'simple' cell falls silent without summation.

'*Complex*' *cells* respond to bars (i.e., broad slits) passing across their receptive fields. They are binocular pyramidal cells receiving from several 'simple' cells having a common slit orientation.

'*Hypercomplex*' *cells* respond to bars at right angles to one another forming an L, and to more elaborate geometrical shapes. They are binocular pyramidal cells receiving simultaneous inputs from 'complex' cells of different orientation response.

Orientation columns

Cells responding to bars of one orientation lie transverse to the axis of the ocular dominance columns. There is an orderly sequence of orientation columns, each one about 10° different from its neighbor (Fig. 29-8).

VISUAL ASSOCIATION AREAS

Areas 18 and 19 of Brodmann are known as the 'peristriate belt'. These areas, and the cortex immediately anterior, have been subdivided into eight areas on architectural grounds, but their structure has yet to be correlated with function.

In monkeys, electrical responses to visual stimuli indicate that area 18 is concerned with fine feature analysis and stereopsis. All responding cells are binocular. Area 19 has specialized subsections: the middle of area 19 is devoted to the macula and responds selectively to object *sizes*; in front of this, area 19 responds to *movement*, often directionally; the inferior part of area 19 is highly responsive to *color*. Human patients with bilateral lesions of the inferior part of area 19 may have reduced color discrimination.

The *inferotemporal cortex* (Fig. 29-9) is the highest visual association area. It receives from areas 7 (serving visual attention, Chapter 32), 18 and 19, and from the entorhinal cortex. It evidently contains highly complex visual memory stores. Stimulation of the inferotemporal cortex during brain surgery may evoke vivid scenes from the patient's past life. Epileptic auras arising here may have the same effect. In monkeys, this area contains 'recognition cells' which discharge only when a meaningful object (such as a monkey's paw) is presented.

The inferior longitudinal fasciculus links the peristriate belt to the inferotemporal cortex. Bilateral lesions of the fasciculus (very rare) may give rise to *visual agnosia*, characterized by inability to name an object presented or to describe its function. If a hammer is presented it is simply not recognized, but if its name is then spoken the patient can immediately indicate its use.

In monkeys, removal of cortex equivalent to area 7 causes an inability to notice the *position* of objects in space. For example, a monkey previously trained to choose a food-containing receptacle (from similar, empty ones) because of another object placed nearby is no longer able to use the cue. Form and color recognition are not affected. The defect may be comparable to the contralateral spatial neglect

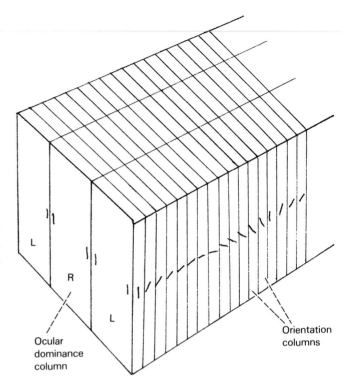

Fig. 29-8   Orientation columns are transverse to dominance columns. (Adapted from Hubel, 1982).

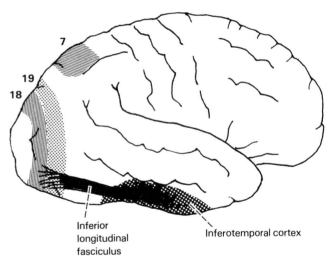

Fig. 29-9   Visual association areas.

observed in humans following parietal lobe lesions (Chapter 25).

In monkeys, removal of the inferotemporal cortex causes an inability to discriminate gross differences in form and color, but spatial ability is retained.

Both areas are richly connected to the entorhinal cortex, which is essential for visual training. They are also richly connected to the frontal cortex, for cognitive and motor responses.

The function of the angular gyrus in transforming the written to the spoken word is mentioned in Chapter 25.

APPLIED ANATOMY

Possible sites of injury to the visual pathway are shown in Fig. 29-10, together with the visual field defects they produce.

Lesions	Field defects
1 Center of optic nerve	Ipsilateral central scotoma
2 Entire optic nerve	Ipsilateral blindness
3 Optic chiasm	Bitemporal hemianopsia
4 Optic tract	Homonymous hemianopsia
5 Meynert's loop	Homonymous upper quadrant anopsia
6 Optic radiation, visual cortex	Homonymous hemianopsia

Visual defects are always described *in terms of the visual fields*.

Notes on lesions

1 Lesions of the macula produce the same visual defect. Eccentric lesions of the retina or optic nerve produce scotomas in the contralateral visual field of that eye.

A patch of demyelination in the optic nerve may be the initial lesion of multiple sclerosis (MS). MS must always be considered when an apparently healthy young adult complains of a 'blind spot' in the visual field of one eye.

2 The optic nerve may be destroyed by a tumor of the meninges surrounding the nerve or by a glioma within it. Secondly, raised intracranial pressure from any intracranial lesion is transmitted in the subarachnoid extension, which ensheathes the entire length of the optic nerve in the orbit. The nerve is uniformly squeezed, and conduction is first blocked in the relatively fine axons coming from the macula. Prolonged pressure (many weeks) may produce blindness in one or both eyes. (Papilledema is considered below.)

3 The optic chiasm usually lies above and behind the pituitary gland (Fig. 29-11). Pituitary tumors rising out of the sella turcica compress intersecting fibers coming from the lower nasal hemiretinas. The result is an upper bitemporal field defect. Later, the bitemporal hemianopsia (Gr., half blindness) becomes complete.

4 Lesions of the optic tract are rare. They result in homonymous hemianopsia, which is usually 'incongruous' – in other words, unequal – because one side of the tract is involved more than the other.

5 Meyer's loop may be compressed by a tumor in the temporal pole. It arises from the lateral part of LGN, and interruption causes a homonymous superior quadrantic field defect.

6 Lesions of the optic radiation or striate cortex are frequent. Causes include vascular disease, tumors, trauma (a blow to the back of the head), and infection (notably temporal lobe abscess caused by middle ear disease in children). Vascular disease may reside in the middle or posterior cerebral arteries. Although the middle cerebral artery does not supply it, the optic radiation may be compressed by edema following hemorrhage from one of the striate branches. It is not uncommon for 'stroke' patients to have a homonymous hemianopsia for one to two weeks, until the edema subsides.

Tumors of the occipital lobe produce complete homonymous defects. Tumors of the parietal lobe may compress the radiation from above and cause bilateral lower quadrant defects. Temporal lobe tumors may attack it from below to produce bilateral upper quadrant defects.

'Macular sparing' (more correctly, sparing of the foveola) in occipital lobe lesions is attributed to a possible projection of the foveola to both occipital lobes. Sparing has been

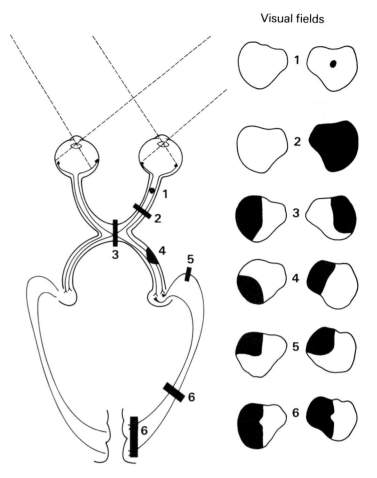

Visual fields

Fig. 29-10 Visual field defects following lesions of the visual pathway.

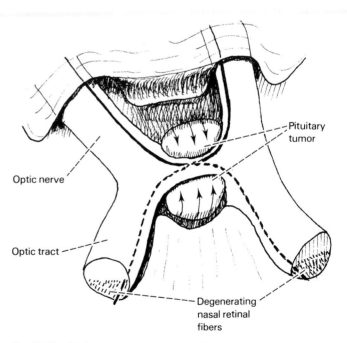

Fig. 29-11 Pituitary tumor compressing the optic chiasm.

207

attributed instead to a supply to the macular cortex from the middle cerebral artery; however, it may be present after excision of the entire primary visual cortex. Sparing is represented in Fig. 29-10, no. 6, by the central notches.

Papilledema

Edema of the optic nerve head, or papilla, may result from disease of the nerve itself or from raised intracranial pressure. The papilla appears swollen and the tributaries of the central vein of the retina become engorged (Fig. 29-12).

The central vessels of the retina arise from the ophthalmic vessels and run forward in the center of the optic nerve (Fig. 29-13). When intracranial pressure is raised, additional blood enters the ophthalmic artery from the internal carotid; it flows into branches of the external carotid surrounding the orbit. This is one of several mechanisms whereby the fluid content of the skull is reduced to compensate for its diminished capacity. The central artery is included in the redistribution of blood, and the increased perfusion in its capillary bed initiates the edema. The edema in turn compresses the central vein, resulting in venous engorgement. Compression of optic nerve fibers also contributes to swelling of the nerve head by interfering with axoplasmic flow.

In animals, compression of the central vein alone does not cause papilledema.

Readings

Alexander, M.P., Cummings, J. and Albert, M.L. (1982) Higher visual functions. In *Neuro-ophthalmology*, Vol. 2 (Lessell, S. and van Dalen, J.T.W., eds.), pp. 88–107. Amsterdam: Excerpta Medica; Princeton: Oxford University Press.

Bender, M.B. and Bodis-Wollner, I. (1978) Visual dysfunction in optic tract lesions. *Ann. Neurol., 3:* 187–193.

Blasdel, G.G. and Lund, J.S. (1983) Termination of afferent axons in macaque striate cortex. *J. Neurosci., 3:* 1389–1413.

Braak, E. (1982) On the structure of the human striate area. *Advances in Anatomy, Embryology and Cell Biology,* 77: 1–86.

Bynke, H. (1984) The visual fields. In *Neuro-ophthalmology*, Vol. 4 (Lessell, S. and van Dalen, J.T.W., eds.), pp. 348–357. Amsterdam: Elsevier; New York: Oxford University Press.

Celesia, G.G., Archer, C.-R., Koroiwa, Y. and Goldfader, P.R. (1980) Visual function of the extrageniculocalcarine system in man. *Arch. Neurol.,* 37: 704–706.

Coleman, P.D. and Flood, D.G. (1982) Studies on the morphological basis of orientation selectivity. *Contrib. Sens. Physiol.,* 7: 75–101.

Crawford, M.L.J., Meharg, L.S. and Johnston, D.A. (1982) Structure of columns in monkey striate cortex induced by luminant-contrast and color-contrast stimulation. *Proc. Natl. Acad. Sci. USA,* 79: 6722–6726.

de Courten, C. and Garey, L.J. (1982) Morphology of the neurons in the human lateral geniculate nucleus and their normal development. *Exp. Brain Res.,* 47: 159–171.

Frisen, L. (1980) The neurology of visual acuity. *Brain,* 103: 639–670.

Giolli, R.A. and Towns, L.C. (1980) A review of axon collateralization in the mammalian visual system. *Brain Behav. Evol.,* 17: 364–390.

Hubel, D.H. (1982) Exploration of the primary visual cortex, 1955–78. *Nature,* 299: 515–524.

Hubel, D.H. and Wiesel, T.N. (1977) Functional architecture of macaque monkey visual cortex. *Proc. R. Soc. Lond. B,* 198: 1–59.

Kaplan, E. and Shapley, R.M. (1982) X and Y cells in the lateral geniculate nucleus of monkeys. *J. Physiol.,* 330: 125–143.

Michael, C.M. (1978) Color vision in monkey striate cortex: single cells with dual-opponent color receptive fields. *J. Neurophysiol., 41:* 1233–1249.

Michael, C.M. (1978) Color-sensitive complex cells in monkey striate cortex. *J. Neurophysiol.,* 41: 1250–1266.

Michael, C.M. (1979) Color-sensitive hypercomplex cells in monkey striate cortex. *J. Neurophysiol.,* 42: 726–743.

Mishkin, M., Ungerleider, L.G. and Macko, K.A. (1983) Object vision and spatial vision: two separate pathways. *Trends Neurosci.,* 6: 414–417.

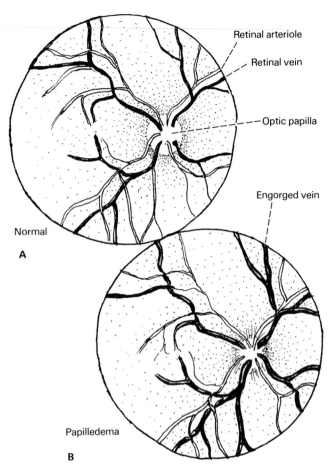

Fig. 29-12 A, normal fundus oculi. B, papilledema.

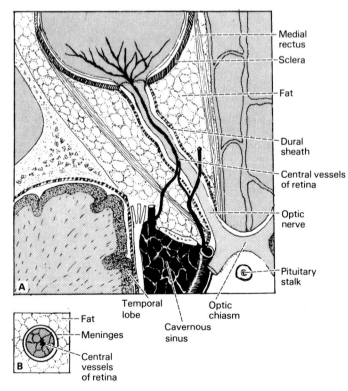

Fig. 29-13 A, horizontal section of the orbit. B, transverse section of the optic nerve.

Pasik, P. and Pasik, T. (1982) Visual functions in monkeys after total removal of visual cerebral cortex. *Contrib. Sens. Physiol., 7:* 147–200.

Richmond, B.J. and Wurtz, R.H. (1982) Inferotemporal cortex in awake monkeys. In *Changing Concepts of the Nervous System*, pp. 411–422. New York: Academic Press.

Roland, P.E. and Skinhøj, E. (1981) Extrastriate cortical areas activated during visual discrimination in man. *Brain Res., 222:* 166–171.

Stone, J. and Dreher, B. (1982) Parallel processing of information in the visual pathways. *Trends Neurosci., 5:* 441–446.

Tootell, R.B., Silverman, M.S., Switkes, E. and De Valois, R.L. (1982) Deoxyglucose analysis of retinotopic organization in primate striate cortex. *Science, 218:* 902–904.

Tusa, R.J. (1982) Visual cortex: multiple areas and multiple functions. In *Changing Concepts of the Nervous System*, pp. 235–259. New York: Academic Press.

Van Essen, D.C. and Maunsell, J.H.R. (1983) Hierarchical organization and functional streams in the visual cortex. *Trends Neurosci., 6:* 370–375.

Wiesel, T.N. and Gilbert, C.D. (1983) Morphological basis of visual cortical function. *Q. J. Exp. Physiol., 68:* 525–543.

Wikström, J., Poser, S. and Ritter, G. (1980) Optic neuritis as an initial symptom in multiple sclerosis. *Acta Neurol. Scand., 61:* 178–185.

Hearing

In the following account it is assumed that the reader is already acquainted with the general structure of the cochlea.

The sound field

The terms *body field*, *visual field*, and *sound field* are illustrated in Fig. 30-1. The terms are used here in respect of the primary sensory cortex concerned in each case. Each primary cortex receives information from the *contralateral hemifield*, whether of personal space (somatosensory) or of extrapersonal space (visual and auditory).

Although hearing is the same as these other two senses with respect to its peripheral territory, it differs from them in that sound, because of its nature, is detected by both ears. A substantial amount of central auditory synaptology is devoted to magnification of the very small differences that exist in the timing and intensity of sounds reaching the ears. The solution to this problem of *binaural hearing* is worked out in the brainstem. Because the problem is unique to hearing, the synaptology of second-order acoustic neurons is far more complex than that of second-order visual or tactile neurons. Only a bare outline of the second-order auditory relays (from cochlear nucleus to thalamus) is given here. The readings listed at the end of this chapter may be consulted for details.

Auditory receptors (Figs. 30-2, 30-3, 30-4)

The receptors for hearing are the *sensory hair cells* of the spiral organ (of Corti). The hair cells are disposed in a single row on the inner side of the tunnel of Corti, and in a triple row on the outer side. Their supporting cells rest on the basilar membrane. Each hair cell has about 100 stereocilia. Those of the inner row lie free in the endolymph, but many in the outer rows touch the tectorial membrane.

Spiral ganglion (Figs. 30-2, 30-3)

The *spiral (cochlear) ganglion* is embedded in the flange-like osseous spiral lamina. It contains about 25 000 bipolar nerve cells and 5000 unipolar nerve cells. The bipolar *cell bodies* have a thin myelin sheath (presumably to speed conduction) and myelinated peripheral and central processes. Their peripheral processes lose their myelin as they emerge from the osseous spinal lamina; they come into direct contact with the inner row of hair cells.

Their central processes form the cochlear nerve proper.

The unipolar neurons are entirely unmyelinated. Their peripheral processes are distributed to the outer hair cells. The destination of their central processes is

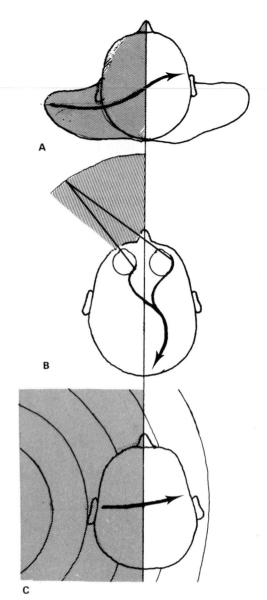

Fig. 30-1　A, body field; B, visual field; C, sound field.

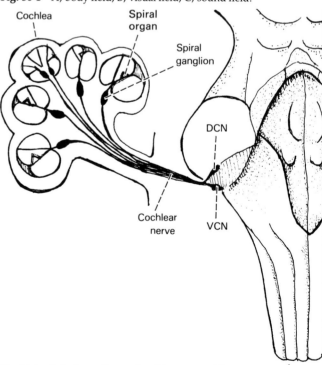

Fig. 30-2　Spiral ganglion and cochlear nerve. The nerve terminates in dorsal (DCN) and ventral (VCN) cochlear nuclei.

uncertain: few if any reach the brain stem. They may terminate upon the nodes of myelinated bipolar neurons. Both their function and that of the outer hair cells are unknown. Action potentials recorded from the main cochlear nerve all appear to be derived from myelinated neurons supplying inner hair cells.

Efferent innervation

The inner and outer rows of hair cells are also supplied with *efferent* nerve fibers that run to the ear from the brain stem. The inner hair cells have small efferent contacts, the outer cells have large ones.

Cochlear nerve (Fig. 30-2)

The *cochlear nerve* is made up of the central processes of spiral ganglion cells. It descends the modiolus and emerges into the internal acoustic meatus. It accompanies the vestibular nerve across the subarachnoid space, pierces the side of the brainstem at the pontomedullary junction, and enters the cochlear nucleus.

From the internal acoustic meatus to the brain stem (a distance of 15–20 mm) the cochlear nerve is invested by central gliocytes (oligodendrocytes and astroglia).

Activation of cochlear nerve

Inward movements of the footplate of stapes (at the oval window) produce *traveling waves* along the basilar membrane. They resemble pulse waves traveling along one side of an arterial wall. The strings of the basilar membrane are transverse to the direction of the waves, and the strings are longer and thinner toward the apex of the cochlea. High-frequency waves, generated by high-pitched tones, are damped out by movement of the short (0.1 mm), thick strings in the basal turn. Low-frequency waves travel to the apex, where they cause displacement of the long (0.4 mm), thin strings. A given tone has a particular site of maximal displacement of the basilar membrane. At this site the spiral organ is shaken and the cilia of the hair cells are dragged against the tectorial membrane or against the endolymph. The drag opens a minute *cuticular pore* adjacent to the longest cilium on each cell, permitting movement of ions through the pore and creating a receptor potential at the cell surface. When the receptor potential reaches the base of the cell, Ca^{2+} ions enter and synaptic vesicles are released to excite the cochlear nerve ending. A major puzzle is the unequal distribution of myelinated and unmyelinated afferent fibers to the inner and outer hair cells.

Each cochlear nerve fiber has a characteristic firing frequency ('tuning curve'), related to the local vibration frequency of the spiral membrane. Like primary afferents in general, all of the afferent cochlear fibers are excitatory at their central synapses. The transmitter may be glutamate or aspartate.

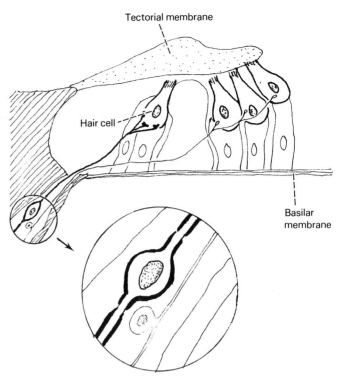

Fig. 30-3 Spiral organ. Inset: myelinated bipolar neuron (left) and unmyelinated unipolar neuron (right) from the spiral ganglion.

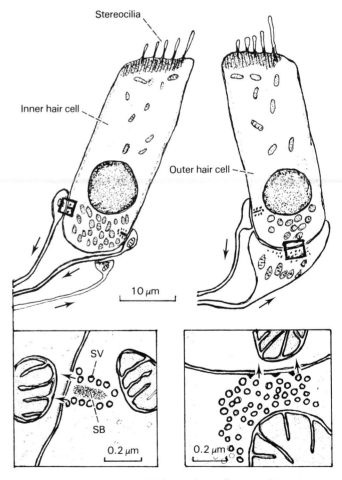

Fig. 30-4 Cochlear neuroepithelium. Three afferent and two efferent nerve fibers are shown. Boxed areas enlarged below: SB, synaptic bar; SV, synaptic vesicles.

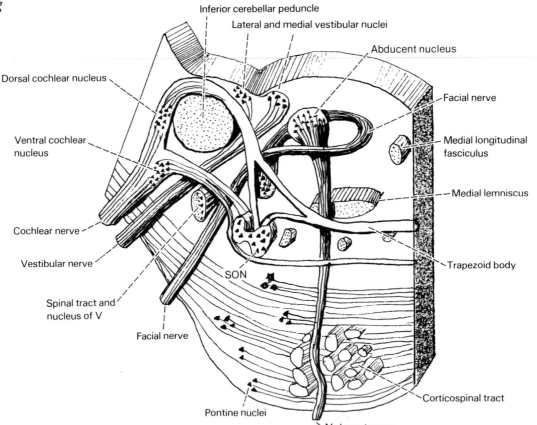

Fig. 30-5 Abducent, facial, and vestibulocochlear nerves. SON, superior olivary nucleus.

Cochlear nucleus (Figs. 30-5, 30-6)

The ventral and dorsal cochlear nuclei (VCN, DCN) lie on the respective sides of the inferior cerebellar peduncle. Each myelinated cochlear fiber divides to enter both nuclei, and the arrangement of terminals is orderly (tonotopic).

Most of the second-order neurons cross in the *trapezoid body*. The trapezoid body is a composite structure straddling the midline at the pontomedullary junction. Its largest component is made up of intersecting second-order cochlear afferents from the right and left sides. The ventral and dorsal *acoustic striae* contain fibers that enter the opposite lateral lemniscus; some of them run all the way to the inferior colliculus.

The trapezoid body also contains intrinsic nuclei which receive afferents from the cochlear nucleus and project to the superior olivary complex.

Function

The ventral cochlear nucleus is relatively simple and nerve impulses undergo little transformation there. For this reason the impulse trains in the ventral acoustic stria are called 'primary-like' (i.e., like those in the primary afferents).

The dorsal cochlear nucleus is complex, containing at least six types of neuron differing in their morphology and electrical behavior. The DCN is evidently involved in *frequency analysis* of primary afferent impulses, but the nature of this analysis is obscure. DCN efferents project to the opposite inferior colliculus.

Superior olivary nucleus

The main nucleus (known from its shape as the S segment) consists of *binaural neurons*, receiving inputs

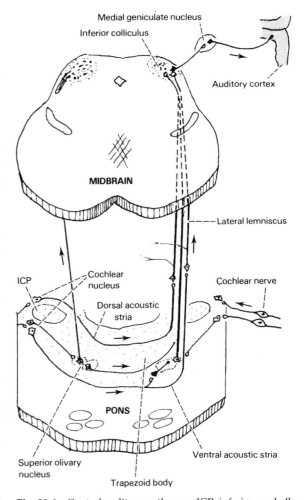

Fig. 30-6 Central auditory pathways. ICP, inferior cerebellar peduncle.

from the VCN of both sides. The ipsilateral DCN input is excitatory; the contralateral is inhibitory. The inhibitory effect derives from impulse passage through the *dorsal nucleus of the trapezoid body*, which projects GABA-secreting axons onto the S segment. The giant synaptic contacts received by the dorsal nucleus are known as the calyces of Held (Fig. 30-7).

The superior olivary nucleus projects to *both* inferior colliculi: *the central auditory pathway is therefore partly uncrossed*. The ipsilateral component of the lateral lemniscus is usually held accountable for the apparent absence of contralateral deafness in patients following a temporal lobectomy (removal of the primary auditory cortex).

Function

The S segment is responsive to intensity differences between the sounds entering the two ears from one side. By exaggerating these differences through the inhibitory internuncials, it is evidently concerned in coding the *direction of sounds in space*. Other cells in the superior olivary complex contribute to this function by responding to the minute time difference of sounds entering the ears from one side.

Lateral lemniscus

The lateral lemniscus ascends through the pons to reach the inferior colliculus (see Figs. 12-7 to 12-11). Its fibers arise (a) in the dorsal and ventral cochlear nuclei of the opposite side, and (b) in the superior olivary complex of both sides. It terminates in the central nucleus of the inferior colliculus. Some of the lemniscal fibers are interrupted by scattered *nuclei of the lateral lemniscus*.

Brain stem reflexes

Fibers derived from the superior olivary and lemniscal nuclei provide the afferent limbs of some acoustic reflexes:
1 Fibers entering the motor nuclei of the trigeminal and facial nerves exert a damping effect on the ossicles of the middle ear (tensor tympani and stapedius muscles). The facial connection accounts for the blinking/flinching response to a loud noise.
2 Fibers entering the parvocellular component of the reticular formation account for the arousal effect of noise (for instance, an alarm clock).
3 The *startle reflex* is the generalized contraction of the voluntary muscles in response to sudden loud noise. Reticulospinal fibers are likely to be involved, but there may be a transcortical loop through the temporal lobe (this is suggested by the fact that in some subjects convulsions may be induced by sudden loud noise).

Inferior colliculus

Spatial information (from the superior olivary nucleus) and frequency information (from the dorsal cochlear nucleus) are integrated in the inferior colliculus. The left and right colliculi are interconnected by commissural fibers and they receive descending fibers from the

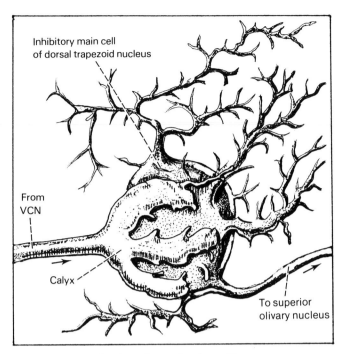

Fig. 30-7 Calyceal ending of second-order cochlear neuron upon inhibitory dorsal trapezoid neuron. VCN, ventral cochlear nucleus. (After Morest, 1965.)

medial geniculate nucleus. Many of the collicular neurons are binaural.

The main (central) nucleus is laminated in a tonotopic manner. The discharge pattern varies from cell to cell within a lamina: some have characteristic tuning curves (they respond to particular tones), some have a wide tonal range, some fire spontaneously but are inhibited by sound, and some respond only to a moving source of sound.

The principal output from the inferior colliclus is the *inferior brachium*, to the medial geniculate body. Other fibers enter the tectobulbar and tectospinal tracts, which originate in the superior colliculus. The auditory input facilitates turning of the head and eyes toward a source of sound.

Function

The capacity of individual inferior collicular neurons for *feature extraction* (to detect particular tonal or directional frequencies) is very advanced for a subcortical structure. In the somatosensory system, such capabilities are found only at the level of the posterior primary sensory cortex (area 2) and in the sensory association cortex (area 5). However, the capabilities of the inferior colliculus are not surprising on phylogenetic grounds: in reptiles, the inferior colliculus is the highest auditory center.

Medial geniculate nucleus

The medial geniculate nucleus (MGN) is the specific thalamic relay center for hearing. The main, ventral nucleus contains transmission cells projecting to the

213

primary auditory cortex. The dendrites of these cells are tufted (Fig. 30-8) and receive synaptic contacts from three sources: the inferior colliculus, the primary auditory cortex, and inhibitory internuncials within the nucleus. The synaptology is very complex. The nucleus is laminated and tonotopic.

Functions

These are at present unknown. No particular feature is known as yet by which the MCN can be described as 'superior' to the inferior colliculus.

The geniculocortical projection forms the *acoustic radiation*, which passes below the posterior limb of the internal capsule and the lentiform nucleus to reach the primary auditory cortex.

Auditory cortex (Fig. 30-9)

The *primary auditory cortex* (areas 41 and 42 of Brodmann) includes the gyrus of Heschl on the upper surface of the superior temporal gyrus, and the adjoining part of the temporal operculum of the insula. 'Columnar organization' is obvious, the 'columns' being in fact stripes disposed mediolaterally. Each stripe is an isofrequency band, and the cortical arrangement is tonotopic: high tones excite the posterior stripes and low tones excite the anterior ones. The stripes are maximally excited from the *contralateral sound field*. Virtually all of the neurons are binaural.

In cats, selective destruction within the primary cortex produces 'sigomas' in the contralateral auditory field, comparable with the contralateral scotomas (blind spots) produced by selective destruction within the primary visual cortex. The auditory cortex would not be expected to show alternating left ear–right ear dominance columns because the left auditory field (for example) has primary access to the left ear whereas the left visual field has equal access to both eyes. Contralateral ear dominance has also been detected in the MGB, inferior colliculus, and superior olivary nucleus. The acoustic striae are the counterparts of the optic chiasm, of the somatosensory decussation in the medulla, and of the spinothalamic decussation in the white commissure of the cord.

The *auditory association cortex* (area 22) occupies the lateral surface of the superior temporal gyrus. It receives short association fibers from the primary cortex and integrates incoming sounds with auditory memory stores.

Area 22 has been subdivided into six cytoarchitectural areas. The most important is Wernicke's sensory speech area (Chapter 25).

Descending pathways

A cascade of descending fibers runs from the primary auditory cortex to the MGB and inferior colliculus, and from the inferior colliculus to the superior olivary nucleus. From the superior olivary nucleus, the *olivocochlear bundle* (OCB) travels to the cochleas of both sides. The crossed fibers end mainly on outer hair cells, the uncrossed fibers on the afferent terminals

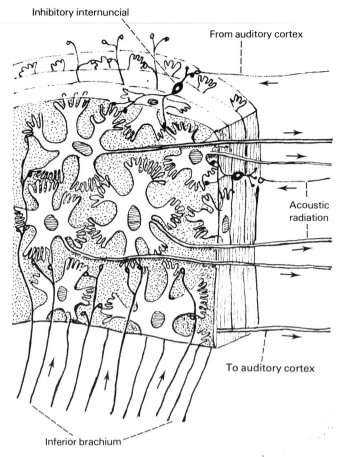

Fig. 30-8 Tufted main cells in medial geniculate body.

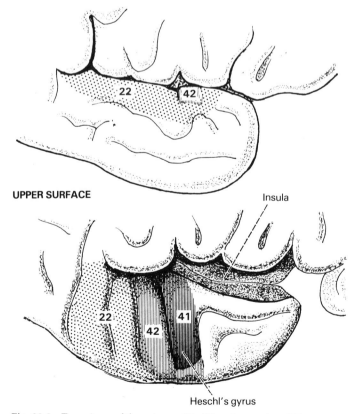

Fig. 30-9 Two views of the primary (41, 42) and secondary (22) auditory cortex.

supplying inner hair cells (Fig. 30-4). The OCB occupies the vestibular nerve at first, then transfers to the cochlear. The entire OCB is cholinergic, and the receptors have both nicotinic and muscarinic characters.

Functions

In the brainstem, the descending cascade is thought to facilitate selective transmission of wanted auditory information while suppressing unwanted information: it may be involved in selective auditory attention whereby, for example, we can single out an individual voice in a crowd (this is known as the 'cocktail party effect'). The evidence for this is largely anecdotal.

The OCB appears on experimental grounds to be concerned with facilitating hair cell transmission when the stimulus is close to threshold – that is, to improve the transduction of low-intensity sounds.

APPLIED ANATOMY

Conductive deafness results from disease in the outer or middle ear. The outer ear may be blocked by congenital atresia of the meatus in infants, or by accumulation of wax in adults. The middle ear is commonly affected by inflammation (otitis media), in which ossicular movement is impaired by fluid accumulation. The ossicles may be immobilized by congenital ankylosis following maternal rubella, or by otosclerosis in the oval window in adults.

Sensorineural deafness arises from disease of the cochlea or of the acoustic nerve. It is relatively rare. Causes include arterial disease in the elderly, ototoxic drugs (such as streptomycin, neocymicin, and quinine), Ménière's disease (Chapter 33), and acoustic neuroma (Chapter 33).

Conductive and sensorineural hearing loss can be differentiated by the Rinné and Weber tests (see clinical textbooks).

Unilateral lesions of the brainstem or temporal lobe produce no obvious reduction in auditory acuity, because sounds continue to be processed by the auditory pathway on the normal side. However, there may be difficulty in estimating the direction and distance of a sound source.

Vascular compression syndromes

The belief is growing that a variety of cranial-nerve clinical syndromes may be caused by compression of the affected nerves by branches of the vertebrobasal arterial system (Chapter 12). The compression is thought to affect particularly the glial investments that extend for a few millimeters along the rootlets of the nerves at risk (but 15–20 mm in the case of the cochlear nerve). Demyelination of the glial elements is thought to elicit ephapsis (cross-talk) among the component axons, including generation of action potentials traveling both proximally and distally. Vascular compression seems to account for some cases of trigeminal neuralgia

(Chapter 34), spasmodic contractions of facial muscles (facial nerve, Chapter 35), glossopharyngeal neuralgia (Chapter 36), and spasmodic torticollis (Chapter 36). Vascular compression has also been cited in some cases of *tinnitus* (a persistent ringing or rushing sound in one ear).

Readings

Brugge, J.F. and Geisler, C.D. (1978) Auditory mechanisms of the lower brain stem. *Annu. Rev. Neurosci., 1:* 363–394.

Carlier, E. and Pujol, R. (1982) Sectioning the efferent bundle decreases cochlear frequency selectivity. *Neurosci. Lett., 28:* 101–106.

Davis, M. (1984) The mammalian startle response. In *Neural Mechanisms of Startle Behavior* (Eaton, R.C., ed.), pp. 287–351. New York: Plenum.

Galaburda, A. and Sandies, F. (1980) Cytoarchitectonic organization of the human auditory cortex. *J. Comp. Neurol., 190:* 597–610.

Guth, P.S. and Melamed, B. (1982) Neurotransmission in the auditory system: a primer for pharmacologists. *Annu. Rev. Pharmacol. Toxicol., 22:* 383–412.

Heffner, H. and Masterson, B. (1978) Contribution of auditory cortex to hearing in the monkey. In *Recent Advances in Primatology, Vol. 1, Behaviour* (Chivers, D.J. and Herbert, J., eds.), pp. 734–754. London & New York: Academic Press.

Hungerbühler, J.P., Saunders, J.C., Greenberg, I. and Reivich, M. (1981) Functional neuroanatomy of the auditory cortex studied with [2-^{14}C]deoxyglucose. *Exp. Neurol., 71:* 104–121.

Jannetta, P.J. (1977) Observations on the etiology of trigeminal neuralgia, hemifacial spasm, acoustic nerve dysfunction, and glossopharyngeal neuralgia. Definitive microsurgical treatment and results in 117 cases. *Neurochirurgica (Stuttgart), 20:* 145–154.

Jenkins, W.M. and Masterson, R.B. (1982) Sound localization: effects of unilateral lesions in central auditory system. *J. Neurophysiol., 47:* 987–1016.

Majorossy, K. and Kiss, A. (1976) Specific patterns of neuron arrangement and of synaptic articulation in the medial geniculate body. *Exp. Brain Res., 26:* 1–17.

Masterson, R.B. (1984) Neural mechanisms for sound localization. *Annu. Rev. Physiol., 46:* 275–287.

Møller, A.R. (1984) Pathophysiology of tinnitus. *Ann. Otorhinolaryngol., 93:* 39–44.

Morest, D.K. (1965) The laminar structure of the medial geniculate body of the cat. *J. Anat., 99:* 143–160.

Phillips, D.P. and Gates, G.R. (1982) Representation of the two ears in the auditory cortex: a re-examination. *Int. J. Neurosci., 16:* 41–46.

Pickles, J.O. (1982) *An Introduction to the Physiology of Hearing.* London & New York: Academic Press.

Seldon, H.L. (1980) Structure of human auditory cortex. 2. Axon distributions and morphological correlates of speech perception. *Brain Res., 229:* 295–310.

Smith, C.A. (1975) The inner ear: its embryological development and microstructure. In *The Nervous System*, Vol. 3 (Tower, D.B., ed.), pp. 1–18. New York: Raven Press.

Spoendlin, H. (1981) Neuroanatomy of the cochlea. In *Audiology and Audiological Medicine, Vol. 1* (Beagley, H.A., ed.), pp. 72–102. Oxford: Oxford University Press.

Thompson, G.C. and Masterson, R.B. (1978) Brain stem pathways involved in reflexive orientation to sound. *J. Neurophysiol., 41:* 1183–1202.

Warr, W.B. (1982) Parallel ascending pathways from the cochlear nucleus. In *Contributions to Sensory Physiology*, Vol. 7, pp. 1–38. New York: Academic Press.

VII
OCULAR MUSCLES AND THEIR CONTROLS

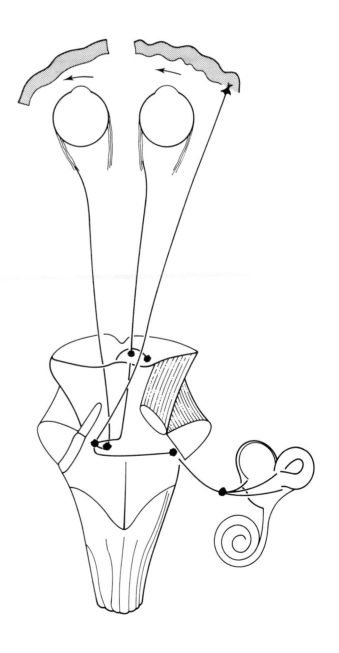

31
Ocular Muscles

The *extrinsic ocular muscles* are the four recti and the two obliques (Fig. 31-1). They all insert into the eyeball and rotate it to control the direction of gaze. They are striated muscles under voluntary control. They also have automatic controls, as described in Chapter 32.

The *intrinsic ocular muscles* are the sphincter and dilator pupillae and the ciliary muscle. They are smooth muscles under autonomic control.

Closely allied to the ocular muscles are the muscles of the eyelids (Fig. 31-2). *Levator palpebrae superioris* is inserted into the superior tarsal plate. It is mostly composed of striated fibers subject to the same controls as the extrinsic ocular muscles. Its lowermost fibers are smooth, and are continuous with Müller's muscle (*orbitalis*), which invests the eyeball and enters both lids. Müller's muscle causes a variable degree of 'popeye' in response to sympathetic stimulation.

OCULAR MOTOR NERVES

The oculomotor, trochlear, and abducent nuclei lie ventral to the central canal. They are in line with the hypoglossal nucleus, which completes the somatic efferent cell column supplying myotomes of cranial origin.

Oculomotor nerve (III)

Nucleus. The nucleus is at the level of the superior colliculus (Fig. 31-3). It is compound, having four

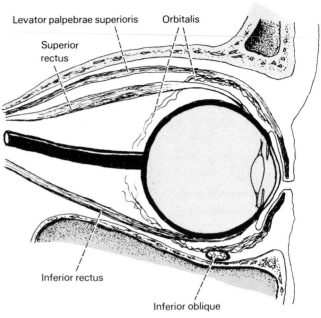

Fig. 31-2 Sagittal section through the orbit.

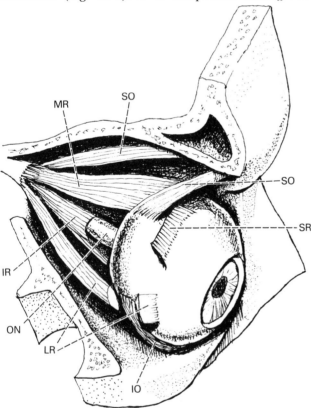

Fig. 31-1 Extrinsic ocular muscles. IO, inferior oblique; IR, inferior rectus; LR, lateral rectus; MR, medial rectus; ON, optic nerve; SO, superior oblique; SR, superior rectus.

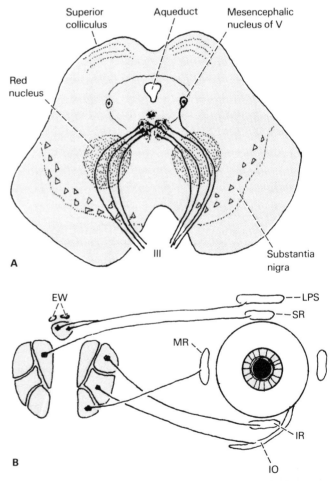

Fig. 31-3 A, oculomotor nerve (III) in midbrain. The mesencephalic nucleus of the trigeminal (V) receives muscle spindle afferents from all of the extrinsic ocular muscles. B, oculomotor supply to extrinsic ocular muscles. EW, Edinger–Westphal nucleus (distribution not shown); IO, inferior oblique; IR, inferior rectus; LPS, levator palpebrae superioris; MR, medial rectus; SR, superior rectus.

218

somatic divisions and one parasympathetic (Edinger–Westphal nucleus). The nuclear group for superior rectus is contralateral.

Course and distribution. The nerve fibers pass through the red nucleus and substantia nigra, uniting as they emerge into the interpeduncular cistern. The nerve runs in the lateral wall of the cavernous sinus and breaks into upper and lower divisions as it traverses the superior orbital fissure. The upper division supplies the levator palpebrae superioris and the superior rectus. The lower division supplies the inferior and medial recti and the inferior oblique.

Trochlear nerve (IV)

Nucleus. The nucleus is at the level of the inferior colliculi (Fig. 31-4).

Course and distribution. The fibers wind around the aqueduct and cross the midline before emerging below the colliculi. The nerve then passes around the crus of midbrain and runs in the lateral wall of the cavernous sinus to reach the superior orbital fissure. Its only target is the superior oblique.

Abducent nerve (VI)

Nucleus. The abducent nucleus occupies the pons, at the level of the facial colliculus.

Course and distribution. The nerve emerges at the lower border of the pons and courses rostrally in the pontine CSF cistern. It angles over the apex of the petrous temporal bone, runs forward in the cavernous sinus beside the internal carotid artery, and passes through the superior orbital fissure. Its only target is the lateral rectus.

Actions of extrinsic muscles

The actions of the extrinsic muscles from the resting, mid-position of the eyeballs are listed in Table 31-1.

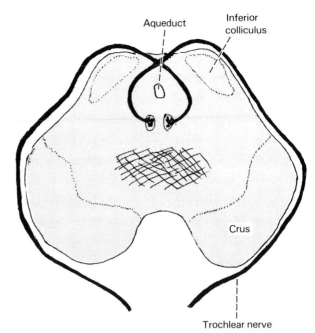

Fig. 31-4 Trochlear nerve (IV).

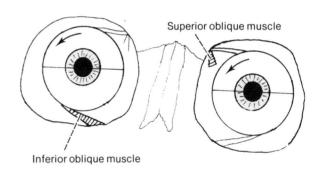

Fig. 31-5 Torsion of the eyeballs. The subject's right eye is undergoing extorsion; the left eye is undergoing intorsion.

Table 31-1 Innervation and actions of extrinsic ocular muscles

| Nerve | Muscle | Actions on eyeball | |
		Primary	Secondary
Oculomotor	Sup. rectus	Elevation	Adduction
	Inf. rectus	Depression	Adduction
	Medial rectus	Adduction	
	Inf. oblique	Elevation	Extorsion
Trochlear	Sup. oblique	Depression	Intorsion
Abducent	Lat. rectus	Abduction	

The movements of extorsion and intorsion are shown in Fig. 31-5. These movements maintain the eyeballs in the horizontal plane during moderate side-to-side tilts of the head.

The motor units

All of the ocular motor units are small, containing about ten muscle fibers (compared with 1000 or more in the tibialis anterior). Most units are divisible into three functional categories, like striated muscles elsewhere (Chapter 4), but two further types have been described. Both receive multiple end plates (a dozen or more) from single nerve fibers spiraling around the individual muscle fibers. One type is slow-twitch; the other is only capable of local, non-propagated contraction beneath each plate. Although there is no direct evidence, one or both may be involved in keeping the two visual axes parallel or slightly convergent. This requires continuous muscular action, even during sleep.

AUTONOMIC NERVES

Sympathetic fibers

The sympathetic pathway from hypothalamus to eyeball is about 50 cm (20 inches) long in adults. It is uncrossed throughout. Its great length makes it vulnerable to disease of the brainstem, spinal cord, upper thorax, and head and neck.

Course (Fig. 31-6)

1 From the posterior hypothalamic area, the *central sympathetic pathway* descends in the posterior longitudinal fasciculus and continues beside the intermediate gray matter of the spinal cord. Fibers controlling the eye synapse in the lateral gray horn in segment T1.

2 The *preganglionic fibers* emerge in the ventral root of the first thoracic spinal nerve and enter the sympathetic chain. The fibers turn upward and pass through the stellate and middle cervical ganglia without interruption before synapsing in the superior cervical ganglion.

3 *Postganglionic fibers* accompany the internal carotid artery through the carotid canal. In the cavernous sinus they form a periarterial plexus in the adventitia of the artery (Fig. 31-7). The ocular fibers enter the superior fissure and run to the eyeball in the long ciliary nerves.

Distribution

Excitatory fibers supply the dilator pupillae, Müller's muscle, and the blood vessels of the eye. Inhibitory fibers supply the ciliary muscle and the sphincter pupillae. The transmitter in both cases is norepinephrine, and the different effects depend upon the type of receptor being activated (Figs. 31-8, 31-9).

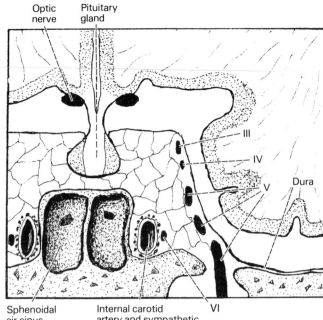

Fig. 31-7 Cavernous sinus, frontal section.

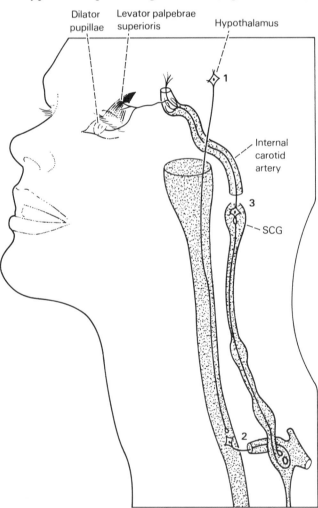

Fig. 31-6 The U-shaped sympathetic pathway from the hypothalamus to the eye. The pathway is ipsilateral throughout. For explanation of numbers see text. SCG, superior cervical ganglion. (Modified from Patten, 1980.)

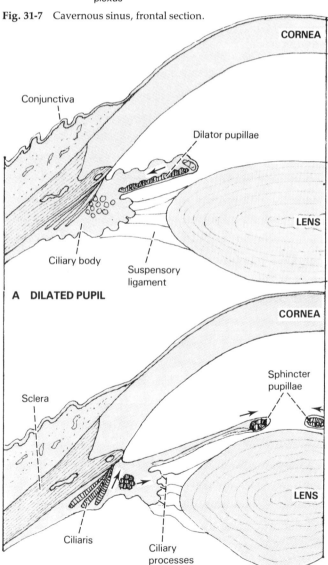

B CONSTRICTED PUPIL + ACCOMMODATION

Fig. 31-8 A, dilator pupillae retracts the iris. B, sphincter pupillae narrows the pupil. The ciliary muscle pulls the ciliary processes forward and centrally, relaxing the suspensory ligament and allowing the lens to bulge.

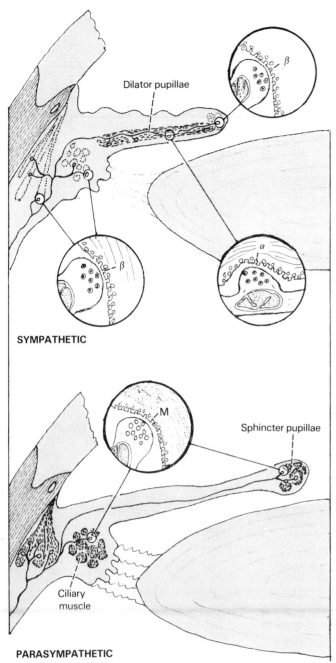

Fig. 31-9 Innervation of intrinsic ocular muscles. Receptor types are indicated: M, muscarinic cholinergic; α, β, adrenergic.

Parasympathetic fibers

From the Edinger–Westphal nucleus, preganglionic fibers accompany the oculomotor nerve to the orbit. They leave the nerve to inferior oblique and synapse in the ciliary ganglion, which lies lateral to the optic nerve (Fig. 31-10). The postganglionic fibers run in the short ciliary nerves, which pierce the lamina cribrosa (L., sieve-like layer) of the sclera. They supply only the ciliary muscle and the sphincter pupillae, which contract in response to activation of muscarinic receptors (Fig. 31-9).

Pupillary light reflex (Fig. 31-11)

Contraction of the pupils in response to light is a four-limb reflex:

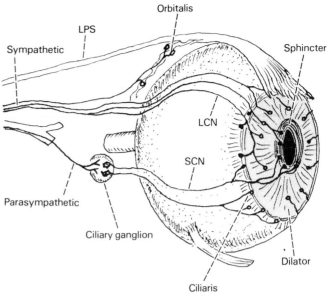

Fig. 31-10 Autonomic supply to intrinsic ocular muscles. Inhibitory sympathetic terminals are shown in black. LCN, SCN, long and short ciliary nerves; LPS, levator palpebrae superioris.

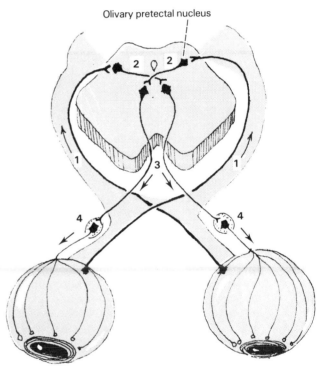

Fig. 31-11 Pupillary light reflex for both temporal fields:
1 Retinopretectal fibers
2 Connection to contralateral Edinger–Westphal nucleus
3 Preganglionic fibers
4 Postganglionic fibers to sphincter pupillae

1 The afferent limb runs from the ganglionic layer of the retina to the midbrain. Conduction rate here is slow (10 meters per second) – indicative of W cell activity (Chapter 28). The fibers from each eye enter both optic tracts and terminate in the *pretectal nucleus*, in the tegmentum ventral to the superior colliculus. The pretectal nucleus has several subdivisions; the *olivary* pretectal nucleus is involved here.

2 The internuncial limb is short: it connects the olivary pretectal nucleus to the Edinger–Westphal

221

(parasympathetic) nucleus of the oculomotor nerve. In monkeys at least, these fibers are all crossed.

3 From the EW nucleus, pupilloconstrictor fibers travel in the oculomotor nerve and synapse in the ciliary ganglion.

4 Postganglionic fibers run in the short ciliary nerves and activate the sphincter pupillae.

Because of the bilateral W cell input to the midbrain both pupils constrict when light is directed into one eye (*consensual reflex*).

Accommodation: the near response

When the eyes view an object close up, as in reading, the ciliary muscle contracts reflexly and allows the lens to become more convex, thus increasing its refractive power. This is *accommodation*. At the same time, the pupils constrict and the two eyes converge so that their visual axes intersect in the plane of the object. The three reactions – ciliary contraction, pupillary constriction, and vergence – constitute the *near response*. The function of pupillary constriction is to prevent spherical aberration effects near the margin of the lens.

Pathway for the accommodation reflex (Fig. 31-12)

Accommodation depends upon stereoscopic analysis of the object by the visual association cortex, where some cortical columns are set aside for this purpose (Chapter 32). This is a bilateral exercise involving cross-talk through the corpus callosum. The efferent pathway from the hemispheres appears to be from the frontal eye fields, since stimulation of area 8 may elicit accommodatory responses. Animal experiments suggest the existence of a specific accommodation center in the caudal midbrain, linked to the Edinger–Westphal nucleus. Accordingly, at least nine sets of neurons are involved, taking the ganglionic layer of the retina as the starting point.

The nature of the adequate stimulus for the accommodation reflex is uncertain. A blurred image alone is insufficient, since the eyes do not accommodate in response to an out-of-focus photograph. Spherical and chromatic aberration effects are probably involved. Only the macular (foveal) retinas are active in initiating the reflex.

At least in the monkey and cat, the *cerebellum* is involved as well. The interpositus and fastigial nuclei both discharge to the oculomotor nucleus while accommodation is taking place. The reason for cerebellar participation is not known. It must be assumed that the cerebellar cortex is informed about the activity of the cerebral cortex, perhaps through corticopontocerebellar connections.

Accommodation: the far response

When the eyes are viewing a blank field, whether in total darkness or in gazing at a clear blue sky, accommodation is not relaxed. In fact, the gaze is fixed at a point only 0.5–1.0 m away. Looking at a distant object requires *sympathetic activity*, which induces (a)

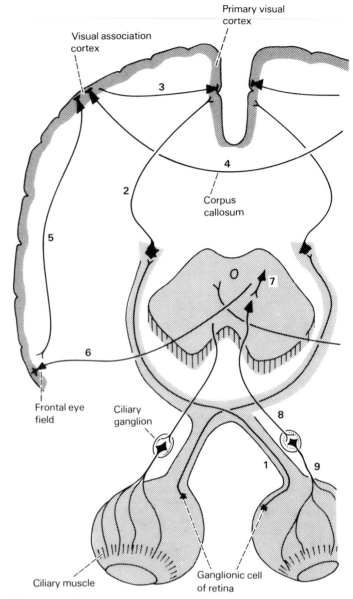

Fig. 31-12 Minimal neuronal circuit for accommodation:
1 Retinogeniculate
2 Geniculocalcarine
3 Primary to association cortex
4 Callosal interconnections for stereopsis
5 Projection to frontal eye field
6 Projection to accommodation center in midbrain
7 Internuncial to Edinger–Westphal cells specified for accommodation
8 Preganglionic fibers to ciliary ganglion
9 Postganglionic fibers to sphincter pupillae and ciliary muscle

complete inhibition of the ciliary muscle, with pronounced flattening of the lens, and (b) moderate inhibition of the pupillary sphincter. It is not yet clear how the relaxation of tonic muscle fibers in the medial recti is brought about.

Cervical sympathectomy, or stellate block (Chapter 6) enhances the speed of contraction of the pupil in the near response. (It diminishes the range of response because the pupil is already small.) Sympathetic stimulation, on the other hand, promotes the far response. Students sitting an important written test may have difficulty in reading the examination paper because of heightened sympathetic activity.

APPLIED ANATOMY

Ocular motor palsies

The oculomotor, trochlear and abducent nerves may be paralyzed individually or collectively, anywhere between the brain stem and the orbit.

Brain stem lesions involving these nuclei are rare. So too, fortunately, is thrombosis of the cavernous sinus. The commonest lesions occur in the subarachnoid space during transit from brain stem to cavernous sinus. The oculomotor or abducent nerve may be paralyzed by herniation of the temporal lobe of the brain into the tentorial notch (Fig. 31-13). The horizontal shift may paralyze *either* of the abducent nerves or the *ipsilateral* oculomotor. Oculomotor paralysis is therefore of 'lateralizing' value in the search for space-occupying lesions inside the head, whereas abducent paralysis is not. The abducent nerve may also be paralyzed by tumors in the posterior cranial fossa.

In addition to the indirect pressures exerted by space-occupying lesions, an ocular motor nerve may be pressed upon by an aneurysm at the base of the brain, or directly involved in meningeal inflammation.

Inequality of the pupils (*anisocoria*) is occasionally seen in normal people. A mild drooping of one or both eyelids, without pupillary changes, may also be encountered. In the elderly, the pupils are usually small and react sluggishly. They *will* react if the light is bright enough.

Oculomotor nerve paralysis

The finest fibers are the first to be paralyzed. These are the parasympathetic ones, and the result of compression is a dilated pupil which may react sluggishly to light (Fig. 31-14A).

As the somatic fibers become involved, the patient progressively loses power to move the eye, except in abduction, and there may be partial ptosis. There is no strabismus (squint) at rest (Fig. 31-14B).

If an oculomotor nerve palsy becomes complete, the unimpeded lateral rectus pulls the eye into fixed abduction. Ptosis is complete, and the pupil is fully dilated and non-reactive (Fig. 31-15).

The pupils and the unconscious patient

The large majority of patients who are found in coma are suffering from drug overdose (including insulin) or diabetic coma. If there has been a head injury, monitoring of the pupils may reveal evidence of an expanding epidural or subdural hematoma needing urgent surgical decompression. The following are important guides:

1 If the pupils are normal and reactive, the patient is in no immediate danger from raised intracranial pressure.

2 If one pupil becomes dilated and is unresponsive to light, uncal herniation (Chapter 2) must be suspected.

3 If both pupils become dilated and fixed in the presence of raised intracranial pressure, the patient will die within 24 hours, regardless of treatment.

4 If both pupils are pin-point in the presence of raised intracranial pressure, the patient will die within 12 hours from compression of the hypothalamus.

It is essential to distinguish brain compression from drug overdose, because one can mimic the other. As examples, amphetamine or cocaine poisoning dilates and fixes the pupils but the patient's life can be saved. (Both of these drugs potentiate the action of the sympathetic system.) In morphine poisoning the pupils are constricted because of a direct action of the drug on the frontal eye fields, stimulating the efferent limb of the accommodation reflex.

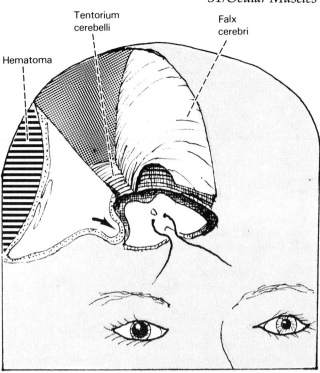

Fig. 31-13 Arrow indicates herniation of temporal lobe into the tentorial notch, causing an early lesion of the parasympathetic fibers in the right oculomotor nerve.

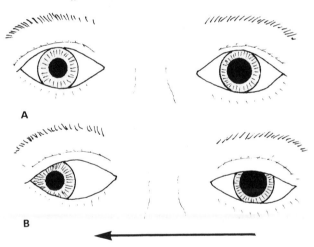

Fig. 31-14 A, early oculomotor nerve lesion on patient's left. Adduction, elevation and depression may be slightly impaired. B, later oculomotor lesion. The affected eye cannot be adducted (arrow); nor can it be elevated or depressed. However, it can be abducted.

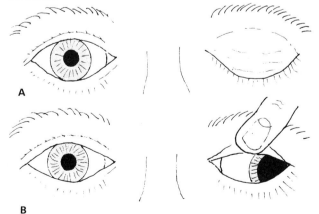

Fig. 31-15 Complete left oculomotor paralysis. A, the left eye is closed (ptosis is complete). B, passive opening shows an abducted pupil (unopposed lateral rectus), which is dilated (unopposed dilator pupillae).

Trochlear nerve paralysis

An isolated trochlear paralysis is rare. When combined with an oculomotor or abducent nerve paralysis it is very hard to detect. With an isolated palsy, the pupils are not at quite the same level (Fig. 31-16). The patient compensates by tilting the head to the other side. The inequality is more pronounced when the patient looks downward. The patient may complain of diplopia (double vision) on going downstairs, or while reading. An isolated trochlear nerve paralysis in a young adult may be the first symptom of multiple sclerosis. The lesion in such cases is probably in the medial longitudinal fasciculus (see below).

Abducent nerve paralysis

In an early abducent lesion, the patient has no strabismus at rest. It appears only when the patient attempts full abduction toward the weak side (Fig. 31-17). Later, the unopposed medial rectus produces a convergent squint (and diplopia) at rest (Fig. 31-18) and in all positions except full abduction of the normal eye.

Note on internuclear ophthalmoplegia

A lesion of one medial longitudinal fasciculus, in the 2 cm interval between the abducent and oculomotor nuclei, produces an isolated paralysis of the medial rectus muscle on that side. This can be explained on the grounds of interruption of axons traveling from the contralateral pontine generator. Classically, internuclear ophthalmoplegia is associated with nystagmus of the contralateral eye during lateral gaze. If the right fasciculus is damaged, therefore, the patient cannot adduct the right eye on looking to the left, and shows a divergent squint on doing so because the left abducent nerve is functional. However, the left lateral rectus is not operating normally because the left eye shows oscillation (nystagmus) during abduction. The reason for this lies in deficient inhibition of the left medial rectus during the saccade, which results in a to-and-fro antagonism between the two left recti concerned.

Horner's syndrome

Unilateral, moderate drooping (ptosis) of the eyelid, together with a small pupil, suggests paralysis of the sympathetic supply to that eye (Fig. 31-19). This pair of signs constitutes *Horner's syndrome*.

Horner's syndrome is of great clinical importance. Unless present from birth (rare) major pathology must be suspected somewhere along the U-shaped sympathetic pathway from the hypothalamus to the eye. In the brainstem or cervical spinal cord, it is most commonly produced by a plaque of multiple sclerosis. In the first thoracic spinal nerve or stellate ganglion, it may be produced by an apical lung cancer or by a cervical rib (an additional rib attached to a cervical vertebra). In the cervical chain, it may be produced by pressure from a thyroid cancer or by lymph nodes enlarged by metastatic cancer. Intracranially, it may be produced by arterial disease.

Anhidrosis – inability to sweat – may be found on the ipsilateral side of the face, but only if the lesion is below the superior cervical ganglion.

It is possible to tell by means of drugs whether or not the pathway from the superior cervical ganglion to the eye is anatomically intact. If it is intact, the dilator pupillae has a normal population of adrenergic endings, which however are silent because they are not being driven by preganglionic neurons. In this case *cocaine* instilled into the eye will cause the pupil to dilate. Cocaine blocks monoamine oxidase and allows the normal leakage of norepinephrine from the dense-cored vesicles to escape from the terminal axoplasm.

If the nerve endings are *absent*, the number of α adrenoceptors in the dilator pupillae will increase (denervation supersensitivity, Chapter 26). A 0.1% solution of

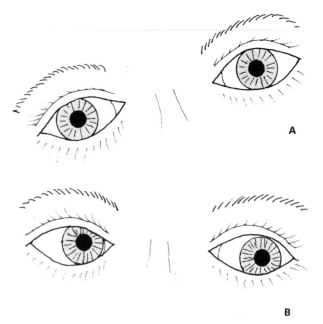

Fig. 31-16 Left trochlear nerve paralysis. A, the patient tilts the head to compensate for the slightly skewed gaze. B, diplopia (double vision) is evident when the head is horizontal.

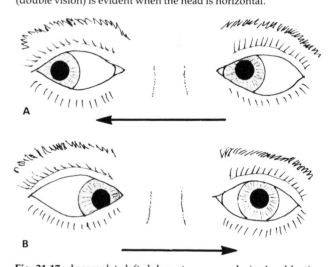

Fig. 31-17 Incomplete left abducent nerve paralysis. A, adduction is normal; so too are elevation and depression. B, strabismus appears when the patient attempts to abduct the affected eye.

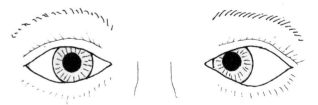

Fig. 31-18 Complete left abducent paralysis, resting position.

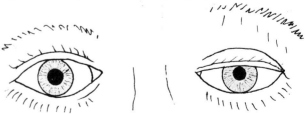

Fig. 31-19 Left Horner's syndrome, revealed by ptosis and miosis. The left eyebrow may be raised by the occipitofrontalis to help lift the eyelid.

epinephrine instilled into the eye will be too weak to stimulate a normally innervated dilator muscle, but it will cause a denervated dilator to contract.

Enophthalmos – a recession of the eyeball into its socket – is sometimes noticeable in Horner's syndrome as a result of paralysis of the orbitalis muscle. The nose may be 'stuffed' on the affected side, because of vasodilatation.

The oculomotor nerve is intact in Horner's syndrome, and the small pupil contracts further in response to light or in accommodation.

The *darkness reflex* is the expansion of the pupil that normally occurs when the ambient light is switched off, because of reduced pupilloconstrictor activity in darkness. After sympathetic denervation the rate of expansion of the pupil is reduced on the affected side.

Horner's syndrome may appear as an isolated disorder in adults, for which no underlying pathology can be found.

Argyll Robertson pupils

Argyll Robertson pupils are small and unreactive to light. They do accommodate (mnemonic: *Accommodation Retained*). Causes include diabetes, tertiary syphilis, and encephalitis. The site of the lesion has been traditionally assigned to the pretectal nuclei. Local disease of the myoepithelial cells of the dilator pupillae is more likely because the patient's pupil dilates sluggishly, or not at all, when the sphincter is paralyzed by atropine. The contraction of the sphincter in accommodation is stronger than that in response to light – sufficient, presumably, to overcome the inertia of a diseased dilator.

Holmes-Adie pupil

A Holmes-Adie pupil is dilated and unresponsive to light. It may react slowly (several minutes) to accommodation. The eye disorder is unilateral as a rule. Complete neurological examination usually reveals loss of tendon reflexes and impairment of sweating. The etiology is unknown, but the cause of the neurological deficits is a widespread degeneration of autonomic ganglion cells (including those of the ciliary ganglion) and of spinal ganglion cells.

Readings

Carpenter, M.B. and Pierson, R.J. (1973) Pretectal region and the pupillary light reflex. An anatomical analysis in the monkey. *J. Comp. Neurol.*, 149: 271–300.

Chiarandini, D.J. and Davidowitz, J. (1979) Structure and function of extraocular muscle fibers. In *Current Topics in Eye Research*, Vol. 1 (Adduniasky, J.A. and Davson, H., eds.), pp. 91–142. New York: Grune & Stratton.

Hulborton, H., Mori, K. and Tsukahara (1978) The neuronal pathway subserving the pupillary light reflex. *Brain Res.*, 159: 255–267.

Kommerell, G. (1984) Supranuclear and nuclear disorders of eye movement. In *Neuro-ophthalmology*, Vol. 3 (Lessell, S. and van Dalen, J.T.W., eds.), pp. 230–239. Amsterdam: Elsevier; New York: Oxford University Press.

Lee, R.J. and Zee, D.S. (1983) *The Neurology of Eye Movements.* Philadelphia: Davis.

Manni, E. and Bortolami, R. (1981) Proprioception in eye muscles. In *Functional Basis of Ocular Motility Disorders* (Lennerstrand, G., Zee, D.S. and Keller, E.L., eds.), pp. 65–70. Oxford & New York: Academic Press.

Namba, T., Nakamura, T. and Grob, D. (1968) Motor nerve endings in human extraocular muscles. *Neurology*, 18: 403–407.

Neufeld, A.H. (1984) The mechanisms of action of adrenergic drugs in the eye. In *Applied Pharmacology in the Medical Treatment of Glaucomas* (Drance, S.M., ed.), pp. 277–301. New York: Grune & Stratton.

Owens, D.A. (1984) The resting state of the eyes. *Am. Sci.*, 72: 378–387.

Patten, J.P. (1980) *Neurological Differential Diagnosis.* London: Harold Starke.

Pierson, R.J. and Carpenter, M.B. (1974) Anatomical analysis of pupillary light reflex pathways in the rhesus monkey. *J. Comp. Neurol.*, 158: 121–144.

Poggio, G.F. (1984) The analysis of stereopsis. *Annu. Rev. Neurosci.*, 7: 379–412.

Sacks, J.G. (1983) Peripheral innervation of extraocular muscles. *Am. J. Ophthalmol.*, 95: 520–527.

Sinnreich, Z. and Nathan, H. (1981) The ciliary ganglion in man. *Anat. Anz.*, 150: 287–297.

Spencer, R.F. and Porter, J.D. (1981) Innervation and structure of extraocular muscles in the monkey in comparison with those of the cat. *J. Comp. Neurol.*, 198: 649–663.

Thompson, H.S. (1984) The pupil. In *Neuro-ophthalmology*, Vol. 3 (Lessell, S. and van Dalen, J.T.W., eds.), pp. 277–289. Amsterdam: Elsevier; New York: Oxford University Press.

Toates, F.M. (1972) Accommodation function of the human eye. *Physiol. Rev.*, 52: 828–863.

Ulrich, J. (1980) Morphological basis of Adie's syndrome. *Eur. Neurol.*, 19: 390–395.

Van der Wiel, H.L. and Van Gijn, J. (1982) Horner's syndrome: criteria for oculosympathetic denervation. *J. Neurol. Sci.*, 56: 293–298.

32
Extrinsic Ocular Muscle Controls

The two eyes always move together. This *conjugate* movement requires that the extrinsic ocular muscles of both sides be simultaneously controlled by neurons acting bilaterally on the ocular motor nuclei. There are local control centers in the brainstem, known as *gaze centers*, and these are controlled in turn by *visuomotor centers* in the superior colliculi and cerebral cortex.

THE GAZE CENTERS

The gaze centers are pattern generators belonging to the reticular formation. There are two in the pons (one for looking to the left, one for looking to the right) and four in the midbrain (two for looking up, two for looking down).

Most important clinically are the pontine gaze centers, formed by the *parabducent nuclei*, which are just lateral to the abducent nuclei. Each parabducent nucleus controls conjugate movement *toward its own side*.

CONJUGATE MOVEMENTS

There are four types of conjugate movements: saccades, tracking, vergence, and the vestibulo-ocular reflexes.

Saccades (Fig. 32-1)

Saccades are the movements used to switch the gaze from one visual target to another. They are the fastest movements of which the neuromuscular system is capable. They are also the most accurate: the switch is made without under- or overshoot.

The key cell type in the gaze centers is the 'burst' neuron, which discharges briefly at up to 1000 impulses per second onto the motoneuron pairs (left and right) producing the saccade. Between saccades the 'burst' neurons are under tonic inhibition. During saccades they disinhibit themselves by means of recurrent collaterals. When a saccade is complete the new position is held by 'tonic' neurons innervated in parallel.

Visuomotor centers

Automatic saccades (such as scanning movements used in reading) are controlled by the superior colliculus (SC). Retinal afferents enter the SC in the medial root of the optic tract. They terminate in a sheet of internuncial neurons arranged in a retinotopic manner for the ipsilateral half retinas. The internuncials

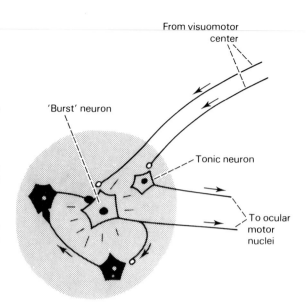

Fig. 32-1 Cell types in a gaze center. The 'burst' cell disinhibits itself when activated by the visuomotor centers.

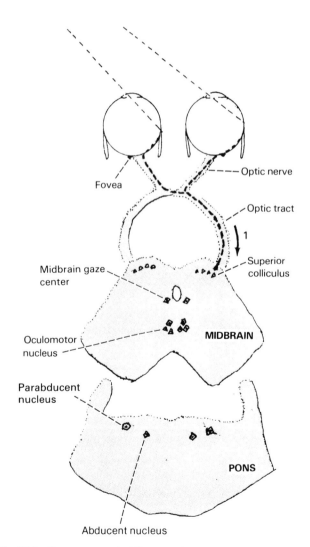

Fig. 32-2 Gaze centers of midbrain and pons.

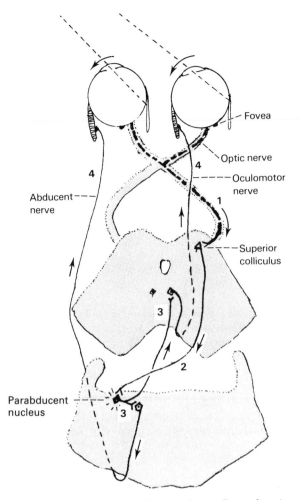

Fig. 32-3 Gaze centers of midbrain and pons. For explanation of numbers see text.

Voluntary saccades are initiated in the *frontal eye field* (FEF), which occupies the cerebral cortex anterior to the face area of the motor cortex (Fig. 32-6). The lamina V pyramidal cells concerned send their axons through the anterior limb of the internal capsule to reach the contralateral gaze centers. Stimulation of the *right* FEF produces a saccade to the *left*. The descending axons give collaterals to the superior colliculus, possibly exciting inhibitory internuncials to 'switch off' the SC during voluntary saccades.

In the presence of a tumor or other lesion involving the FEF, the patient may be unable to look toward the opposite side on request. Upward or downward movements are not affected because the midbrain centers (embedded in the medial longitudinal fasciculi) operate in bilateral pairs.

Tracking (smooth pursuit)

The eyes can follow a target moving across the visual field, using a relatively slow conjugate movement to keep the target imaged on the foveas. Calculation of the distance and velocity of the object requires *stereoscopic analysis* (see later) by the visual association areas of both sides. The association areas project to the superior colliculi. The tracking movements are controlled by 'tonic' neurons in the brainstem gaze centers.

synapse upon a sheet of deeply placed effector neurons, some of which project to the contralateral gaze centers. In monkeys, stimulation of these neurons on the right side produces a saccade to the left, and vice versa. The saccade-related neurons discharge to correct the error between present and intended eye position. This is a complex computation requiring feedback signaling the present position of the eyes in the orbit. Eye position may be coded in recurrent branches of the ocular motoneurons. Information about the position of the head in space is fed directly to the gaze centers from the vestibular nuclei, and from the neck muscles.

Two steps are shown in Figs. 32-2 and 32-3. In Fig. 32-2 the eyes are directed forward. A signal enters from the left visual field and is relayed (1) to the right superior colliculus. In Fig. 32-3 the SC responds by stimulating (2) 'burst' cells in the left parabducent nucleus. The burst cells excite (3) the left abducent nucleus and the right oculomotor cells serving the medial rectus. The two nerves (4) pull the eyes toward the signal. The saccade stops when the foveas are on target. The connections are shown more schematically in Fig. 32-4.

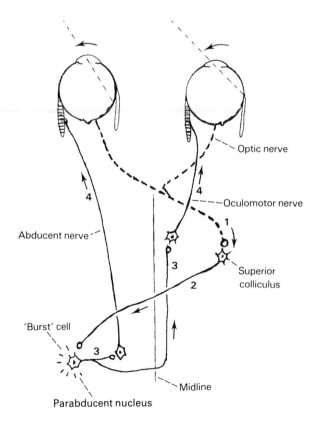

Fig. 32-4 Diagram derived from Fig. 32-3. The movement (arrows) will place the foveas on target.

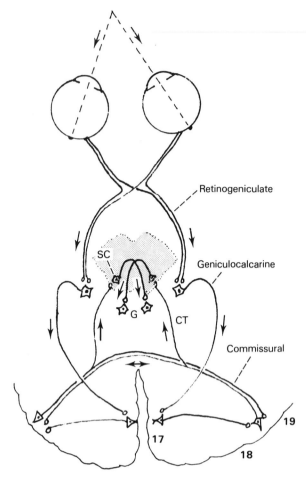

Fig. 32-5 Six neuron pairs link the retina to the pontine gaze center (G) for vergence (two more are required to activate the medial rectus muscles). CT, corticotectal neuron; SC, superior colliculus.

Vergence (Fig. 32-5)

When an object is viewed in close-up the two medial rectus muscles make the visual axes converge (the near response, Chapter 31). During the far response, the lateral rectus muscles make the visual axes parallel. For these *vergence* movements the distance of the object is computed by areas 18 and 19 of both sides. The result is transmitted widely – to the frontal eye fields, superior colliculi, and brainstem gaze centers.

Stereopsis

Stereopsis is the process whereby the brain measures the disparity between the two retinal images, thereby constructing a three-dimensional image. Many neurons in the peristriate belt ('binocular depth cells') are uniquely sensitive to simultaneous stimulation of the two eyes. Included here are 'far' neurons which respond to objects beyond the point of fixation, and 'near' neurons which respond to objects that are closer than that point.

Stereopsis appears to be fully developed by the end of the fifth postnatal month.

Plasticity of visuomotor centers

The three visuomotor centers each have one primary function: frontal eye fields for voluntary saccades,

superior colliculi for automatic saccades, and visual association cortex for stereopsis. However, their functions are to some extent interchangeable. In monkeys, ablation of *either* area 8 or the superior colliculus on one side does not abolish contralateral conjugate gaze. Ablation of both, or of either one together with ablation of the visual association areas, does paralyze contraversive gaze. In humans, lesions of area 8 or of its descending projection paralyzes contraversive gaze for a few hours.

Vestibulo-ocular reflexes

These keep the gaze fixed on a target during movements of the head. They originate in the labyrinth and are described in Chapter 33.

VISUAL ATTENTION (Fig. 32-6)

In the posterior parietal cortex (area 7) of monkeys, some cells become active when an 'object of interest' appears in the visual field. Their activity is enhanced if the animal makes a saccade in the direction of the object, but not otherwise. They are not saccade neurons (unlike those of the frontal eye field and SC). However, they project to the FEF and presumably facilitate a saccade in the appropriate direction. Area 7 receives substantial inputs from the limbic system (entorhinal and cingulate cortex) and from visual association cortex. It probably provides the substrate for *visual attention*, whether to satisfy primitive needs (food and sex) or specific needs (for example, to signal objects of a particular shape or color).

Normal humans are more readily alerted to visual stimuli from the left visual field than from the right. Also, lesions of area 7 on the right are more likely to result in neglect of the contralateral visual field. Therefore, the right area 7 seems to be dominant for visual attention.

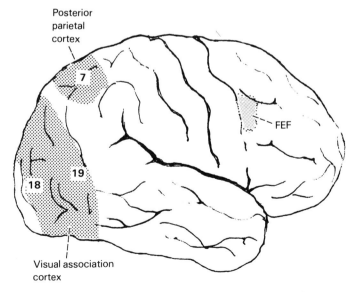

Fig. 32-6 Frontal eye field (FEF), posterior parietal cortex, and visual association cortex.

Readings

Alpern, M. (1969) Types of movement. In *The Eye, Vol. 3, Muscular Mechanisms*, 2nd ed. (Davson, H., ed.), pp. 65–174. New York: Academic Press.

Edwards, S.B. and Henjel, C.H. (1978) Superior colliculus connections with the extraocular motor nuclei in the cat. *J. Comp. Neurol., 179:* 451–468.

Goldberg, M.E. (1981) Supranuclear control of saccadic eye movements. In *Functional Basis of Ocular Motility Disorders* (Lennerstrand, G., Zee, D.S. and Keller, E.L., eds.), pp. 489–496. Oxford & New York: Academic Press.

Hepp, K. and Henn, V. (1981) Physiology of horizontal gaze. In *Functional Basis of Ocular Motility Disorders* (Lennerstrand, G., Zee, D.S. and Keller, E.L., eds.), pp. 247–256. Oxford & New York: Academic Press.

Hikosaka, O. and Wurtz, R.H. (1981) The role of substantia nigra in the initiation of saccadic eye movements. In *Progress in Oculomotor Research* (Fuchs, A.F. and Becker, W., eds.), pp. 145–152. New York, Amsterdam & Oxford: Elsevier/North-Holland.

Keller, E.L. (1981) Brain stem mechanisms in saccadic control. In *Progress in Oculomotor Research* (Fuchs, A.F. and Becker, W., eds.), pp. 57–62. New York, Amsterdam & Oxford: Elsevier/North-Holland.

Kommerell, G. (1984) Supranuclear and nuclear disorders of eye movement. In *Neuro-ophthalmology, Vol. 3* (Lessell, S. and van Dalen, J.T.W., eds.), pp. 230–239. Amsterdam: Elsevier; New York: Oxford University Press.

Leichnetz, G.R. (1980) An anterogradely-labelled prefrontal cortico-oculomotor pathway in the monkey demonstrated with HRP gel and TMB neurohistochemistry. *Brain Res., 198:* 440–445.

Mays, L.E. (1984) Neural control of vergence eye movements: convergence and divergence neurons in midbrain. *J. Neurophysiol., 51:* 1091–1108.

Petrides, M. and Pandya, D.N. (1984) Projections to the frontal cortex from the posterior parietal region in the Rhesus monkey. *J. Comp. Neurol., 228:* 105–116.

Robinson, D.A. and Zee, D.S. (1981) Metrics and models of saccadic eye movements. In *Progress in Oculomotor Research* (Fuchs, A.F. and Becker, W., eds.), pp. 3–12. New York, Amsterdam & Oxford: Elsevier/North-Holland.

Roucoux, A. and Crommelinck, M. (eds.) (1982) *Physiological and Pathological Aspects of Eye Movements*. The Hague: Junk.

Sparks, D.L. and Mays, L.E. (1981) The role of the monkey superior colliculus in the control of saccadic eye movements: a current perspective. In *Progress in Oculomotor Research* (Fuchs, A.F. and Becker, W., eds.), pp. 137–144. New York, Amsterdam & Oxford: Elsevier/North-Holland.

Spector, R.H. and Troost, B.T. (1981) The ocular motor system. *Ann. Neurol., 9:* 517–525.

Takemori, S., Aiba, T. and Shiozawa, R. (1983) Saccade and pursuit eye movements. *Acta Otorhinolaryng., 30:* 80–82.

Trojanoswski, J.Q. and Lafontaine, M.H. (1981) Neuroanatomical correlates of selective downgaze paralysis. *J. Neurol. Sci., 52:* 91–101.

Vender, M.B. (1980) Brain control of conjugate horizontal and vertical eye movements: a survey of the structural and functional correlates. *Brain, 103:* 23–69.

Vilis, T. and Hore, J. (1981) Characteristics of saccadic dysmetria in monkeys during reversible lesions of medial cerebellar nuclei. *J. Neurophysiol., 46:* 828–838.

Wurtz, R.H., Goldberg, M.E. and Robinson, D.L. (1982) Brain mechanisms of visual attention. *Sci. Am., 246:* 100–107.

Zee, D.S. (1984) Ocular motor control: the cerebral control of saccadic eye movements. In *Neuro-ophthalmology, Vol. 3* (Lessell, S. and van Dalen, J.T.W., eds.), pp. 141–156. Amsterdam: Elsevier; New York: Oxford University Press.

33
Balance, Including Vestibulo-ocular Reflexes

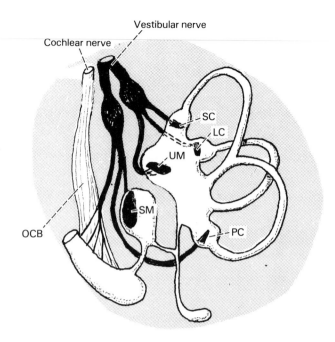

Fig. 33-1   Medial view of right vestibular labyrinth. UM, SM, utricular and saccular maculae; SC, LC, PC, superior, lateral, posterior cristae. OCB, olivocochlear bundle.

The sensory end organs of balance occupy the membranous labyrinth. They are the maculae of the utricle and saccule and the cristae of the semicircular ducts (Fig. 33-1).

The specific receptor throughout is a hair cell which synapses upon a bipolar neuron of the vestibular nerve.

VESTIBULAR HAIR CELLS (Fig. 33-2)

The vestibular epithelium consists of hair cells and supporting cells. The hair cells resemble those of the cochlea, but in addition to stereocilia each displays a long *kinocilium*; this has the ultrastructure of a true cilium. The hair cells have a resting receptor potential sufficient to cause constant discharge of vesicles from basal synaptic bars. The transmitter (nature unknown) excites the underlying vestibular nerve afferents.

Morphologic orientation

The kinocilium is attached to one margin of the cell surface. Displacement of the kinocilium *away* from the stereocilia opens an ion pore on its inner aspect and facilitates (increases) the discharge rate. Displacement *toward* the stereocilia disfacilitates the cell. The position of the kinocilium indicates the *morphologic orientation* of the hair cell.

The hair cells have two innervation patterns (the significance of this is not understood). Type 1 innervation resembles that of inner hair cells in the cochlea. Type 2 innervation resembles that of outer cochlear hair cells.

THE MACULAE (Fig. 33-3)

Each macula consists of a table of hair cells and supporting cells resting on a lamina propria, and covered by a gelatinous matrix containing crystals of protein-bound calcium carbonate. The crystals are called *statoconia*, or otoliths (Gr., ear stones). The hair cells have opposite morphologic orientation on each side of a central groove called the *striola*.

Static labyrinth

When the head is tilted the statoconia exert drag on the underlying cilia. The drag persists as long as the head is tilted. The hair cells are facilitated in one half of the

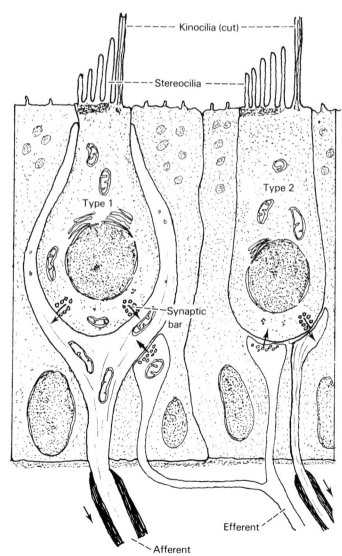

Fig. 33-2   Vestibular hair cells. (Adapted from Spoendlin, 1966.)

230

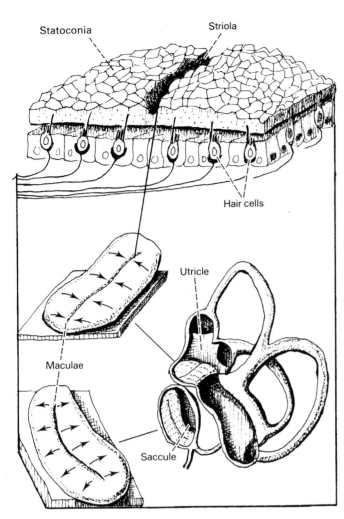

Fig. 33-3 The two maculae. Arrows indicate morphological orientation of hair cells.

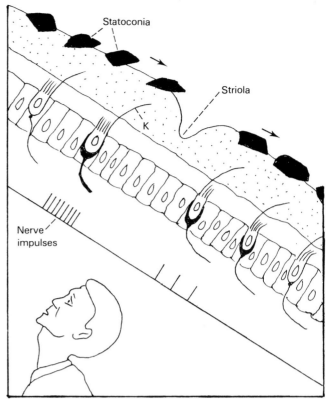

Fig. 33-4 Head tilting facilitates one half of the macula, and disfacilitates the other half. K, kinocilium.

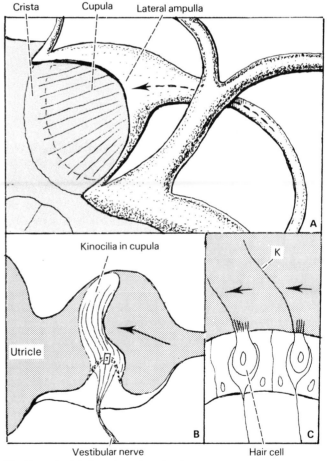

Fig 33-5 A, right lateral semicircular duct. Turning the head to the right displaces endolymph toward the utricle (arrow). B, fluid displacement toward the utricle bends the cupula. C, displacement of kinocilia (K) away from the stereocilia activates vestibular nerve endings.

macula and disfacilitated in the other half. The utricular macula is mainly horizontal and changes its firing pattern when the head is held in the flexed or extended position (Fig. 33-4). The saccular macula is mainly vertical and responds when the head is tilted to one side. Left and right maculae operate in matching pairs.

THE CRISTAE (Fig. 33-5)

The three cristae occupy the ampullae of the semicircular ducts. The vestibular epithelium lies astride a ridge of lamina propria laid across each ampulla, and this is topped by a 'sail' of gelatinous matrix (without crystals) called the *cupula*.

Dynamic labyrinth

Movement of the head causes the cupulae to be deflected passively (like sails). The morphologic orientation of the hair cells is uniform throughout each crista. The orientation is such that the lateral ampullary crista is facilitated by movement of endolymph *into* the utricle from the lateral semicircular duct. The superior and posterior cristae are facilitated by movement of endolymph *out of* the utricle. These

231

directional selectivities form the basis of the vestibulo-ocular reflexes (see later).

VESTIBULAR NERVE (Fig. 33-1)

The *vestibular nerve* comprises the central processes of the vestibular bipolar ganglion cells, which are lodged in the internal acoustic meatus. The nerve crosses the subarachnoid space in company with the cochlear and facial nerves. It pierces the brain stem at the pontomedullary junction and ends in the vestibular nucleus. A few fibers bypass the nucleus and synapse in the flocculus of the cerebellum instead.

Vestibular efferents

Cholinergic neurons located in the tegmentum of the pons send axons to the labyrinth in the vestibular nerve. They synapse upon vestibular afferent terminals and upon hair cells (Fig. 33-2). Their function is uncertain.

VESTIBULAR NUCLEUS (Fig. 33-6)

The *vestibular nucleus* is made up of four individual nuclei: lateral, medial, superior, and inferior. Little is known about the inferior nucleus. The lateral and medial are involved in static labyrinthine reflexes, the medial and superior in dynamic, vestibulo-ocular reflexes.

Static labyrinthine reflexes (Fig. 33-7)

The lateral vestibular (Deiters') nucleus receives afferents from the maculae. When the head is tilted to one side, the ipsilateral vestibulospinal tract increases extensor tone to compensate for the weight of the head. (Try this.) When the head is tilted forward or backward, the maculae of both ears are activated and both vestibulospinal tracts increase extensor or flexor tone, as required. The necessary computations are carried out by the cerebellum. Purkinje cells modulate the discharges of Deiters' nucleus both directly and via the fastigial nuclei. (Contralateral fastigial fibers loop over the superior cerebellar peduncle in the *hook bundle* of Russel and leave in the *juxtarestiform body*, medial to the inferior cerebellar peduncle.)

Head-righting reflexes operate to maintain a level gaze when the body is craned forward or to one side. The nodal point of these reflexes is the medial vestibular nucleus (MVN). Afferents reach the MVN from the spindle-rich neck muscles, from the neck joints, and from the maculae. Efferents from the MVN run up and down the ipsilateral medial longitudinal fasciculus:

1 Up to the nuclei controlling torsion of the eyeballs (Chapter 31);

2 Down to neck motoneurons in order to rectify the head. Being ipsilateral, these neurons ('medial vestibulospinal') are inhibitory.

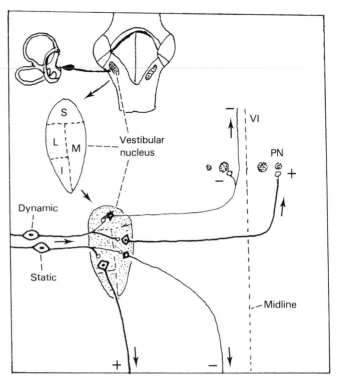

Fig. 33-6 Superior (S), lateral (L), medial (M), and inferior (I) vestibular nuclei. PN, parabducent nucleus.

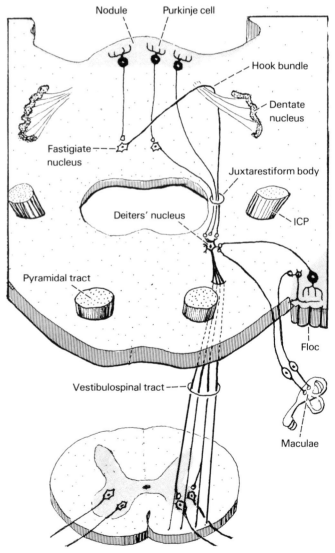

Fig. 33-7 Connections of lateral vestibular nucleus. Floc, flocculus; ICP, inferior cerebellar peduncle.

Dynamic labyrinthine reflexes

The vestibulo-ocular reflexes are designed to maintain the gaze on any selected target, regardless of the position of the head. They are amazingly delicate, compensatory reflexes: these lines can be read while the head is moving from side to side or up and down. (Try this.)

The effect of rotating the head to the *left* is shown in Fig. 33-8. The endolymph has inertia, and it remains relatively stationary during backward rotation of the lateral semicircular canal. It displaces the lateral cupula in the direction of morphologic orientation of the underlying hair cells, thereby facilitating them. The afferents (1) play upon the medial vestibular nucleus (MVN). The MVN excites (2) the *contralateral* parabducent nucleus, which responds (3, 4) by pulling the eyes to the right. The pathway from MVN to medial rectus crosses the midline twice.

When the neck is flexed, endolymph enters the superior ampullae on both sides. When the neck is extended, endolymph enters the inferior ampullae. These head movements excite the corresponding cristae, causing the MVN to act upon the midbrain generators controlling vertical gaze.

Tilting of the maculae during head movements has a small synergistic effect through convergence onto crista-responsive neurons in the MVN.

The superior vestibular nucleus is also excited by head movement. Via the medial longitudinal fasciculus, it leaks inhibitory transmitter onto motoneurons antagonistic to the particular movement.

The *cerebellum* is informed both by the MVN and by the retinas:
1 Fibers from the MVN enter the flocculonodular cortex.
2 Some ganglion cells in the medial retinal halves act as *slip detectors* to prevent the visual image from slipping off the foveas. Their axons cross in the optic chiasm and are relayed by the midbrain reticular formation to the ipsilateral inferior olive. Olivocerebellar fibers play on the *same* Purkinje cells receiving from the MVN. The fastigial nucleus plays upon the MVN and even sends fibers directly to the individual ocular motor nuclei (via the medial longitudinal fasciculus).

The vestibulo-ocular is an 'open loop' reflex, the effector organ being distinct from the source of stimulation. The retinocerebellar, *optokinetic* reflex is 'closed loop'.

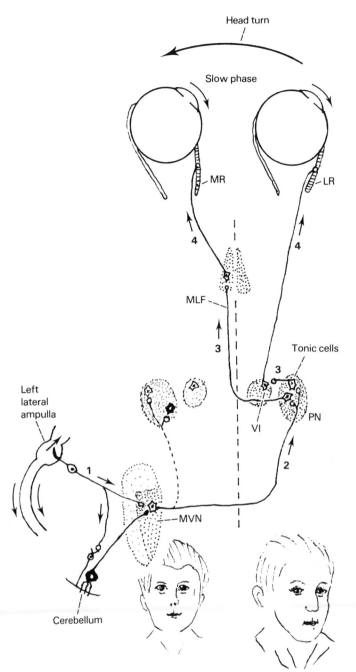

Fig. 33-8 Four neurons of the vestibulo-ocular reflex (slow phase). LR, MR, lateral and medial recti; MLF, medial longitudinal fasciculus; MVN, medial vestibular nucleus; PN, parabducent nucleus.

Iatrogenic nystagmus (Gr., iatros, doctor)

Endolymph can be induced to move forward (toward the utricle) in the lateral semicircular duct by running warm water (44°C) into the outer ear canal. The subject is placed with the head tilted back 60°, bringing the lateral canal into the vertical plane and allowing the heated endolymph to produce upward convection currents (Fig. 33-9). This is the warm-water *caloric test* of vestibular function. A vestibulo-ocular reflex is induced, as if the head were turning to that side: the labyrinth is fooled. The eyes turn slowly away ('slow phase'), snap back to a central position ('fast phase'),

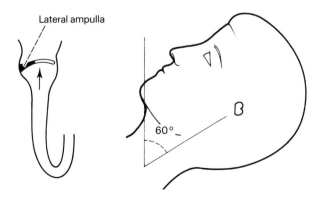

Fig. 33-9 Head position for warm-water caloric test.

and resume a slow phase. The alternating slow and fast phases are known as *nystagmus*. Unfortunately, the direction of the nystagmus is named after its fast-phase component: the subject in Fig. 33-9 will have 'nystagmus to the left'. The fast phase is in fact the recovery phase. Its mechanism is shown in Fig. 33-10. Stimulation of the vestibular nerve progressively arouses the ipsilateral pontine gaze center, and when threshold is reached, excitatory 'burst' cells snap the left lateral and right medial recti into action.

Vestibulocortical connections

The superior temporal gyrus seems to contain a (?contralateral) center for balance perception, because auras (warnings) of vertigo may precede anterior temporal lobe epilepsy. In monkeys, a 'standard' projection has been found from the vestibular nucleus to the contralateral sensory face area via the thalamic ventroposteromedial nucleus. In humans, there may be another center in area 7 (posterior parietal cortex).

APPLIED ANATOMY

Disorders of the labyrinth are manifested by *vertigo*: a sense of rotation in relation to the external world. The clinician's first task is always to distinguish true vertigo from dizziness, blackouts, and so on, which may have quite different origins.

Both labyrinths are tonically active. In the standing position, the maculae stimulate the vestibulospinal tracts via Deiters' nuclei to maintain antigravity tone. The cristae of the two lateral ampullae interact at the level of the ocular nuclei to keep the gaze directed forward.

Attack

If one labyrinth is struck by disease it ceases to function, and *symptoms are produced by continued activity of the other, intact labyrinth*. In sudden disorder of the right labyrinth, the standing patient will fall to the right, and he will veer to the right if he walks. He experiences acute vertigo and shows nystagmus to the left. The active ocular connections are those of Figs. 33-8 and 33-10. The direction of nystagmus being named after the fast phase, our patient has 'nystagmus to the left' – that is, away from the side of the lesion.

In addition to vestibular ataxia and nystagmus, repeated vomiting is usual because of abnormal impulse patterns descending to the vomiting center.

Recovery

After several hours the vertigo, vomiting and nystagmus subside. The improvement is brought about by the *clamping action of the cerebellum*. The flocculonodular lobe rectifies the mismatched input to the brainstem by suppressing the normal, uninjured vestibular nucleus. The patient is then devoid of labyrinthine function and free of symptoms when lying down. When upright, he can compensate for lost vestibular proprioception by making full use of his eyes, and of his trunk and limb proprioceptors, to provide an adequate sense of position. However, he will fall over if he closes his eyes, or looks up, and he will be unable to get about in semi-darkness.

Causes of vertigo

Benign positional vertigo
In this condition the room spins when the patient lies down.

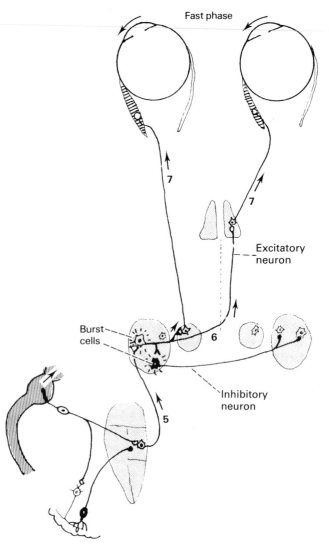

Fig. 33-10 Vestibulo-ocular reflex, fast phase. Compare with Fig. 33-8.

Vestibular neuronitis
This is an inflammatory disorder thought to be kindred to Bell's palsy (Chapter 35).

Benign positional vertigo and vestibular neuronitis are the commonest labyrinthine disorders.

Drug side-effects

Arterial disease
Attacks are common among elderly people whose labyrinthine arteries are diseased.

Multiple sclerosis
Vestibulo-ocular fibers in the medial longitudinal fasciculus may be injured by plaques of demyelination in multiple sclerosis (internuclear ophthalmoplegia, Chapter 31). Nystagmus of brainstem origin does not subside like labyrinthine nystagmus because the cerebellar clamping mechanism cannot reach it.

Ménière's disease
This is an uncommon disorder of the elderly, characterized by attacks of intense vertigo, tinnitus (in the form of a rushing or hissing sound) and deafness. The exact cause is not known but there is overproduction of endolymph (with abnormal chemistry) by the stria vascularis.

Cerebellar disease

Nystagmus sometimes occurs in cerebellar disease. Nystagmus is toward the lesion, because of lost tonic cerebellar inhibition of the ipsilateral vestibular nucleus.

Acoustic neuroma

This is a benign, Schwann-cell glioma of the acoustic nerve. It arises in the vestibular division within the internal acoustic meatus and gradually extends into the posterior cranial fossa. Pin-head tumors of the vestibular nerve are to be found in about 1% of routine autopsies, but tumors large enough to produce clinical symptoms are rare. Early diagnosis is very important because surgical removal of large tumors from the posterior cranial fossa is hazardous, and substantial, permanent functional deficits are certain. *The presence of a tumor must be suspected in every middle-aged or elderly patient presenting with auditory or vestibular symptoms.*

Although it arises in the vestibular nerve, the first symptoms are usually cochlear. *Tinnitus* (high-pitched) is accompanied by *deafness* which increases slowly over a period of months or years. Episodes of *vertigo* occur as deafness progresses, and nystagmus may appear. The *corneal reflex* must always be tested in patients presenting with deafness and/or vertigo for which there is no obvious explanation. The fine fibers supplying the cornea enter the pons in the sensory root of the trigeminal nerve, and they are very susceptible to pressure as the tumor emerges into the posterior cranial fossa. In advanced cases the patient may report pain over one or more divisions of the trigeminal, and response to pin-prick may be dulled on the affected side. The *facial* nerve is surprisingly resistant to stretching, but a typical infranuclear facial palsy is a feature with large tumors. As the growth extends downward (Fig. 33-11), the *glossopharyngeal* nerve is compressed, causing pain in the throat (oropharynx) followed by ipsilateral sensory loss. Compression of *cranial accessory* nerve filaments may cause difficulty in swallowing, and hoarseness.

Pressure on the *cerebellum* may produce ipsilateral cerebellar signs, and compression of the *brainstem* may compromise one or both pyramidal tracts. Raised intracranial pressure is a late feature because the tumor is slow-growing (taking up to ten years).

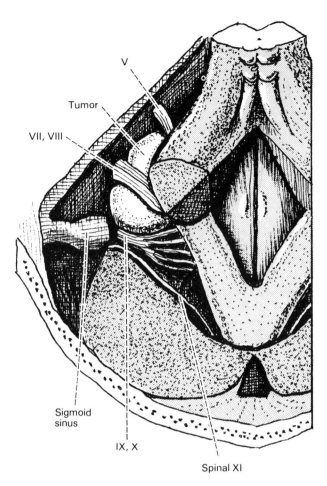

Fig. 33-11 Acoustic neuroma in posterior cranial fossa.

Readings

Baker, R., Evinger, C. and McCrea, R.A. (1981) Some thoughts about the three neurons in the vestibular ocular reflex. *Ann. NY Acad. Sci.*, 374: 171–188.

Büttner, V. and Dichgans, J. (1984) The vestibulo-ocular reflex and related functions. In *Neuro-ophthalmology, Vol. 3* (Lessell, S. and van Dalen, J.T.W., eds.), pp. 205–229. Amsterdam: Elsevier; New York: Oxford University Press.

Büttner, V. and Lang, W. (1975) The vestibulocortical pathway: neurophysiological and anatomical studies in the monkey. In *Reflex Control of Posture and Movement* (Granit, R. and Pompeiano, O., eds.), pp. 581–588. Amsterdam, New York & Oxford: Elsevier/North-Holland.

Buttner-Ennever, J.A. (1981) Vestibulo-oculomotor organization. In *Progress in Oculomotor Research* (Fuche, A.F. and Beeker, W., eds.), pp. 361–370. New York, Amsterdam & Oxford: Elsevier/North-Holland.

Carleton, S.C. and Carpenter, M.B. (1983) Afferent and efferent connections of the medial, inferior and lateral vestibular nuclei in the cat and monkey. *Brain Res.*, 278: 29–51.

Fredrickson, J.M. and Schwarz, W.F. (1975) Vestibulocortical projection. In *The Vestibular System* (Naunton, R.F., ed.), pp. 203–210. New York: Academic Press.

Gacek, R.R. (1975) The innervation of the vestibular labyrinth. In *The Vestibular System* (Naunton, R.F., ed.), pp. 21–30. New York: Academic Press.

Galey, F.R., Ylikoski, J., Lundquist, P., Bagger-Sjöbäck, D. and Smith, C. (1981) Human vestibular epithelia: prospects for future study. *Am. J. Otol.*, 3: 126–133.

Goldberg, J.M. (1979) Vestibular receptors in mammals: efferent discharge characteristics and efferent control. In *Reflex Control of Posture and Movement* (Granit, R. and Pompeiano, O., eds.), pp. 355–367. Amsterdam, New York & Oxford: Elsevier/North Holland.

Hallpike, C.S. (1966) Some observations on the character and mechanism of spontaneous nystagmus in subjects with tumors of the VIII nerve. In *The Vestibular System and its Diseases* (Wolfson, R.J., ed.), pp. 390–403. Philadelphia: University Press.

Maekawa, K. and Simpson, J.I. (1973) Climbing fiber responses evoked in the vestibulo-cerebellum of rabbit from the visual system. *J. Neurophysiol.*, 35: 649–666.

Nyberg-Hansen, R. (1975) Anatomical aspects of the functional organization of the vestibulo-spinal pathways. In *The Vestibular System* (Naunton, R.F., ed.), pp. 71–98. New York: Academic Press.

Parker, D.E. (1980) The vestibular apparatus. *Sci. Am.*, 243: 98–111.

Precht, W. (1979) Labyrinthine influences on the vestibular nuclei. In *Reflex Control of Posture and Movement* (Granit, R. and Pompeiano, O., eds.), pp. 369–381. Amsterdam, New York and Oxford: Elsevier/North Holland.

Precht, W. (1981) Functional organization of optokinetic pathways in mammals. In *Progress in Oculomotor Research* (Fuche, A.F. and Beeker, W., eds.), pp. 425–433. New York, Amsterdam & Oxford: Elsevier/North Holland.

Roberts, R.D.M. (1977) The relationship of gravity to vestibular studies. In *Proceedings of the European Symposium on Life Sciences Research in Space*, pp. 139–145. Cologne: ESASP-130.

Schuknecht, H.F. (1974) Neoplastic growth. In *Pathology of the Ear*, pp. 415–452. Cambridge, Massachusetts: Harvard University Press.

Smith, C.A. and Tanaka, K. (1975) Some aspects of the structure of the vestibular apparatus. In *The Vestibular System* (Naunton, R.F., ed.), pp. 3–20. New York: Academic Press.

Spoendlin, H.H. (1966) Ultrastructure of the vestibular sense organ. In *The Vestibular System and its Diseases* (Wolfson, R.J., ed.), pp. 39–68. Philadelphia: University Press.

Tonndorf, J. (1983) A mechanical view of peripheral vestibular function. *Adv. Otorhinolaryngol., 30:* 34–39.

Wilson, V.J. and Peterson, B.W. (1981) Central pathways for vestibular reflexes. In *Handbook of Physiology, Section 1, The Nervous System, Vol. 2, Part 1* (Brooks, B.V., ed.), pp. 671–678. Bethesda, Maryland: American Physiological Society.

VIII
CRANIAL NERVES
V–XII

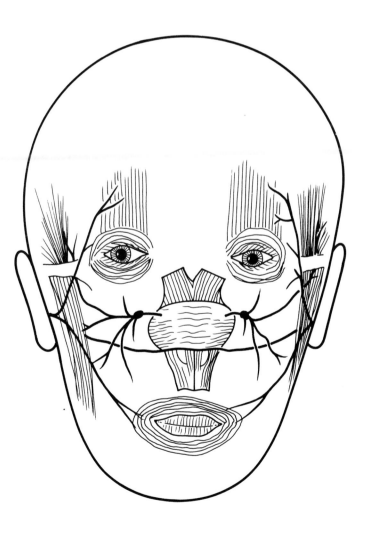

Trigeminal Nerve

The trigeminal nerve provides the motor supply to the muscles of mastication. It provides sensation to the skin of the face, to the oronasal mucous membranes, and to the teeth. The sensory fibers of the nerve have their cell bodies in the trigeminal ganglion, and the sensory root corresponds to a spinal posterior nerve root.

The trigeminal has three separate sensory nuclei in the brainstem. The most caudal (in the medulla) is of particular clinical interest because it receives nociceptive terminals from areas additional to the trigeminal area: from the ear, pharynx, and dura mater of the posterior cranial fossa.

MOTOR NUCLEUS (Fig. 34-1)

The *motor nucleus* is the branchial efferent nucleus supplying the muscles of the mandibular arch. These muscles comprise the six masticatory muscles attached to the mandible on each side, and the tensor tympani and tensor palati. The nucleus occupies the lateral pontine tegmentum.

The *motor root* emerges from the nucleus and enters the mandibular division of the trigeminal for distribution.

Mastication (Fig. 34-2)

Mastication is a complex activity requiring integrated contractions and relaxations of muscles of the jaw, cheeks (facial nerves), tongue (hypoglossal nerves) and infrahyoid muscles (cervical spinal nerves). Integration is controlled by the *supratrigeminal nucleus*, a pattern generator partly embedded in the motor nucleus. The rhythm and force of mastication depend on the consistency of the food and are regulated by feedback from the oral mucous membrane and teeth.

Supranuclear control

Masticatory movements can be elicited by stimulation of the premotor cortex (area 6) anterior to the face area of the motor cortex.

Masticatory movements can also be elicited by stimulation of the orbital cortex of the frontal lobe, or of the cortical amygdala; both receive olfactory inputs.

SENSORY NUCLEI (Fig. 34-3)

The *sensory root* of the trigeminal is composed of the central processes derived from the unipolar cells of the trigeminal ganglion (gasserian ganglion). It contains equal numbers of myelinated and unmyelinated axons, which enter the trigeminal sensory nuclei. One

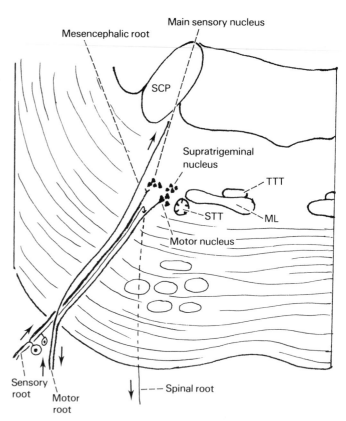

Fig. 34-1 Transverse section of pons showing trigeminal nerve components. ML, medial lemniscus; SCP, superior cerebellar peduncle; STT, spinothalamic tract; TTT, trigeminothalamic tract.

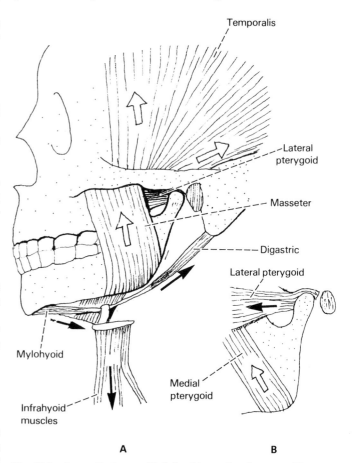

Fig. 34-2 A, masticatory and infrahyoid muscles. B, pterygoid muscles of right side, medial view. Clear arrows: elevators; black arrows: depressors.

sensory nucleus occupies the midbrain, one the pons, and one the medulla oblongata.

Mesencephalic nucleus

The midbrain nucleus is a ribbon of unipolar cells lying beside the aqueduct of the midbrain and rostral end of the fourth ventricle, the *only* group of unipolar neurons within the CNS. Their peripheral processes supply sensory fibers to muscle spindles over a wide area: the extrinsic ocular muscles (rich in spindles), the facial muscles (poor), and the masticatory muscles (rich).

Their central processes (which may enter the pons in the motor root) run in three directions: to the supratrigeminal nucleus, cerebellum, and contralateral thalamus.

Pontine nucleus

The pontine (*main sensory*) nucleus receives tactile information from the facial skin. It is homologous with the nucleus gracilis and nucleus cuneatus of the medulla, and it projects mainly into the contralateral trigeminal lemniscus (see later).

Spinal nucleus

The spinal nucleus is so called because it blends with the posterior gray horn of the spinal cord. It extends the full length of the medulla oblongata and is divided into three parts:

1 The *pars oralis* receives tactile information from the mouth.
2 The *pars interpolaris* receives nociceptive fibers from the teeth.
3 The *pars caudalis* comprises a ribbon of small cells homologous with the substantia gelatinosa of the posterior gray horn and a ribbon of larger cells homologous with the nucleus proprius. Fine (Aδ and C) fibers signaling painful and thermal sensations synapse upon the small cells. Coarser afferents serving tactile sensation synapse upon the larger cells.

The principal sensory territories of the pars caudalis are the epithelia of the entire trigeminal area: corneal, facial (epidermis), nasal and oral. The modalities served are pain, temperature, and touch (the tactile fibers are collaterals of those entering the pontine nucleus). Topographical representation in the nucleus is onion-like (Fig. 34-4).

The pars caudalis also receives afferents (a) from the external acoustic meatus, middle ear, and eustachian tube, (b) from the skin of the neck, via the dorsal rami of C2 and C3, (c) from the dura mater, which is innervated above the tentorium cerebelli by the ophthalmic nerve and below the tentorium by C2, C3, and the vagus, and (d) from the pharynx and esophagus.

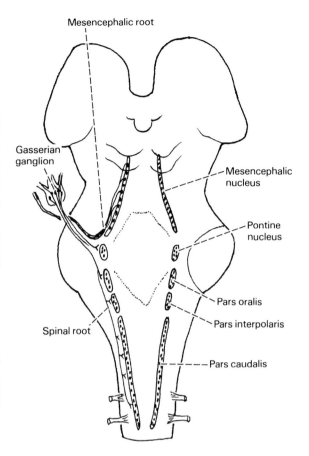

Fig. 34-3 Brainstem from behind showing the sensory nuclei of the trigeminal nerve.

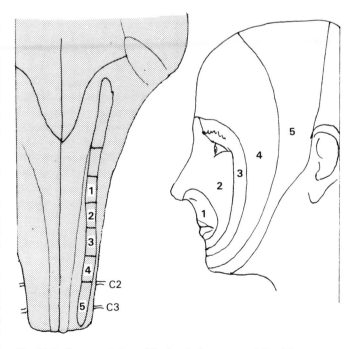

Fig. 34-4 Representation of the face in the pars caudalis of the spinal nucleus of trigeminal nerve. (C1 often has no posterior nerve root.) (Adapted from Sears and Franklin, 1980.)

239

SECOND-ORDER AFFERENTS (Fig. 34-5)

The small-celled component of the pars caudalis has complex synaptic configurations resembling those of the substantia gelatinosa. It sends excitatory and inhibitory fibers to the large-celled component. The large cells give rise to the *trigeminothalamic tract* (TTT), which is the homologue of the spinothalamic tract. The TTT ascends the contralateral brain stem, where it is joined by crossing fibers from the pontine nucleus to complete the *trigeminal lemniscus*. The lemniscus terminates in the ventroposteromedial nucleus of thalamus (see Fig. 17-3). Third-order sensory neurons pass to the face area of the somesthetic cortex, and to SII.

Trigeminoreticular fibers are counterparts of the spinoreticular system. They synapse in the reticular formation, where they are responsible for the arousal effect of stroking or slapping the face, and of the old-fashioned 'smelling salts' (the ammonia irritates trigeminal endings in the nose).

Modulation of transmission in the pars caudalis is a replica of that found in the posterior gray horn of the spinal cord (Chapter 15).

Innervation of the teeth

From the superior and inferior alveolar nerves, Aδ and C fibers enter the root canals of the teeth and form a dense plexus within the pulp. Individual fibers terminate in the pulp, in the predentin, and in dentinal tubules. Fifty to seventy per cent of dentinal tubules underlying the occlusal surfaces of the teeth contain single nerve fibers. However, the nerves are confined to the innermost 0.1 mm of the tubules, whereas pain can be elicited at the outer surface of dentin when the enamel has been removed. Hydrodynamic and chemical factors have been invoked, as well as possible participation of odontoblasts in pain transduction. The odontoblasts reach far into the tubules, but only desmosomal contacts have been seen between them and the nerve fibers.

The *periodontal ligaments* suspend the teeth within the bone-walled alveoli. The ligaments are richly innervated by the nerves supplying the oral epithelium including the gums. The periodontal nerve endings function as tension recorders because the ligaments are arranged like hammocks around the roots of the teeth.

Mandibular reflexes

The *jaw-opening reflex* is usually initiated by dental occlusion. The periodontal afferents reach the mesencephalic nucleus of the trigeminal, which synapses in the supratrigeminal nucleus and puts this generator into a jaw-opening mode.

The *jaw-closing reflex* is triggered by passive stretching of muscle spindles in the temporalis, masseter, and medial pterygoid muscles. The supratrigeminal nucleus is stimulated to enter a jaw-closing mode by the spindle afferents.

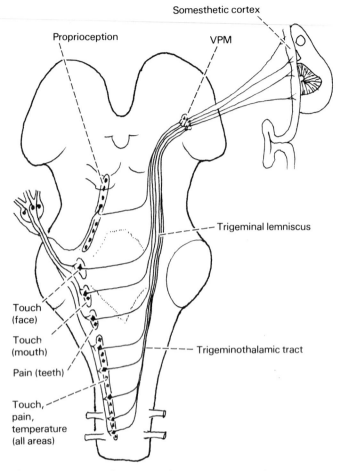

Fig. 34-5 Trigeminal sensory pathways. VPM, ventral posteromedial nucleus of thalamus.

Corneal reflex

The corneal reflex is considered with the facial nerve, in the next chapter. The afferent limb of the reflex is the ophthalmic nerve, which synapses in the pars caudalis of the spinal nucleus.

APPLIED ANATOMY

The motor nucleus and motor root are rarely affected by disease, but the root will be included if the mandibular nerve is divided in treating trigeminal neuralgia. Motor paralysis is revealed by deviation of the jaw toward the weak side on opening the mouth. The deviation is caused by the unopposed action of the healthy lateral pterygoid.

The *jaw-jerk* reflex (elicited by tapping the chin with a downward stroke) is routinely tested when the cranial nerves are being examined. Exaggeration of the jaw-jerk reflex signifies bilateral supranuclear lesions.

If the supranuclear supply to the motor nucleus is mainly contralateral, the jaw of a hemiplegic patient will deviate to the affected side when the mouth is opened.

Trigeminal neuralgia is a rare but important condition, characterized by attacks of excruciating pain in the territory of one or more divisions of the trigeminal nerve. The patients are able to map out the affected division(s) accurately. Since the condition has to be distinguished from many other causes of facial pain, the clinician must be able to draw the trigeminal sensory map (Fig. 34-6).

Most patients respond to drug therapy, but a minority require surgery. A common practice is to insert a needle electrode through the foramen ovale from below, and to note the distribution of tingling sensations caused by passing a low current. When the affected division has been located, it is injured by raising the voltage until sensation is almost lost from the skin. The small, C-fiber neurons are destroyed first, and the intention is to preserve some tactile sense. The corneal reflex can also be preserved in this way.

An alternate approach is the Sjöqvist operation, in which the spinal root of the trigeminal is sectioned through the dorsolateral surface of the medulla.

Some cases of trigeminal neuralgia are caused by vascular compression of the nerve (Chapter 30).

Meningitis

Acute bacterial meningitis is characterized by severe, generalized headache, and neck rigidity. The headache is caused by irritation of nociceptive nerve endings in the dura mater; the fibers terminate in the pars caudalis of the spinal nucleus. The neck rigidity is caused by reflex stimulation of the muscles supplied by spinal segments C1–C3, in response to irritation of cervical posterior root fibers in the posterior cranial fossa (Fig. 34-7).

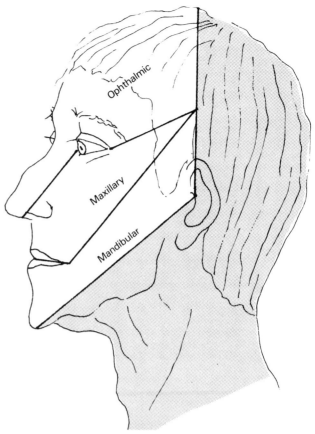

Fig. 34-6 The five lines required to make a trigeminal sensory map.

Readings

Abrahams, V.C. and Richmond, F.J.R. (1977) Motor role of the spinal projections of the trigeminal system. In *Pain in the Trigeminal System* (Anderson, M.E. and Matthews, B., eds.), pp. 405–411. Amsterdam: Elsevier/North Holland Biomedical Press.

Baumel, J.J. (1974) Trigeminal–facial communications. Their function in facial innervation and reinnervation. *Arch. Otolaryngol., 99:* 34–44.

Bratzlavsky, M. (1976) Human brainstem reflexes. In *The Motor System: Neurophysiology and Muscle Mechanisms* (Shahani, M., ed.), pp. 135–154. New York: Raven Press.

Byers, M.R. and Matthews, B. (1981) Autoradiographic demonstration of ipsilateral and contralateral sensory nerve endings in cat dentin, pulp, and periodontium. *Anat. Rec., 201:* 249–260.

Byers, M.R., Neuhaus, S.J. and Gehrig, J.D. (1982) Dental sensory receptor structure in human teeth. *Pain, 13:* 221–235.

Dubner, R., Sessle, B.J. and Storey, A.T. (1978) Jaw, facial, and tongue reflexes. In *The Neural Basis of Oral and Facial Function* (by Dubner, R., Sessle, B.J. and Storey, A.T.), pp. 246–310. New York: Raven Press.

Ganchrow, D. (1978) Intratrigeminal and thalamic projections of nucleus caudalis in the squirrel monkey (*Saimiuri sciurius*): a degeneration and autoradiographic study. *J. Comp. Neurol., 178:* 281–312.

Gobel, S. and Binck, J.M. (1977) Degenerative changes in primary trigeminal axons and in neurons in nucleus caudalis following tooth pulp extirpations in the cat. *Brain Res., 132:* 347–354.

Hayashi, H. (1982) Differential terminal distribution of single large cutaneous afferent fibers in the spinal trigeminal nucleus and in the cervical spinal dorsal horn. *Brain Res., 244:* 173–177.

Hussein, M., Wilson, L.A. and Illingworth, R. (1982) Patterns of sensory loss following fractional posterior fossa Vth nerve section for trigeminal neuralgia. *J. Neurol. Neurosurg. Psychiatry, 45:* 786–790.

Jannetta, P.J. (1967) Arterial compression of the trigeminal nerve in patients with trigeminal neuralgia. *J. Neurosurg., Suppl. 26:* 159–162.

Kruger, L. (1971) A critical review of theories concerning the organization of the sensory trigeminal nuclear complex of the brain stem. In *Oro-facial Sensory and Motor Mechanisms* (Dubner, R. and Kawamura, Y., eds.), pp. 135–158. New York: Appleton-Century-Crofts.

Lund, J.P. and Olsson, K.A. (1983) The importance of reflexes and their control during jaw movement. *Trends Neurosci., 5:* 458–463.

Nakamura, Y., Takatori, M., Kubo, Y., Nozaki, S. and Enomoto, S. (1979) Masticatory rhythm formation: facts and a hypothesis. In *Integrative Control Functions of the Brain*, Vol. 2 (Ito, M., Kubota, K., Tsukahara, N. and Yagi, K., eds.), pp. 321–331. Tokyo: Kondasha; Amsterdam: Elsevier/North Holland Biomedical Press.

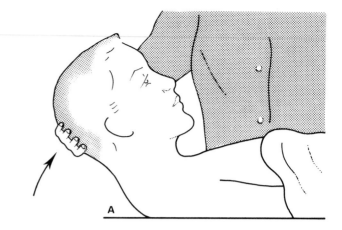

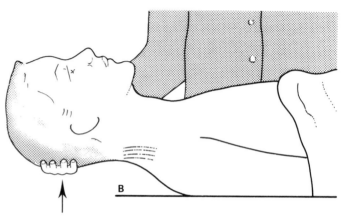

Fig. 34-7 Neck sign in posterior fossa meningitis: A, normal; B, neck rigidity.

Nugent, G.R. (1982) Technique and results of 800 percutaneous radiofrequency thermocoagulations for trigeminal neuralgia. *Appl. Neurophysiol.*, *45:* 504–507.

Price, D.D., Dubner, R. and Hu, J.W. (1976) Trigeminothalamic neurons in nucleus caudalis responsive to tactile, thermal, and nociceptive stimulation of monkey's face. *J. Neurophysiol.*, *39:* 936–953.

Sears, E.S. and Franklin, G.M. (1980) Diseases of the cranial nerves. In *Neurology* (Rosenberg, R.N., ed.), pp. 471–494. New York: Grune & Stratton.

Sumal, K.K., Pickel, V.M., Miller, R.J. and Reis, D.J. (1982) Enkephalin-containing neurons in substantia gelatinosa of spinal trigeminal complex: ultrastructure and synaptic interaction with primary sensory afferents. *Brain Res.*, *248:* 223–236.

Tolgart, L., Hokfelt, T., Nilsson, G. and Pernow, B. (1977) Localization of substance P-like immunoreactivity in nerves in the tooth pulp. *Pain*, *4:* 153–159.

Young, R.F. (1978) Unmyelinated fibers in the trigeminal motor root: posible relationship to the results of trigeminal rhizotomy. *J. Neurosurg.*, *49:* 538–543.

Young, R.F. and Stevens, R. (1979) Unmyelinated axons in the trigeminal motor root of human and cat. *J. Comp. Neurol.*, *183:* 205–214.

Facial Nerve

The facial is the most frequently paralyzed of all the peripheral nerves. It has four component parts, or roots (Table 35-1).

Table 35-1 Facial nerve components

Root	Nucleus	Territory
Branchial efferent	Principal	Mimetic muscles
Parasympathetic	Superior salivatory	Lacrimal glands, salivary glands
Special sense	Nucleus solitarius	Taste buds of tongue and palate
Somatic sensory	Spinal V	Skin of outer ear

BRANCHIAL EFFERENT ROOT

The branchial efferent root (main facial nerve) supplies the muscles derived from the second branchial arch. They include all of the muscles inserting into the skin of the face, together with the stapedius and stylohyoid muscles and the posterior belly of the digastric muscle.

Origin (Fig. 35-1)

The main motor nucleus occupies the lateral pontine tegmentum. Before emerging, the axons wind around the nucleus of the abducent nerve (VI), giving rise to the facial colliculus in the floor of the fourth ventricle.

Course and distribution

The main facial nerve leaves the pons at its lower border and crosses the subarachnoid space to enter the temporal bone. It passes above the vestibule of the labyrinth, bends backward at the genu (L., knee) and descends to the stylomastoid foramen in the interval between the middle ear and the mastoid process. Before emerging from the skull it supplies the stapedius muscle. When it emerges it gives branches to the occipitalis, digastric (posterior belly), and stylohyoid muscles. Finally, it divides within the parotid gland into six branches to the mimetic muscles (muscles of facial expression) (Fig. 35-2).

Supranuclear connections

Pyramidal connections

All of the cells of the principal nucleus receive a monosynaptic supply from corticobulbar neurons arising in the 'face' area of the contralateral motor cortex. In addition, the cells supplying the upper half of the face (the occipitofrontalis and orbicularis oculi muscles) receive an equal, ipsilateral supply; this bilateral supply may be a reflection of the normally paired action of the upper facial muscles. It makes it

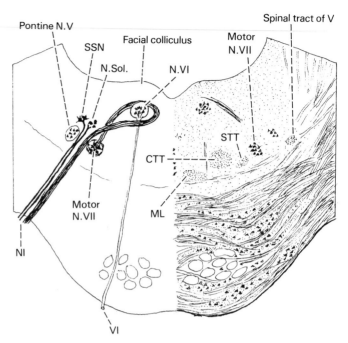

Fig. 35-1 Facial nerve in pons. CTT, central tegmental tract; ML, medial lemniscus; Motor N.VII, motor nucleus of facial nerve; NI, nervus intermedius; N.Sol., nucleus solitarius; N.VI, abducent nucleus; Pontine N.V, pontine nucleus of trigeminal nerve; SSN, superior salivatory nucleus; STT, spinothalamic tract.

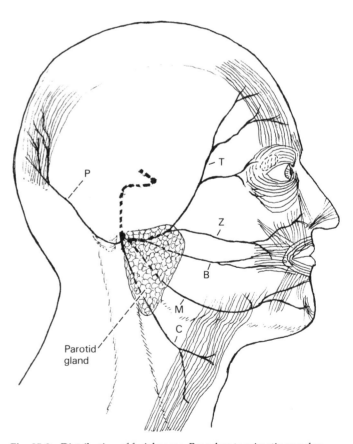

Fig. 35-2 Distribution of facial nerve. Branches to mimetic muscles: B, buccal; C, cervical; M, mandibular; P, posterior auricular; T, temporal; Z, zygomatic.

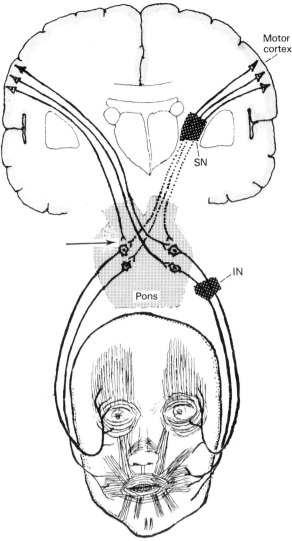

Fig. 35-3 In a supranuclear lesion (SN) of VII, the upper facial muscles escape because of ipsilateral corticobulbar innervation of the upper part of the nucleus (arrow). In an infranuclear lesion (IN) the entire face is paralyzed on the same side. (Adapted from Sears and Franklin, 1980.)

easy to distinguish a supranuclear from an infranuclear lesion of the nerve (Fig. 35-3).

Limbic connections

A hemiplegic patient may use the paralyzed lower face during a spontaneous smile (Fig. 35-4). The 'emotional' supranuclear fibers presumably travel from the limbic cortex. Their course is uncertain but it may include the basal ganglia; this is suggested by the absence of emotional expression in patients with Parkinson's disease.

Nuclear connections

These are listed in Table 35-2. The most important clinically is that from the spinal trigeminal nucleus, serving the corneal reflex.

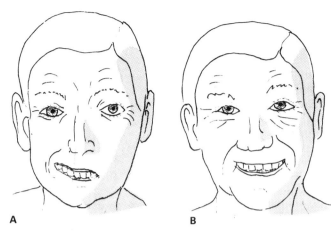

Fig. 35-4 A, supranuclear lesion of the left facial nerve. B, the patient can smile spontaneously.

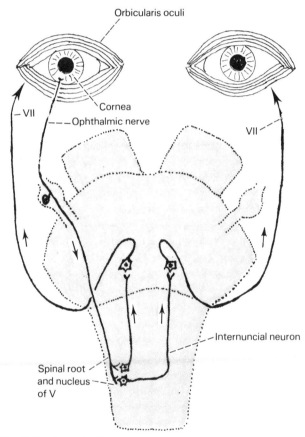

Fig. 35-5 Corneal reflex.

Corneal reflex (Fig. 35-5)

Touching the cornea with a cotton wisp elicits a bilateral blink response. The afferent limb is the ophthalmic nerve (its nasociliary branch supplies the cornea); the efferent limb is the facial, to the palpebral (eyelid) fibers of the orbicularis oculi muscle.

Table 35-2 Brainstem reflexes involving the facial nerve

	Corneal reflex	*Sucking reflex*	*Blinking to light*	*Blinking to noise*	*Sound attenuation*
Receptor	Cornea	Lips	Retina	Cochlea	Cochlea
Afferent	Ophthalmic nerve	Mandibular nerve	Optic nerve	Cochlear nucleus	Cochlear nucleus
First synapse	Spinal nucleus of trigeminal	Pontine nucleus of trigeminal	Superior colliculus	Inferior colliculus	Superior olive
Second synapse	Facial nucleus	Facial nucleus	Facial nucleus	Facial nucleus	Facial nucleus
Effector	Orbicularis oculi	Orbicularis oris	Orbicularis oculi	Orbicularis oculi	Stapedius

PARASYMPATHETIC AND SPECIAL SENSE ROOTS (Fig. 35-6)

The nervus intermedius (NI) intervenes between the main facial nerve and the vestibulocochlear nerve in the internal acoustic meatus. It joins the facial nerve proximal to the genu.

The *parasympathetic root* of the NI arises in the superior salivatory nucleus. It contributes to the greater petrosal and chorda tympani nerves. The greater petrosal fibers synapse in the pterygopalatine ganglion, whose postganglionic fibers supply the lacrimal and nasal glands (Fig. 35-7). The chorda tympani fibers synapse in the submandibular ganglion, whose postganglionic fibers supply the submandibular, sublingual, and intralingual glands.

The *special sense root* of NI has its unipolar cell bodies in the geniculate ganglion of the facial nerve. The peripheral processes of the ganglion enter the greater petrosal nerve to supply the palatal taste buds and enter the chorda tympani to supply the taste buds of the anterior two-thirds of the tongue, being carried there by the lingual nerve.

SOMATIC SENSORY ROOT

A few cells of the geniculate ganglion send their peripheral processes to skin in the external acoustic meatus and behind the ear. Their central processes terminate in the pars caudalis of the spinal nucleus of the trigeminal nerve.

APPLIED ANATOMY

Supranuclear lesions

Supranuclear lesions of the facial nerve are caused by damage to the contralateral pyramidal tract. Weakness of the lower face is a classical feature of a 'stroke' (thrombosis or hemorrhage in the internal capsule).

Nuclear lesions

These are rare. Best known is the medial pontine syndrome, in which facial paralysis is accompanied by a contralateral hemiplegia (Millard–Gubler syndrome, Chapter 12).

Infranuclear lesions (Fig. 35-8)

Infranuclear lesions are relatively frequent. Much the commonest is *Bell's palsy*, caused by neuritis (?viral) of the facial nerve. More than one-third of patients have diabetes; pathology of small arteries in the nerve may be a contributory factor here. There is usually initial pain in the ear on the affected side, but the condition is otherwise painless.

Facial paralysis in Bell's palsy is complete. On the affected side the patients is unable to raise the eyebrow, close the eye, purse the lips, or retract the lip. Tears may spill from the lax conjunctival sac, and saliva may drool from one corner of the mouth. During mastication the hand may be pressed against the cheek to prevent food falling into the vestibule of the mouth. Nystagmus can usually be elicited at the onset of illness, if the eye is brought into full abduction. The nystagmus may be caused by pressure of the swollen facial nerve upon the vestibular nerve in the internal acoustic meatus.

The chorda tympani is nearly always paralyzed on the affected side. (Taste function is usually tested electrically, and submandibular function by the clearance rate of

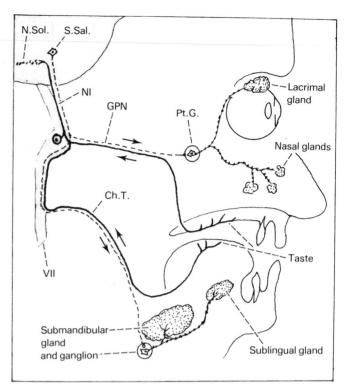

Fig. 35-6 The nervus intermedius. Ch.T., chorda tympani; GPN, greater petrosal nerve; Pt.G., pterygopalatine ganglion; NI, nervus intermedius; N.Sol., nucleus solitarius; S.Sal., superior salivatory nucleus.

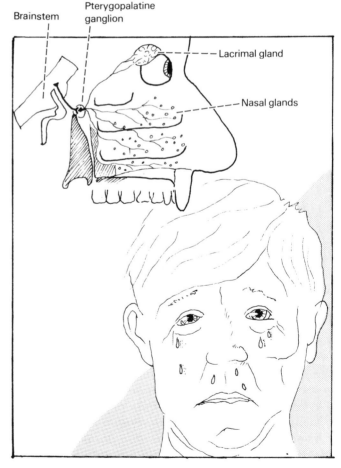

Fig. 35-7 Pterygopalatine ganglion ('ganglion of hay fever').

technetium-99m from the gland following systemic injection).

The lacrimal gland is sometimes affected, leading to dryness of the eye. Lacrimal flow can be compared on the two sides by measuring the rate of wetting of a strip of filter paper inserted into the outer corner of each eye.

Paralysis of the stapedius muscle may result in *hyperacusis*, with unpleasant intensification of loud sounds.

Four out of five cases recover completely in two to six weeks, because the nerve has only suffered a conduction block ('neuropraxia'). In the remainder, the nerve undergoes Wallerian degeneration; recovery then takes about three months and is usually incomplete. Some preganglionic fibers may regenerate in the wrong direction and stimulate the lacrimal gland at mealtimes (producing the so-called 'crocodile tears').

Facial paralysis in the *newborn* is caused by compression of one or both nerves by the obstetrician's forceps. The facial nerve is vulnerable at birth because of the absence of the protective mastoid process at this time; the stylomastoid foramen opens in a lateral direction.

Other causes of infranuclear palsy in adults include tumors of the parotid gland, tumors in the cerebellopontine angle, and surgical procedures within the middle ear or mastoid process. *Herpes zoster oticus* is a rare but well recognized viral infection of somatic sensory neurons of the facial nerve. Very severe pain in the ear for one to two days precedes the appearance of a vesicular rash in and around the external acoustic meatus. Swelling of the geniculate ganglion may be sufficient to cause a complete facial palsy (Ramsay Hunt syndrome).

Table 35-3 Stimulus–response characteristics for the corneal reflex

Lesion* (Right side)	Stimulus (Cornea)	Response (Orbicularis oculi)
1 (Afferent)	R	—
	L	L + R
2 (Internuncials)	R	—
	L	L
3 (Effector)	R	L
	L	L

*Locations as indicated in Fig. 35-9.

Corneal reflex

Three kinds of lesions may interrupt the corneal reflex (1, 2, and 3 in Fig. 35-9). The need for bilateral testing is evident from the figure and Table 35-3.

Readings

Brtazlavsky, M. (1976) Human brainstem reflexes. In *The Motor System: Neurophysiology and Muscle Mechanisms* (Shahani, M., ed.), pp. 135–154. Amsterdam: Elsevier.

Dubner, R., Sessle, B.J. and Storey, A.T. (1978) Jaw, facial, and tongue reflexes. In *The Neural Basis of Oral and Facial Function* by Dubner, R., Sessle, B.J. and Storey, A.T., pp. 246–310. Amsterdam: Elsevier.

Groves, J. (1976) Facial nerve. In *Scientific Foundations of Otolaryngology* (Hinchcliffe, R. and Harrison, D., eds.), pp. 429–459. London: Heinemann.

Ongeboer de Visser, B.W. (1980) The corneal reflex: electrophysiological and anatomical data in man. *Prog. Neurobiol.*, 15: 71–82.

Rinn, W.E. (1984) The neuropsychology of facial expression: a review of the neurological and psychological mechanisms for producing facial expressions. *Psychol. Bull.*, 95: 52–77.

Sears, E.S. and Franklin, G.M. (1980) Diseases of the cranial nerves. In *Neurology* (Rosenberg, R.N., ed.), pp. 471–494. New York: Grune & Stratton.

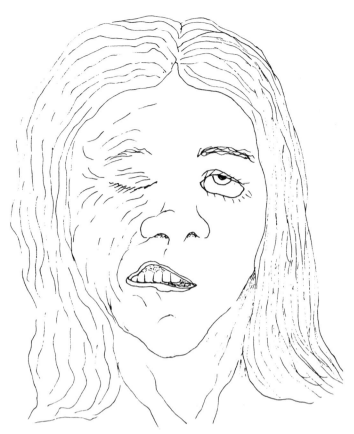

Fig. 35-8 Bell's palsy, left side. Response to the request, 'Close your eyes and show your teeth'.

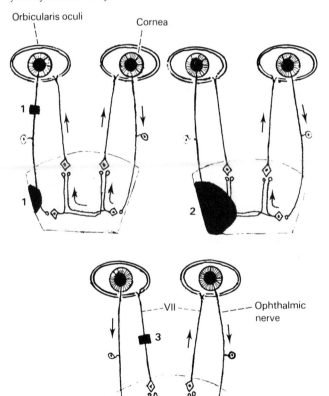

Fig. 35-9 Lesions of corneal reflex pathway. 1, lesion of ophthalmic nerve, or its spinal root within the medulla oblongata; 2, deep lesion of medulla; 3, facial nerve lesion. (Adapted from de Visser, 1980).

Cranial Nerves IX, X, XI, and XII

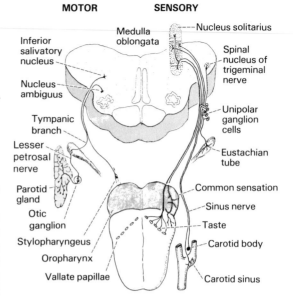

Fig. 36-1 Plan of the glossopharyngeal nerve.

GLOSSOPHARYNGEAL NERVE

The glossopharyngeal (cranial nerve IX) is a composite nerve, with diverse functions (Table 36-1, Fig. 36-1).

The nerve accompanies the vagus through the jugular foramen, then passes forward to enter the oropharynx in company with the stylopharyngeus muscle. Before entering the pharynx it gives off the slender *sinus nerve*, which supplies the carotid sinus and carotid body. The main nerve supplies the walls of the oropharynx – the pharyngeal mucous membrane, tonsil, and posterior third of tongue – and the eustachian tube. Taste fibers cross the sulcus terminalis to reach the vallate papillae.

Within the jugular foramen the glossopharyngeal nerve gives off a tympanic branch, which ramifies on the tympanic membrane before emerging into the middle cranial fossa as the *lesser petrosal nerve*. The lesser petrosal supplies preganglionic fibers to the otic ganglion; the postganglionic fibers are secretomotor to the parotid gland.

The glossopharyngeal afferents have unipolar cell bodies in the superior (somatic) and inferior (visceral) ganglia, in and below the jugular foramen. The great majority terminate in the *nucleus solitarius*.

Nucleus solitarius (Fig. 36-2)

This nucleus is the most densely packed in the entire CNS. It fuses with its opposite number at the level of the nucleus gracilis, forming the *commissural nucleus*. Its upper end reaches the lowermost part of the pons. Its center is at the level of the obex (lower tip of fourth ventricle). In its core is the *tractus solitarius*, which contains afferents from the facial, glossopharyngeal, and vagus nerves.

Chemically, the nucleus solitarius is highly diverse. It houses cell bodies of epinephrine and norepinephrine neurons, and nerve endings of substance-P-, enkephalin-, and GABA-containing neurons.

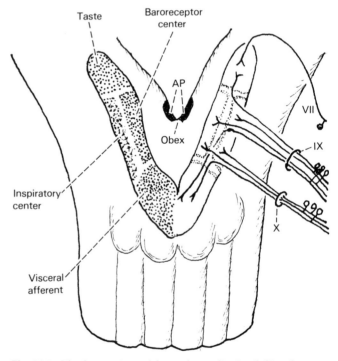

Fig. 36-2 The four regions of the nucleus solitarius (left) and their afferents (right). Area postrema (AP) is also indicated.

Table 36-1 Components of the glossopharyngeal nerve

Component	Distribution	Nucleus	Function
Visceral afferent	1 Carotid sinus	Nucleus solitarius	Control of blood pressure
	2 Carotid body	Nucleus solitarius	Control of respiration
	3 Oropharynx	Nucleus solitarius	Initiates swallowing reflex
Branchial afferent	Vallate papillae	Nucleus solitarius	Bitter taste
Somatic afferent	Middle ear	Trigeminal (pars caudalis)	Middle ear pain
Visceral efferent	Parotid gland	Inferior salivatory nucleus	Salivary secretion
Branchial efferent	Stylopharyngeus	Nucleus ambiguus	Unimportant

Anatomically, the nucleus is divided into eight subsections, but it is convenient to describe four *regions*: the rostral region, medial and lateral midregions, and a caudal region (Fig. 36-2).

1 The rostral region is the *gustatory nucleus*. It receives primary taste afferents from the facial nerve (tongue and palate), glossopharyngeal (vallate papillae), and vagus (taste buds in the epiglottis). It projects to the contralateral ventrobasal complex of thalamus.

2 The medial midregion receives baroreceptor afferents from the carotid sinus and aortic arch. Projections from this region are widespread (Chapter 37).

3 The lateral midregion has a structure typical of the reticular formation. It is the *inspiratory center*. It receives chemoreceptor afferents and it projects to the contralateral muscles of inspiration. Respiratory reflexes are detailed in Chapter 38.

4 The caudal region is a visceral afferent nucleus. It receives primary afferents from the alimentary and respiratory tracts. It projects to the hypothalamus, and to the swallowing and vomiting centers (see 'Vagus Nerve' later).

APPLIED ANATOMY: GLOSSOPHARYNGEAL NERVE

Glossopharyngeal neuralgia is a rare condition in which very severe pain occurs in the throat, tongue, and ear on swallowing. Reflex bradycardia with fainting attacks may result from involvement of nerve fibers supplying the carotid sinus. The neuralgia may be 'spontaneous', or it may be secondary to a local condition such as oropharyngeal carcinoma or an ossified stylohyoid ligament. *Whenever an adult complains of constant pain in one ear, and has no evidence of middle ear disease, a cancer of the pharynx must be suspected.*

'Spontaneous' glossopharyngeal neuralgia is usually caused by pressure from a vascular loop in the posterior cranial fossa. Removal of such pressure is sufficient for cure. Alternatively, the nerve may be cut intracranially, or tractotomy of the spinal root of the trigeminal may be performed. Section of the glossopharyngeal nerve on one side produces some anesthesia of the fauces, and loss of the gag reflex on the same side (stroking the fauces with a spatula normally elicits contraction of the pharyngeal constrictors). (See also 'Group lesions of the vagus, spinal accessory and hypoglossal nerves'.)

VAGUS NERVE

Like the glossopharyngeal, the vagus (cranial nerve X) is a composite nerve (Table 36-2, Fig. 36-3). Its most important components are:

1 Visceral afferents, which make up 80% of the entire nerve. The afferents come from the aortic arch, lower

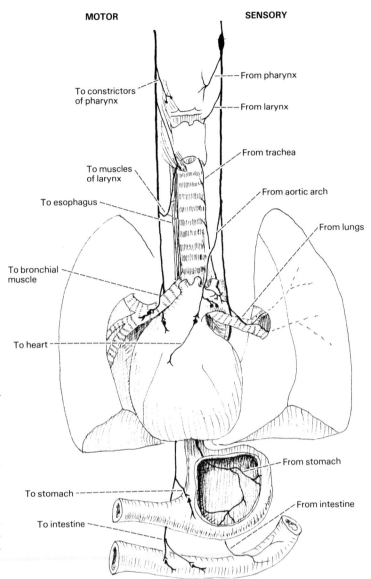

Fig. 36-3 Plan of the vagus nerve.

Table 36-2 Components of vagus nerve

Component	Distribution	Nucleus	Function
Visceral afferent	1 Aortic arch	Nucleus solitarius	Control of blood pressure (Chapter 37)
	2 Aortic bodies	Nucleus solitarius	Control of respiration (Chapter 38)
	3 Laryngopharynx, respiratory tract	Nucleus solitarius	Control of respiration
	4 Esophagus, GI tract	Nucleus solitarius	Control of GI motility (Chapter 39)
Branchial afferent	Taste (epiglottis)	Nucleus solitarius	? Control of respiration
Somatic afferent	External ear	Trigeminal nucleus (pars caudalis)	Sensation
Visceral efferent	1 Heart	Nucleus ambiguus	Cardiac slowing
	2 Bronchi	Dorsal nucleus of vagus	Bronchoconstriction
	3 Alimentary tract	Dorsal nucleus of vagus	Peristalsis, secretion
Branchial efferent	Levator palati, muscles of larynx and pharynx	Nucleus ambiguus	Vocalization, swallowing

respiratory tract, and alimentary tract. All of these afferents terminate in appropriate parts of the nucleus solitarius.

2 Parasympathetic preganglionic fibers to the heart, bronchi, and alimentary tract. In the cat (the only species studied in detail) the fibers arise partly in the nucleus ambiguus and partly in the dorsal motor nucleus of the vagus.

3 Branchial efferent fibers supplying the levator palati, larynx (intrinsic muscles), pharynx, and upper esophagus. These fibers arise in the nucleus ambiguus. Most emerge behind the sensory and parasympathetic rootlets of the vagus. They are sometimes called the *cranial (bulbar) accessory nerve* (cranial XI) and they join the vagal trunk below the jugular foramen. They are distributed by the pharyngeal and laryngeal nerves (Fig. 36-4). Although the cranial and spinal accessory nerves share a dural sheath for one centimeter, there is no exchange of fibers.

REFLEXES INVOLVING GLOSSOPHARYNGEAL AND VAGUS NERVES

Swallowing (Fig. 36-5)

Deglutition (swallowing) is a complex sequence of movements controlled by a specific generator in the reticular formation. The sequence has oral, pharyngeal, and esophageal phases.

Oral phase. The bolus of food is forced into the oropharynx by elevation of the tongue against the palate, the shape of the tongue being molded by its own intrinsic muscles. Elevation and retraction of the tongue are carried out by the mylohyoid and digastric muscles (the infrahyoid muscles being inhibited at the same time), and by the palatoglossus and styloglossus.

Pharyngeal phase. Afferents from the oropharynx terminate in the caudal nucleus solitarius, whose cells synapse upon the nucleus ambiguus and cause it to activate the pharyngeal constrictors from above downward. Regurgitation into the *mouth* is prevented by the maintenance of phase 1 contractions until the food has entered the esophagus. Regurgitation into the *nasopharynx* is prevented by contraction of the levator and tensor palati, which pull the palate against the pharyngeal wall. Regurgitation into the *larynx* is prevented by firm adduction of the vocal folds and by constriction of the laryngeal inlet.

Esophageal phase. The peristaltic wave that propels food into the esophagus continues all the way to the stomach. The upper third of the esophagus contains striated muscle innervated by fine motor axons from the vagus; several small end plates are applied to each muscle fiber. The middle third contains a mixture of striated and smooth muscle. The lower third contains only smooth muscle. Myenteric and submucous nerve plexuses are found in the lower two-thirds, and secondary peristaltic waves are produced by local myenteric reflexes (Chapter 39).

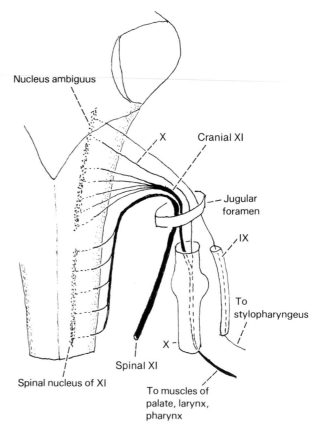

Fig. 36-4 The nucleus ambiguus contributes motor fibers to the glossopharyngeal, vagus and cranial accessory nerves. The cranial accessory nerve is distributed by the vagus.

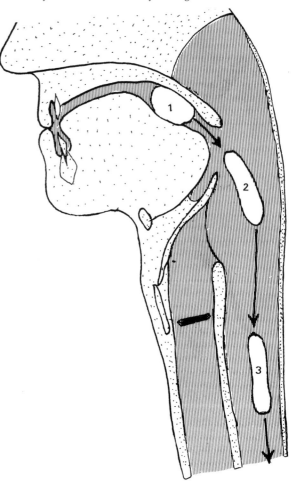

Fig. 36-5 Deglutition. The numbers indicate the position of the food bolus at the commencement of the oral (1), pharyngeal (2), and esophageal (3) phases.

The pattern generator

A *swallowing center* occupies the reticular formation of the medulla oblongata on each side; it is partly embedded in the midregion of nucleus solitarius. It receives afferents from this nucleus and from the spinal nucleus of the trigeminal nerve. In animals, stimulation of either swallowing center produces complete swallowing movements. Supranuclear control resides in the same areas that initiate masticatory movements, namely the premotor cortex, orbital cortex, and amygdala.

Vomiting

The vomiting center is a separate node of medullary reticular formation lying beside the swallowing center. It projects into the vagus nerve as well as to spinal cord neurons supplying the abdominal muscles. The initial event in vomiting is a relaxation of the esophagus and stomach. This is followed by mass contraction of the abdominal muscles, and by reverse peristalsis in the small intestine.

The four sources of stimulation of the center are shown in Fig. 36-6:

1 Descending fibers in the reticular formation carry impulses from the limbic cortex. They account for the nausea that may be associated with unpleasant sights and odors.

2 Ascending, spinoreticular fibers account for the nausea that accompanies acute physical injury.

3 Fibers from the nucleus solitarius complete the arc for the gag reflex. The afferent limb is provided by glossopharyngeal nerve fibers supplying the oropharynx. The efferent limb passes to the pharyngeal constrictors, but a complete vomiting sequence can be initiated in an emergency by firm stroking of the oropharynx.

4 The area postrema (Figs. 36-2, 36-6) is the *chemoreceptor trigger zone*. It is outside the blood–brain barrier and its rich capillary bed is fenestrated. It contains a small number of neurons of primitive appearance, as well as astrocytes (also primitive). The neurons synapse upon the vomiting center. In animals, the powerful emetic apomorphine is ineffective if the area has been destroyed. Its presence accounts for the emetic action of many drugs which cannot penetrate the blood–brain barrier. Its neurons contain abundant receptors for dopamine (reason unknown). Levodopa in high doses produces nausea. Conversely, dopamine antagonists are powerful antiemetic drugs.

APPLIED ANATOMY: VAGUS NERVE

The vagus is rarely paralyzed alone. The symptoms and signs of vagal interruption are listed in Table 36-3, and two signs are shown in Fig. 36-7.

SPINAL ACCESSORY NERVE

The spinal accessory nerve (cranial nerve XI) is a purely motor nerve. Its nucleus is a ribbon of α and γ

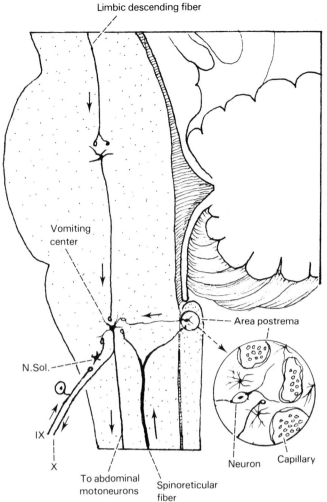

Fig. 36-6 Vomiting center and area postrema. N. Sol., nucleus solitarius.

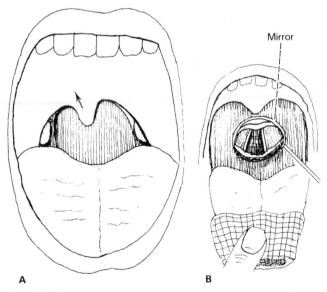

Fig. 36-7 Paralysis of left vagus. A, uvula moves to normal side (arrow). B, left vocal fold fails to abduct on deep inspiration.

Table 36-3 Effects of unilateral infranuclear vagal paralysis

Symptom	Paralyzed element
Nasal speech, nasal regurgitation of fluids	Soft palate
Movement of uvula to normal side	Soft palate
Hoarseness of speech	Larynx
Paralysis of vocal cord	Larynx
Cardiac, alimentary irregularity	Parasympathetic

motoneurons extending through the upper five segments of the spinal cord, in the base of the anterior horn.

The nerve runs upward to enter the cranial cavity through the foramen magnum. It leaves the skull through the jugular foramen. In the neck, it passes through the sternomastoid muscle and supplies it, then terminates in the trapezius. The longest part of the nerve extends from the neck to the lower thoracic level, lying at first deep to the trapezius and then within it.

Proprioceptive fibers enter the sternomastoid from cervical spinal nerves. They enter the trapezius from cervical and thoracic spinal nerves.

APPLIED ANATOMY: SPINAL ACCESSORY NERVE

Isolated paralysis of the spinal accessory nerve may result from a stab wound in the neck, or from surgical injury during removal of cancerous lymph nodes. If the lesion is proximal to the sternomastoid this muscle will waste and there will be diminished resistance to rotation of the head toward the opposite side. Wasting of the trapezius causes characteristic scalloping of the contour of the neck (Fig. 36-8).

Spasmodic torticollis is characterized by spasmodic contractions of the sternomastoid, often accompanied by neck pain. It is usually caused by pressure on the spinal accessory nerve within the vertebral canal, by a low-lying vertebral or posterior spinal artery (Fig. 36-9).

HYPOGLOSSAL NERVE

The hypoglossal nerve (cranial nerve XII) is a purely motor nerve supplying the extrinsic and intrinsic muscles of the tongue. Its nucleus (somatic efferent) underlies the hypoglossal triangle near the lower apex of the fourth ventricle.

The nerve emerges between the pyramid and the olive. It passes through the hypoglossal canal before descending in company with the vagus as far as the angle of the jaw. It then turns forward above the mylohyoid to supply the lingual musculature.

In the neck, proprioceptive fibers enter the hypoglossal nerve from the cervical plexus, for distribution to about 100 neuromuscular spindles in the tongue on the same side.

APPLIED ANATOMY: HYPOGLOSSAL NERVE

A nuclear or infranuclear lesion of the hypoglossal nerve is characterized by wasting of the affected side of the tongue, and deviation of the tongue to that side on protrusion (unopposed forward pull of the healthy genioglossus). Fasciculation of wasting muscle fibers is best seen when the tongue is only slightly protruded (Fig. 36-10).

APPLIED ANATOMY: GROUP LESIONS OF VAGUS, SPINAL ACCESSORY AND HYPOGLOSSAL NERVES

Supranuclear lesions

These are often detectable following vascular damage to the internal capsule. The nucleus ambiguus and hypoglossal nucleus may have a supply from the ipsilateral pyramidal tract that is adequate to preserve normal movements; otherwise the palate, larynx, and tongue are weak. This

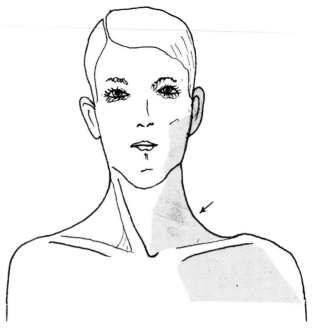

Fig. 36-8 Long-standing paralysis of the left spinal accessory nerve. The trapezius (arrow) and sternomastoid have wasted and the clavicle is lower on the affected side. (The trapezius normally helps to support the weight of the limb.)

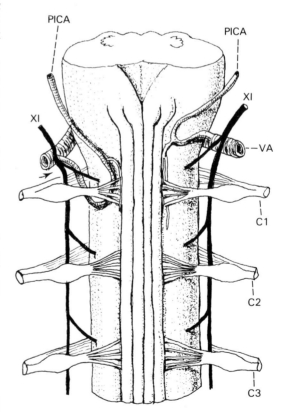

Fig. 36-9 Posterior view of medulla and spinal cord. A low-lying posterior inferior cerebellar artery (PICA) is stretching the left spinal accessory nerve (arrow). VA, vertebral artery. (Adapted from Hagenah et al., 1983).

weakness is on the same side as the weakness of the limbs and lower face. The trapezius *always* shows weakness (on shrugging the shoulders against resistance) on the same side as the affected limbs. The *opposite* sternomastoid may also be weak (see Chapter 20).

Pseudobulbar palsy is caused by widespread but incomplete vascular disorder of both pyramidal tracts, as part of a generalized atherosclerosis of brainstem arteries. Supranuclear disorders of the motor cranial nerves of the pons and medulla are revealed by slurring of speech and difficulty in mastication and swallowing. The gait is slow and shuffling because of involvement of pyramidal tract fibers to the limbs.

Nuclear lesions

These are seen in terminal stages of motor neuron disease, and in syringomyelia with bulbar extension.

Infranuclear lesions

Long-standing tumors at the cerebellopontine angle (for example, acoustic neuroma) may cause infranuclear lesions. Extracranial lesions are caused by malignant lymph nodes or other growths near the jugular foramen. Pain is felt in the neck or ear. The tongue and larynx may be paralyzed on the same side. A Horner's syndrome (ptosis and small pupil) appears should the cervical sympathetic be trapped near the carotid canal.

Readings

Aleksic, S.N., Budzilovich, G.N. and Budzilovich, A.G. (1973) Herpes zoster oticus and facial paralysis (Ramsay Hunt syndrome). Clinico-pathologic study and review of literature. *J. Neurol. Sci., 20:* 149–159.

FitzGerald, M.J.T., Comerford, P.T. and Tuffery, A. (1982) Sources of innervation of the neuromuscular spindles in sternomastoid and trapezius. *J. Anat., 134:* 471–490.

FitzGerald, M.J.T. and Sachithanandan, S.R. (1979) The structure and source of lingual proprioceptors in the monkey. *J. Anat., 128:* 523–552.

Freckmann, N., Hagenah, R., Herrmann, H.-D. and Müller, D. (1981) Treatment of neurogenic torticollis by microvascular lysis of the accessory nerve roots – indication, technique, and first results. *Acta Neurochir., 59:* 167–175.

Hagenah, R., Kosak, M. and Freckmann, N. (1983) Anatomical topography of the spinal accessory nerve roots to the vessels of the cranial cervical region. *Acta. Anat., 115:* 158–167.

Kalia, M. and Mesulam, M.-M. (1980) Brain stem projections of sensory and motor components of the vagus complex in the cat:

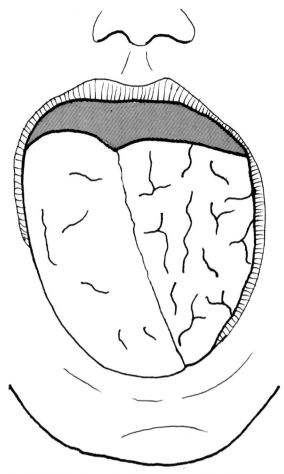

Fig. 36-10 Effect of long-standing paralysis of the left hypoglossal nerve.

the cervical vagus and nodose ganglion. *J. Comp. Neurol., 193:* 435–465.

Kerr, F.W.L., Hendler, N. and Bowron, P. (1969) Viscerotopic organization of the vagus. *J. Comp. Neurol., 138:* 279–290.

Leslie, R.A. and Guyn, D.G. (1984) Neuronal connections of the area postrema. *Fed. Proc., 43:* 2941–2943.

Sawchenko, P.E. (1983) Central connections of the sensory and motor nuclei of the vagus nerve. *J. Auton. Nerv. Syst., 9:* 13–26.

Weerasuriya, A., Bieger, D. and Hockman, C.H. (1980) Interaction between primary afferent nerves in the elicitation of swallowing. *Am. J. Physiol., 239:* R407–R414.

IX
VISCERAL REFLEXES

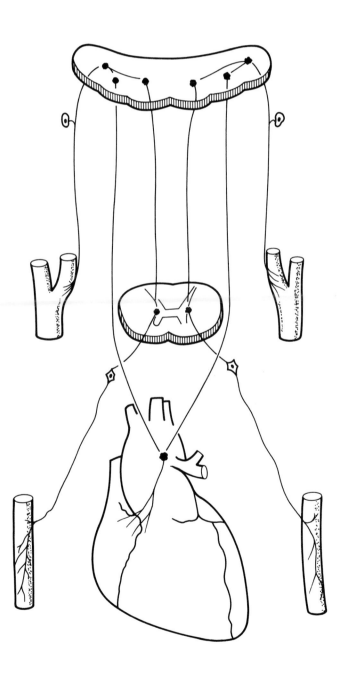

37

Cardiovascular Reflexes

THE HEART

Sympathetic innervation (Fig. 37-1)

Cardiac sympathetic fibers emerge from spinal cord segments T1–T5 on each side. They synapse in the three cervical sympathetic ganglia and in the upper five thoracic sympathetic ganglia. The postganglionic fibers pass through the cardiac plexuses (see later) and form varicosities on the sinoatrial and atrioventricular nodal tissue, conducting tissue, and ventricular myocardium. Stimulation of the sympathetic increases nodal firing rate, conduction rate, and ventricular force. The receptors are mostly β_1, although α receptors participate as well. The receptors have several effects on the flow of Ca^{2+}, Na^+ and K^+ through ion channels in the muscle membrane.

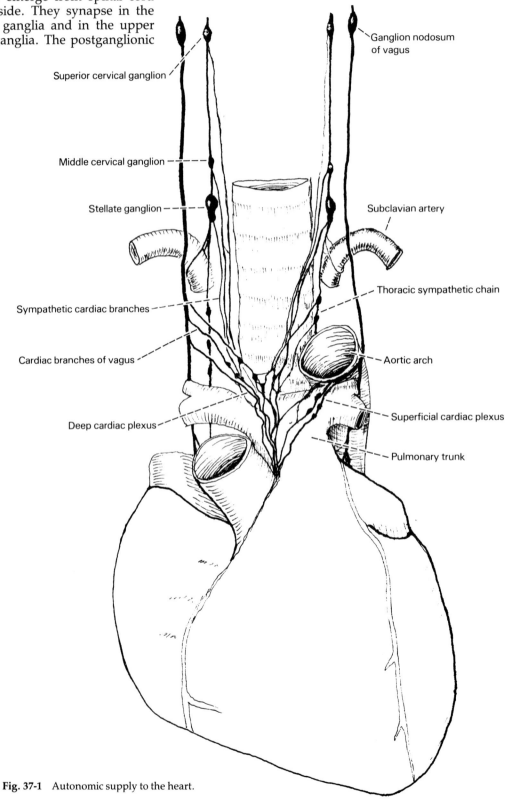

Fig. 37-1 Autonomic supply to the heart.

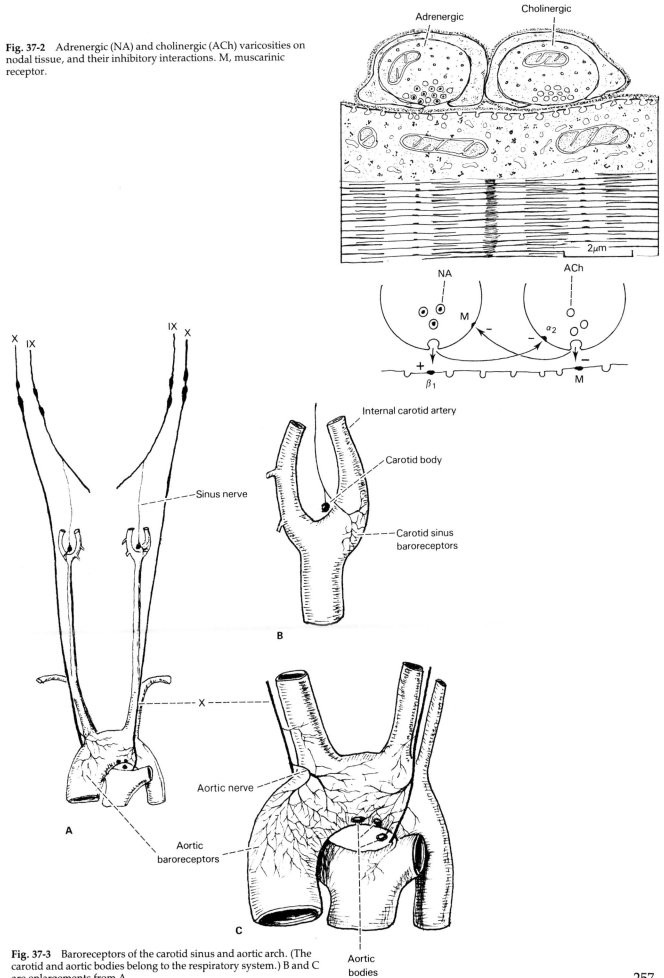

Fig. 37-2 Adrenergic (NA) and cholinergic (ACh) varicosities on nodal tissue, and their inhibitory interactions. M, muscarinic receptor.

Fig. 37-3 Baroreceptors of the carotid sinus and aortic arch. (The carotid and aortic bodies belong to the respiratory system.) B and C are enlargements from A.

The coronary arteries are rich in β_2 receptors and they relax in response to circulating epinephrine. They also have receptors responsive to muscle metabolites.

Parasympathetic innervation (Fig. 37-1)

Cardiac parasympathetic fibers arise from a node of the reticular formation embedded in the nucleus ambiguus. They leave the vagus just above the heart and synapse in the cardiac plexuses and in ganglia located on the posterior wall of the heart. (The superficial cardiac plexus lies between the aortic arch and the bifurcation of the pulmonary trunk. The deep cardiac plexus lies behind and above the pulmonary bifurcation. Both plexuses contain sympathetic, parasympathetic and afferent fibers but the ganglia are all parasympathetic.)

Postganglionic fibers from the right vagus form varicosities on the sinoatrial node and both atria. Postganglionic fibers from the left vagus form varicosities on conducting tissue and ventricular myocardium. Vagal stimulation inhibits nodal, conducting and myocardial tissue, thereby slowing the heart and reducing its contractile force. The receptors are all muscarinic, and the ionic changes are in general the opposite of those produced by sympathetic stimulation.

Axo-axonal interactions (Fig. 37-2)

Vagal and sympathetic fibers often lie side by side on nodal tissue. The vagal fibers inhibit the release of norepinephrine from the sympathetic fibers via prejunctional muscarinic receptors on the sympathetic fibers. The sympathetic fibers inhibit release of acetylcholine from the vagal fibers via prejunctional α_2 receptors on the vagal fibers.

Afferent innervation

1 The myocardium contains C fibers, which follow the sympathetic system to the cervical and upper five thoracic sympathetic ganglia. The C fibers reach their parent unipolar cell bodies in the second to fifth thoracic spinal ganglia and they enter the posterior gray horn of the spinal cord. These afferents are sensitive to myocardial ischemia and they are responsible for the pain of angina pectoris and coronary thrombosis (Chapter 7). There is reason to believe that under physiological conditions the myocardial afferents reflexly increase sympathetic tone, counterbalancing the inhibitory effects of the baroreceptor reflex.
2 The subendocardial connective tissue of the right atrium contains afferent nerve endings whose parent cells occupy the ganglion nodosum of the vagus. Distension of the right atrium causes reflex cardiac acceleration (the Bainbridge reflex), but the physiological importance of this reflex is uncertain.

GREAT ARTERIES (Figs. 37-3, 37-4)

The great arteries are rich in *baroreceptors* (Gr., *baros*, weight). The receptors are spatulate nerve endings

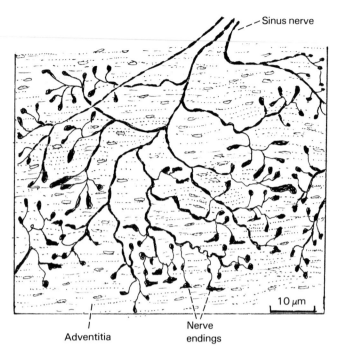

Fig. 37-4 Stretch afferents in the adventitia of the carotid sinus.

located in the adventitial coat. They are especially numerous in the carotid sinus – the bulbous expansion at the root of the internal carotid artery – and in the aortic arch. The carotid sinus is more sensitive than the aorta because the tunica media of the sinus is very thin.

Sinus and aortic nerves

The baroreceptors feed into the sinus branch of the glossopharyngeal nerve and into the small *aortic nerve* (a branch of the vagus). Centrally, the nerves synapse in the medial part of the nucleus solitarius, at the level of the obex.

Baroreceptor reflex

The sinus and aortic nerves are called the *buffer nerves* because they have a buffering effect on the arterial blood pressure: they operate to keep it within the physiological range. The receptors are tonically active. A rise in pulse pressure increases their firing rate and a fall reduces it; these effects are seen in experimental recordings from the sinus nerve, even during normal systole and diastole.

The buffer nerves reflexly *slow the heart* by means of excitatory internuncials passing from the nucleus solitarius to cardioinhibitory neurons embedded in the nucleus ambiguus.

The buffer nerves reflexly *reduce sympathetic tone* in the small peripheral arteries, by lowering the firing rate of cells in the lateral gray horn of the spinal cord. There are several pathways connecting the nucleus solitarius to the lateral horn (Fig. 37-5):
1 Solitarospinal axons run direct to the intermediolateral cell column (IML). They include epinephrine neurons of the C2 group and norepinephrine neurons of the A2 group (see Fig. 15-2); both are embedded in the nucleus solitarius.

2 Internuncials pass from the nucleus solitarius to the 'pressor' and 'depressor' areas of the medullary reticular formation (see Fig. 15-1). These areas send excitatory and inhibitory fibers, respectively, to the IML. The paired 'pressor' and 'depressor' areas have been called, collectively, the 'vasomotor center'. Many workers now believe that the IML has a greater claim to this title because some reflex arcs either bypass or traverse the 'pressor' and 'depressor' areas on their way to the cord.

3 Internuncials pass from the nucleus solitarius to aminergic cell groups elsewhere in the brainstem: to noradrenergic group A5 at the lower border of the pons, noradrenergic group A6 (nucleus ceruleus), and serotonin-cells close to the medullary midline. All three send aminergic fibers direct to the IML. Inactivation of A5 or of its descending fibers severely impairs the sympathetic depressor response to baroreceptor stimulation.

4 Some nucleus solitarius neurons project to the hypothalamus. Some hypothalamic neurons project all the way to the IML (Chapter 16).

5 Finally, some nucleus solitarius axons travel to the amygdala, apparently without interruption. The amygdalar projection to the hypothalamus has major sympathetic effects (Chapter 22).

APPLIED ANATOMY

Essential hypertension arises without any overt cause such as severe renal impairment or tumor of the suprarenal medulla. Demographic factors including race, inheritance, diet, and stress appear to act as triggers. The hypertension is labile (periodic) initially and permanent later. The sympathetic system is unquestionably overactive in established cases, and the thrust of present-day treatment is to reduce sympathetic activity by pharmacological methods. Drugs may act on the sympathetic supply in several parts of its course from brainstem to arteriolar walls, and their exact mode of action is often uncertain.

In addition to the increased sympathetic drive, the baroreflex is 'reset' in essential hypertension. Its threshold is raised. The resetting is selective for the heart: reflex slowing of the heart is impaired, whereas reflex vasodilatation is not impaired. This differential response suggests that the defect is unlikely to be due to structural changes in the great arteries or afferent nerve endings. Attention has focused on the nucleus solitarius because an experimental lesion of the baroreceptor area of the nucleus results in severe, *neurogenic hypertension*.

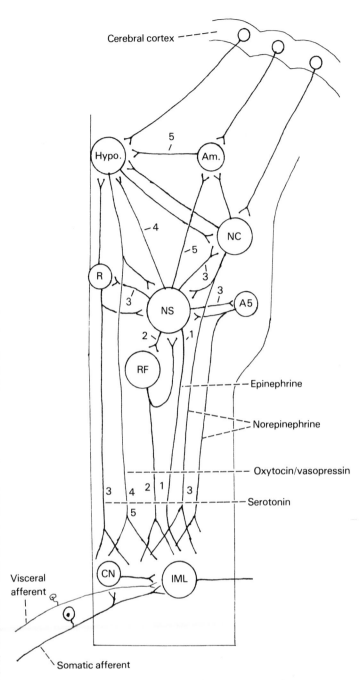

Fig. 37-5 Pathways from the nucleus solitarius to sympathetic centers in the spinal cord. For numbers see text. Am., amygdala; CN, central nucleus (internuncial sympathetic nucleus); Hypo., hypothalamus; IML, intermediolateral cell column; NC, nucleus ceruleus; NS, nucleus solitarius; R, raphe nucleus; RF, reticular formation.

Central effects

The baroreceptor area of the nucleus solitarius receives inputs from baroreceptor afferents, from the hypothalamus, and from adrenergic, noradrenergic, GABAergic and other neurons in the brainstem:

1 The baroreceptor afferents comprise myelinated fibers with glutamate as a verified transmitter, and some unmyelinated fibers with substance P as transmitter. Infusion of minute amounts of glutamate into the nucleus solitarius of experimental animals produces cardiac deceleration and peripheral vasodilatation. A defect either in glutamate liberation, or in glutamate receptor function in secondary neurons, could account for reduced baroreceptor function. Deficiency of substance P is unlikely to be significant because substance P infusion produces a hypertensive response.

2 The two-way connection between the nucleus solitarius and hypothalamus may be important because stimulation of the posterior hypothalamus or of the vasopressin- and oxytocin-synthesizing areas of the anterior hypothalamus produces sympathetic responses in the heart and blood vessels. The initial change in neural activity could even be at cortical level, since the hypothalamus receives several inputs from the limbic system (Chapter 22).

3 The epinephrine and norepinephrine neurons of the brainstem appear to be reciprocally inhibitory, both on one another and on sympathetic tone. The *epinephrine hypothesis* of hypertension regards a reduction in epinephrine content of the nucleus solitarius as a primary causative factor.

4 GABAergic nerve endings and receptors are found in the nucleus solitarius and in the dorsal (motor) nucleus of the vagus. Activation of these receptors by GABA agonists produces bradycardia and vasodilation.

Peripheral effects

A variety of changes in the peripheral effector system have been noted in hypertensives.

1 The amount of circulating norepinephrine is increased. This has been explained by a reduction in the number of prejunctional α_2 receptors, resulting in increased norepinephrine release.

2 The α_1 postjunctional response to norepinephrine is increased in hypertensives, suggesting that the number of α_1 receptors is increased.

3 Ion conductance across the membrane of smooth muscle cells (and of other cells) is altered in hypertensives. The depolarization threshold is lowered, and the amount of intracellular calcium is also raised.

4 Sympathetic nerves normally have a trophic action on smooth muscle. Sympathetic denervation in normal animals causes a reduction of the wall-to-lumen ratio of arteries. In hypertension, increased sympathetic activity is associated with generalized muscular hypertrophy in the arterial walls. The relative contributions of sympathetic action and raised blood pressure have been assessed in a genetic strain of spontaneously hypertensive rats, by carrying out a unilateral superior cervical ganglionectomy when hypertension has set in. The muscular hypertrophy in the denervated cerebral arteries is only half as great as that in the intact side, although both sides are equally exposed to the elevated blood pressure.

Readings

Abboud, F.M. (1982) The sympathetic nervous system in hypertension. *Hypertension*, suppl. 2, *4:* 208–225.

Antonaccio, M.J. (1984) Central transmitters: physiology, pharmacology, and effects on the circulation. In *Cardiovascular Pharmacology*, 2nd ed. (Antonaccio, M.J., ed.), pp. 155–195. New York: Raven Press.

Broadley, K.I. (1982) Cardiac adrenoceptors (review). *J. Auton. Pharmacol.*, 2: 119–145.

Creazzo, T., Titus, L. and Hartzell, C. (1983) Neural regulation of the heart. *Trends Neurosci.*, 6: 430–433.

Goldstein, S. (1983) The beta-blocker heart trial in perspective. *Cardiology*, 70: 255–262.

Hilton, S.M. and Spyer, K.M. (1980) Central nervous regulation of vascular resistance. *Annu. Rev. Physiol.*, 42: 399–411.

Langhorst, P., Schulz, B., Schulz, G. and Lambertz, M. (1983) Reticular formation of the lower brainstem. A common system for cardiorespiratory and somatomotor functions: discharge patterns of neighboring neurons influenced by cardiovascular and respiratory afferents. *J. Auton. Nerv. Syst.*, 9: 411–432.

Levy, M.N. (1984) Cardiac sympathetic–parasympathetic interactions. *Fed. Proc.*, 43: 2598–2602.

Malliani, A., Pagani, M., Pizzinelli, P., Furlan, R. and Guzzetti, S. (1983) Cardiovascular functions mediated by sympathetic afferent fibers. *J. Auton. Nerv. Syst.*, 7: 295–301.

Mathias, C.J. (1984) Blood pressure control and the peripheral sympathetic nervous system. In *Mild Hypertension* (Weber, M.A. and Mathias, C.J., eds.), pp. 24–30. Darmstadt: Steinkopff Verlag.

McCloskey, D.I. and Potter, E.K. (1981) Excitation and inhibition of cardiac vagal motoneurones by electrical stimulation of the carotid sinus nerve. *J. Physiol.*, 316: 163–175.

Peart, W.S. (1984) Some neurological aspects of blood pressure control. In *Mild Hypertension* (Weber, M.A. and Mathias, C.J., eds.), pp. 1–10. Darmstadt: Steinkopff Verlag.

Polinsky, R.J. (1984) Central nervous system control of blood pressure. In *Mild Hypertension* (Weber, M.A. and Mathias, C.J., eds.), pp. 11–23. Darmstadt: Steinkopff Verlag.

Reis, D.J., Perrone, M.H. and Talman, W.T. (1981) Glutamic acid as the neurotransmitter of baroreceptor afferents in the nucleus tractus solitarii: possible relationship to neurogenic hypertension. In *Central Nervous System Mechanisms in Hypertension* (Buckley, J.P. and Ferrario, P.M., eds.), pp. 37–47. New York: Raven Press.

Stock, G., Schmelz, M., Knuepfer, M.M. and Forssman, W.G. (1983) Functional and anatomic aspects of central nervous cardiovascular regulation. In *Central Cardiovascular Control* (Ganten, D. and Pfaff, D., eds.), pp. 1–30. Berlin: Springer-Verlag.

Respiratory Reflexes

Respiration is under the immediate control of the respiratory centers of the brain stem. The *respiratory centers* are three paired nuclei: the inspiratory and expiratory nuclei in the medulla oblongata, and the pneumotaxic center in the pons. All belong to the reticular formation, and contain 'respiration-related' neurons which alter their firing rate during the respiratory cycle. The medullary respiratory centers are pattern generators: their axons supply the many separate groups of anterior horn cells serving respiratory movements.

INSPIRATORY CENTER (Fig. 38-1)

The inspiratory center comprises the *dorsal respiratory nuclei*, located in the lateral part of the nucleus solitarius on each side, at the level of the obex. The neurons of the center discharge in complete synchrony during inspiration, being linked by electronic synapses (gap junctions). Their axons cross the midline before descending to terminate monosynaptically on the motoneurons supplying the inspiratory muscles: the phrenic nucleus (C3–C5) and intercostal nuclei (T1–T12). The nuclei serving accessory muscles of inspiration and the abductors of the vocal cords are also supplied.

EXPIRATORY CENTER (Fig. 38-1)

The expiratory center comprises the *ventral respiratory nuclei*, which lie alongside the nucleus ambiguus. Like the inspiratory center, its neurons have inherent rhythmicity and discharge synchronously. They project contralaterally to the motoneurons serving the internal intercostals and accessory muscles of expiration. During quiet breathing, discharges are insufficient to activate these muscles: normal expiration is produced by the elastic recoil of the lungs. The ventral respiratory nuclei appear to function only in forced expiration.

The inspiratory and expiratory centers are not as distinct as the above account implies. 'Respiration-related neurons' are also found between them, with considerable spatial overlap of inspiratory and expiratory functions. There is no clear evidence of any inhibitory interaction between dorsal and ventral respiratory groups.

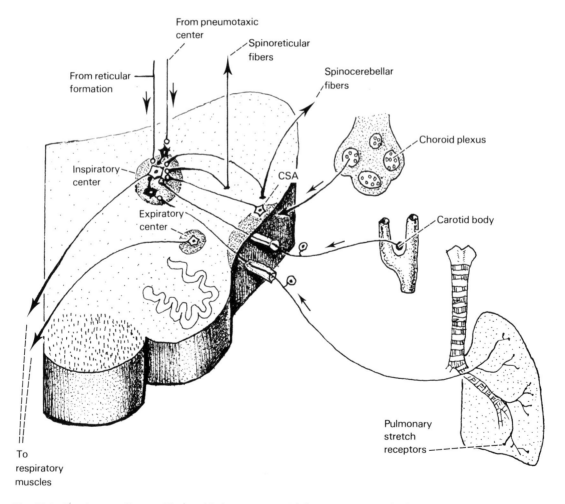

Fig. 38-1 Respiratory afferents. The two black neurons are inhibitory internuncials. CSA, chemosensitive area.

PNEUMOTAXIC CENTER

As its name suggests, the pneumotaxic center influences the *rate of breathing*. The center consists of paired nuclei lying medial to the superior cerebellar peduncles, or brachia conjunctiva – hence the alternative name, *parabrachial nuclei*.

The function of the parabrachial nuclei is not well understood. Some of its neurons discharge only during inspiration, others during expiration, and still others during both phases. Physiological experiments indicate that the pneumotaxic center inhibits dorsal respiratory neurons, tending therefore to shorten the respiratory cycle. Transection of the lower pons severs the descending inputs and results in deep respiratory cycles.

RESPIRATORY AFFERENTS

Afferents influencing respiratory rate

Chemoreceptors

Two sets of chemoreceptors play upon the inspiratory center: the arterial chemoreceptors, and chemosensitive cells at the surface of the medulla oblongata.

The *arterial chemoreceptors* are the carotid and aortic bodies (Fig. 38-2). The *carotid bodies* (one on each side) occupy the bifurcation of the common carotid artery. Each weighs only 2 mg, and is supplied by a twig from the internal carotid. Two or three *aortic bodies* are found on the aortic arch and are supplied by twigs from the arch. The aortic bodies are not important for respiratory control in humans.

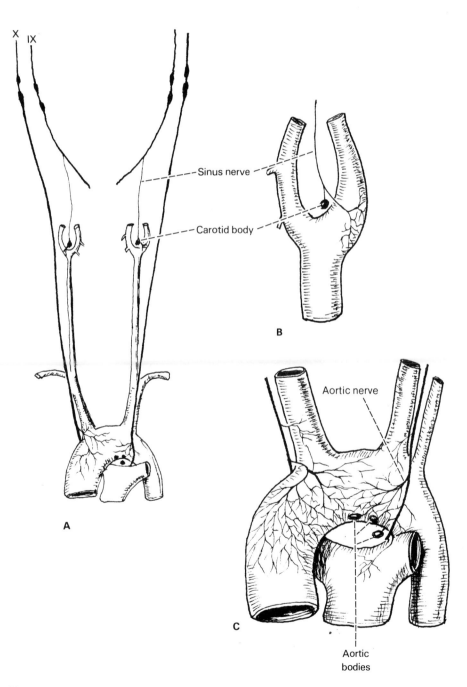

Fig. 38-2   Carotid and aortic bodies. B and C are enlarged from A.

The carotid bodies have the richest blood flow of any tissue in the body – five times more per milligram than the kidney. They are riddled with capillaries and the blood flow is so intense that the arteriovenous partial pressure of oxygen (Po_2) changes by less than 1% during passage. The carotid chemoreceptors effectively sample the arterial blood.

The primary function of the carotid bodies is to monitor arterial Po_2 and to increase pulmonary ventilation reflexly whenever Po_2 falls. Afferent nerve fibers enter the sinus nerve and synapse centrally in the inspiratory center. A fall in arterial Po_2 increases impulse traffic in the sinus nerve, and the inspiratory center responds by increasing the depth and then the rate of breathing.

The peripheral chemoreceptors are also sensitive to a rising H^+ concentration resulting from hypercapnia (increased CO_2 levels in the blood).

Structure of the carotid body (Figs. 38-3, 38-4). The bulk of the parenchyma is made up of round, *glomus cells* with dopamine-containing dense-cored vesicles. The glomus cells make synaptic contacts with sensory fibers from the sinus nerve (IX) or vagus. Some of the synapses are glomo-axonal, some are axo-glomal, and some have both features – they are reciprocal (Chapter 1).

A fall in Po_2 or a rise in Pco_2 causes the afferent fibers to discharge direct to the inspiratory center.

The site of the Po_2/Pco_2 receptors is unsettled. They could be in the nerve endings, in which case the glomus cells may exert a negative feedback effect through dopamine liberation. In this view, depolarization of the nerve endings activates the axo-glomal synapses, and the glomus cells respond by activating the inhibitory glomo-axonal synapses (dopamine).

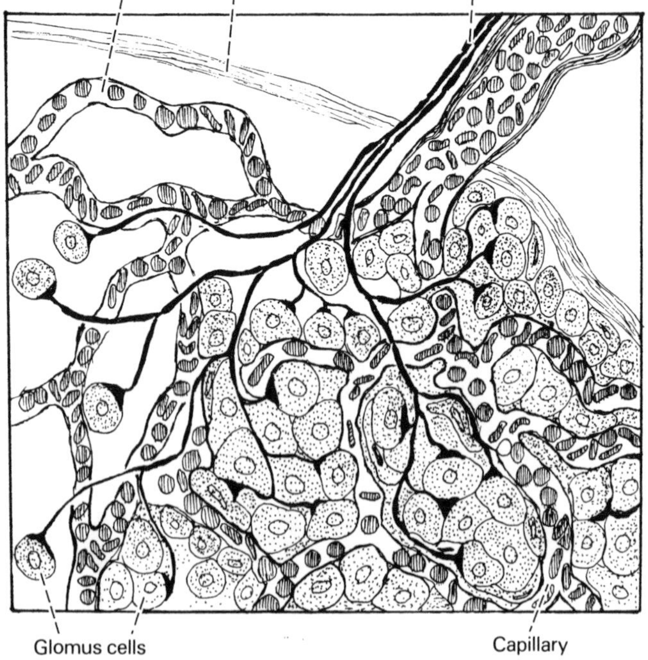

The *chemosensitive area* (CSA) of the medulla oblongata is a strip of reticular formation close to the rootlets of the glossopharyngeal nerve (Fig. 38-1). It is bathed by cerebrospinal fluid passing from the lateral aperture of the fourth ventricle into the basal cistern. A tuft of choroid plexus emerges through each lateral aperture and lies beside the medulla oblongata (Fig. 38-5).

The neurons of the CSA are exquisitely sensitive to a rise of H^+ ions from any cause. They are not sensitive to hypoxia. Blood CO_2 crosses the choroidal epithelium without interference. It is immediately hydrated and dissociates into H^+ and CO_3^- ions, which diffuse through the

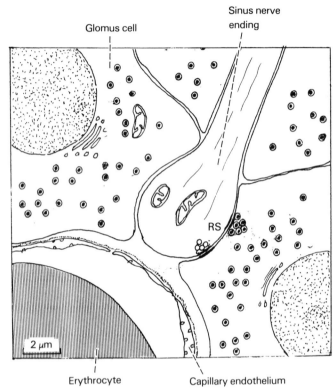

Fig. 38-4 A nerve ending in the carotid body. RS, reciprocal synapse.

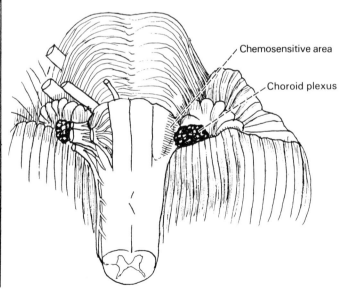

Fig. 38-5 A tuft of choroid plexus protrudes through the lateral aperture of the fourth ventricle, to lie beside the chemosensitive area of the medulla oblongata.

Fig. 38-3 Innervation of the carotid body.

pia–glial membrane covering the surface of the medulla. The CSA responds by stimulating the inspiratory center.

Proprioceptors

Respiratory rate increases at the commencement of exercise, before metabolic changes have had time to produce their effects. Even passive movements of a recumbent individual stimulate respiration. The afferents concerned are collaterals from the spinocerebellar tracts (Fig. 38-1).

Afferents influencing respiratory rhythm

1 *Pulmonary stretch receptors* are vagal nerve endings in the perilobular and subpleural connective tissue. They excite inhibitory internuncials in the inspiratory center. If the vagi are cut (in animals), deep respiratory cycles follow. If the lower pons is sectioned as well as the vagi, 'apneustic' breathing sets in: a deep breath every two to three minutes, separated by intervals of apneusis (no breathing).

In humans, the pulmonary stretch receptors are less important than in lower mammals. They only come into action during deep ventilation.

2 *Irritant receptors* are supplied by the vagus to the epithelium of the trachea. They respond to foreign matter in the airway by inhibiting the inspiratory center and exciting the *coughing center*, a nuclear subgroup within the expiratory center. Another subgroup, the *sneezing center*, responds to particulate matter in the nose. The exact location of these two centers is uncertain.

3 *J (juxtacapillary) receptors* in the lungs produce tachypnea (rapid breathing) and bradycardia (cardiac slowing) in response to pulmonary vascular congestion. In acute failure of the left ventricle of the heart (most often in severely hypertensive patients), blood accumulates in the pulmonary capillaries and produces rapid, gasping respiration known as *cardiac asthma*.

4 The *spinoreticular tract* gives branches to the inspiratory center. They account for the sharp intake of breath caused by cold or painful stimuli.

5 During normal breathing, muscle spindle afferents from the intercostal and abdominal muscles act *during inspiration* to inhibit the inspiratory center. (The diaphragm has very few spindles.)

6 The *load compensation reflex* (Chapter 10) becomes vitally important when the airway is obstructed by foreign material. Such obstruction produces a mismatch between on-going fusimotor contraction and arrested extrafusal contraction, resulting in powerful α motoneuron activation of the external intercostals. This is a purely spinal reflex.

Afferents influencing both rate and rhythm

1 *Pyramidal tract* fibers terminate monosynaptically upon the anterior horn cells supplying the inspiratory and expiratory muscles. Rhythm and rate can be altered at will.

2 The *limbic system* has two-way connections with the pneumotaxic center. Afferents from the septum and amygdala synapse directly on the parabrachial nuclei. The limbic connections account for changes in rhythm and rate during bouts of anger or fear.

Opiate receptors

Morphine is a classical respiratory depressant. At least part of its action is upon the inspiratory center, which contains opiate receptors in high concentrations. These receptors are also responsive to endogenous opiates (the endorphins), which may exert a tonic inhibitory effect on the inspiratory center.

APPLIED ANATOMY

The central and peripheral respiratory reflexes and manifestly important in respiratory pathology and in anesthesia. Discussions of these topics are to be found in textbooks of applied physiology and biochemistry.

Readings

Cohen, M.J. (1981) Central determinants of respiratory rhythm. *Annu. Rev. Physiol., 43:* 91–104.

Coleridge, J.C.G. and Coleridge, H.M. (1984) Afferent vagal C fibre innervation of the lungs and airways and its functional significance. *Rev. Physiol. Biochem. Pharmacol., 99:* 1–110.

Eldridge, F.L. and Millhorn, D.E. (1981) Central regulation of respiration by endogenous neurotransmitters and neuromodulators. *Annu. Rev. Physiol., 43:* 121–135.

Gillis, R.A., Helke, C.J., Hamilton, B.L., Norman, W.P. and Jacobowitz, D.M. (1980) Evidence that substance P is a neurotransmitter of baro- and chemoreceptor afferents in nucleus tractus solitarius. *Brain Res., 181:* 476–481.

Hellström, S., Hanbauer, I., Commissiong, J., Karoum, F. and Kislow, S. (1984) Role and regulation of catecholamines in the carotid body. In *Dynamics of Neurotransmitter Function* (Hannin, I., ed.), pp. 31–38. New York: Raven Press.

Kalia, M.P. (1981) Anatomical organization of central respiratory neurons. *Annu. Rev. Physiol., 43:* 105–120.

Kalia, M.P. (1981) Localization of aortic and carotid baroreceptor and chemoreceptor primary afferents in the brain stem. In *Central Nervous Mechanisms in Hypertension* (Buckley, J.P. and Ferrario, C.M., eds.), pp. 9–24. New York: Raven Press.

Levitzky, M.G. (1982) *Pulmonary Physiology.* New York: McGraw-Hill.

Nilsestuen, J.O., Coon, R.L., Woods, M. and Kampine, J.P. (1981) Location of lung receptors mediating the breathing frequency response to pulmonary CO_2. *Resp. Physiol., 45:* 343–355.

Pack, A.I. (1981) Sensory inputs to the medulla. *Annu. Rev. Physiol., 43:* 73–90.

Pack, R.J. and Richardson, P.S. (1984) The aminergic innervation of the human bronchus: a light and electron microscopic study. *J. Anat., 138:* 493–502.

Shannon, R. and Freeman, D. (1981) Nucleus retroambigualis respiratory neurons: responses to intercostal and abdominal muscle afferents. *Resp. Physiol., 45:* 357–375.

Widdicombe, J. and Davies, A. (1983) *Respiratory Physiology.* London: Arnold.

39
Enteric Nervous System

The enteric nervous system (Gr., *enteron*, gut) extends from the middle third of the esophagus to the anorectal junction – a distance of about ten meters. It has intrinsic and extrinsic components.

The *intrinsic* innervation is provided by some 100 million neurons embedded in the wall of the gut. This population is equivalent to that of the entire spinal cord. They exert a high degree of local control. For example, if the extrinsic nerves are removed the gut is still capable of propagating peristaltic waves in response to local distension. The contraction waves are ring-like and ahead of them are waves of relaxation (Bayliss–Starling Law).

The *extrinsic* innervation is provided by sympathetic (postganglionic) fibers and by parasympathetic (preganglionic) fibers.

INTRINSIC NERVE SUPPLY (Fig. 39-1)

Myenteric plexus

The *myenteric plexus* (of Auerbach) lies between the longitudinal and circular coats of smooth muscle. A large-meshed *primary plexus* contains multipolar ganglion cells and receives the extrinsic nerves. A finer, *secondary plexus* contains axons and dendrites of the ganglion cells. A *tertiary plexus* distributes axons to the smooth muscle coats and digestive glands.

Submucous plexus

The *submucous plexus* (of Meissner) is in the submucous coat. Most of its ganglion cells are unipolar or bipolar, suggesting a sensory function. Their peripheral processes extend to the mucous membrane, and their central processes synapse upon myenteric neurons.

Transmitters

More than 20 transmitter-type substances have been demonstrated in intrinsic neurons, mainly by immunocytochemistry. Excitatory transmitters include acetylcholine, substance P, and cholecystokinin. Inhibitory transmitters include adenosine triphosphate (ATP) and enkephalins. Vasoactive intestinal polypeptide (VIP) inhibits intestinal and vascular smooth muscle and stimulates intestinal secretion. Serotonin inhibits colonic segmentation but stimulates segmentation in the small intestine.

The myenteric reflex

The *myenteric reflex* is the wave of contraction that follows local intestinal distension. As already noted, it

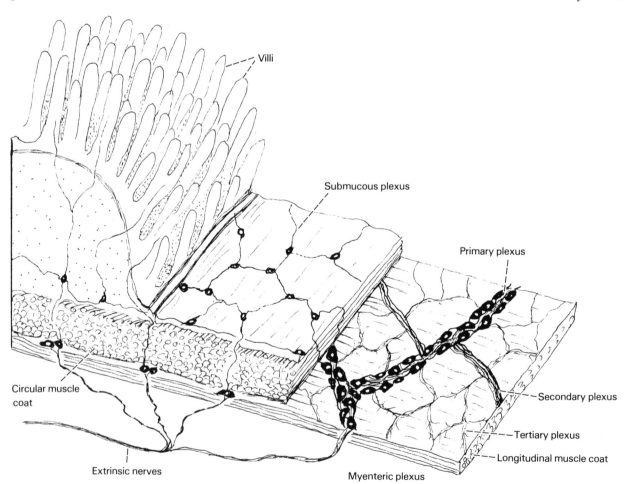

Fig. 39-1 The myenteric and submucous plexuses in the intestine.

is preceded by a wave of relaxation and is independent of the extrinsic nerve supply. Bayliss and Starling found that the reflex was abolished by nicotine, and therefore involved cholinergic transmission. It is also abolished if an anesthetic is applied to the mucous membrane; therefore mucosal fibers from the submucous plexus are also involved.

A model of the myenteric reflex can be made by postulating one set of afferent neurons and two sets of internuncials: one internuncial set driving inhibitory effector neurons and another driving excitatory effector neurons (Fig. 39-2). The inhibitory transmitter may be ATP. The excitatory transmitter is acetylcholine. Cholinergic varicosities are numerous on the surface of the longitudinal and circular muscle coats. Excitation is propagated through gap junctions (Fig. 39-3).

EXTRINSIC NERVE SUPPLY

Sympathetic supply

Preganglionic fibers for the foregut and midgut (stomach to splenic flexure of colon) emerge from spinal cord segments T5–T12. They pass through the thoracic sympathetic chain without relay, emerging as the thoracic splanchnic nerves (Chapter 6). They synapse in the abdominal splanchnic (preaortic) ganglia. Postganglionic fibers accompany the gastrointestinal arteries.

The hindgut (descending and sigmoid colon, and rectum) receives fibers from the splanchnic ganglia, but it is supplied mainly from the lumbar ganglia of the sympathetic chain. The postganglionic fibers accompany the inferior mesenteric artery.

Sympathetic stimulation causes the alimentary sphincters to contract, and the detrusor (emptying) musculature to relax. The sphincters are supplied direct by postganglionic fibers activating α_1 receptors. The detrusor muscle is inhibited both directly via β_2 receptors and indirectly via α_2 receptors located on cholinergic nerve endings (Fig. 39-4). The α_2 effect is to inhibit the tonic release of acetylcholine.

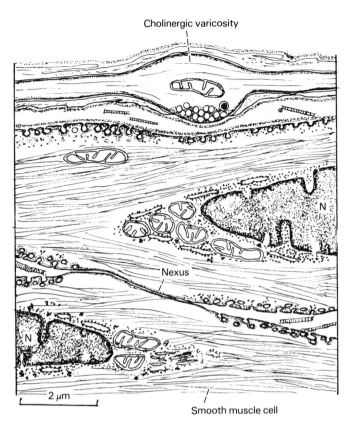

Fig. 39-3 Parasympathetic innervation of intestinal muscle. Two muscle cells are shown (N, nucleus). Excitation is propagated via nexuses.

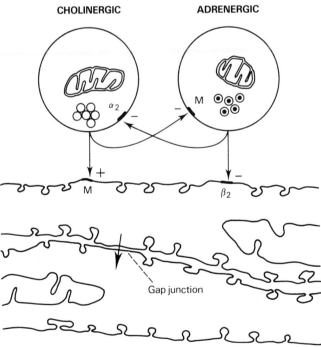

Fig. 39-4 Cholinergic and adrenergic varicosities in the intestine, and their inhibitory interactions. M, muscarinic receptor.

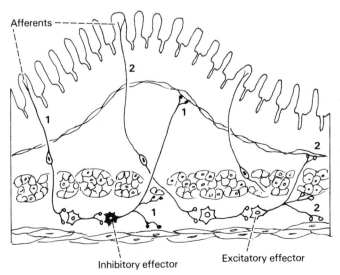

Fig. 39-2 Propagation of a peristaltic wave. 1, inhibitory reflex arc; 2, excitatory reflex arc.

If the celiac and mesenteric ganglia are removed the adrenergic innervation of the intestine degenerates completely: there are no sympathetic nerve cells in the intestinal wall.

Structure of splanchnic ganglia

Although the great majority of the ganglion cells are adrenergic neurons receiving preganglionic, cholinergic boutons, a variety of other neurons are also present – some cholinergic, others peptidergic (somatostatin, substance P, enkephalin). In addition, some sensory fibers running from gut to spinal cord give collaterals to ganglion cells. Some myenteric neurons also give collaterals to the splanchnic ganglia. These collaterals may initiate the *entero-enteric reflex* – relaxation of coils of intestine remote from a site of intestinal distension.

Parasympathetic supply

The two vagus nerves exchange fibers on the outer surface of the esophagus. They enter the abdomen as the *anterior and posterior vagal trunks* (Fig. 39-5). About two-thirds of the vagal fibers are distributed to the stomach. The intestine (as far as the splenic flexure of colon) is supplied by branches of the posterior trunk. Some fibers synapse in the splanchnic ganglia but most are preganglionic until they synapse upon neurons of the myenteric plexus.

The descending colon and rectum receive their parasympathetic innervation from spinal cord segments S2, S3 and S4 (pelvic splanchnic nerves, Chapter 40).

Vagal stimulation has marked effects on the stomach (see later). In the intestine, although stimulation of the cut distal ends of the human vagi produces peristaltic waves, vagotomy (section of both vagal trunks) is not followed by intestinal stasis. Instead, it may be followed by bouts of diarrhea, perhaps because of changes in the bacterial flora.

Visceral afferents

Finely myelinated and unmyelinated afferents travel to the CNS from all layers of the wall of the gut. Their nerve endings are free, and no structure/function correlation has been detected as yet. Electrical records from splanchnic nerves have revealed four classes of sensory units:
1 Mechanoreceptors in the muscle and mucous membrane;
2 Chemoreceptors responsive to pH changes, to the presence of glucose, or to amino acids;
3 Thermoreceptors (cold, warm, and mixed) capable of influencing central thermal regulation;
4 Osmoreceptors, responding to changes in the tonicity of intestinal contents.

From the stomach and proximal intestine the vagus is the predominant pathway for afferents of all four classes. The sympathetic pathway predominates for the more distal intestine. (Afferents from Pacinian corpuscles located in the root of the mesentery of the

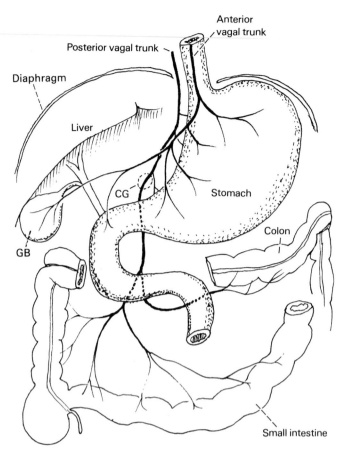

Fig. 39-5 Distribution of the vagal nerve trunks. CG, celiac ganglion; GB, gallbladder.

small intestine also reach the CNS by following the splanchnic nerves. The corpuscles may participate in the regulation of blood flow to the intestine.)

Clinically, intense stimulation of visceral afferents by distension, vigorous contraction, or ulceration gives rise to visceral pain (Chapter 7). Blockage of splanchnic or other sympathetic ganglia may afford dramatic relief by interrupting the afferents.

Paraneurons

Endocrine cells of neural origin (Chapter 17) are scattered among the basal cells of the gastric glands and in the crypts of Lieberkühn throughout the intestine. They secrete polypeptides into the local tissue fluid (in some cases, into the capillary bed). Cells having local ('paracrine') effects include argentaffin (L., silver-affinity) cells releasing serotonin and VIP cells releasing vasoactive intestinal polypeptide.

STOMACH

The vagus is important for control of gastric motility and secretion. The sympathetic system is of minor significance: stimulation of the splanchnic nerves merely causes contraction of the pyloric sphincter.

Motility

Weak electrical stimulation of the human vagal nerve trunks causes peristaltic waves to pass smoothly from fundus to pylorus. The smooth progression of peristaltic waves is initiated by *pacemaker* muscle cells in the fundus. Normal pacemaker activity is vagus-dependent. Following vagotomy, other pacemaker sites appear, and peristalsis becomes disorganized: gastric contents accumulate in the antrum, a phenomenon known as 'dumping'.

Secretion

The initial, *psychic phase* of gastric secretion is induced by the sight or smell of food. It is mediated by the vagi. The cholinergic neurons concerned run from the local myenteric plexus to the glandular cells secreting acid (oxyntic cells), pepsinogen (peptic cells), and mucus (surface epithelium and mucous neck cells). In the *gastric phase*, initiated by entry of food into the stomach, secretion is reinforced through reflex arcs (afferent limb, Meissner's plexus; efferent limb, Auerbach's plexus). The secretogogue hormone, gastrin, is liberated by vagal action on the antrum and by the local reflex arcs.

Gastroesophageal junction

The lower esophageal sphincter is a physiological rather than an anatomical entity. During digestion the lower end of the esophagus is tonically contracted, preventing regurgitation of food. The circular muscle coat is not thickened but the innermost, oblique muscle coat of the stomach forms an 'oblique sphincter' around the gastroesophageal inlet (Fig. 39-6). This muscle is excited by circulating gastrin at mealtimes.

Striated muscle from the right crus (mainly) of the diaphragm loops around the gastroesophageal junction. This loop exerts a pinchcock effect when intra-abdominal pressure is elevated during exercise.

APPLIED ANATOMY

Vagotomy is frequently performed on patients having a chronic duodenal (peptic) ulcer. The operation greatly reduces hydrochloric acid secretion and promotes healing of the ulcer. Three kinds of vagotomy are possible (Fig. 39-7): truncal, selective, and highly selective.

Truncal vagotomy
Both vagal trunks are cut. Disadvantages are gastric stasis (dumping), dilation of the gallbladder (which normally contracts in response to vagal stimulation), and impaired pancreatic secretion.

Selective vagotomy
Only the gastric branches are cut. Its disadvantage is that dumping is so frequent that a surgical bypass of the antrum must be performed as well (gastrojejunostomy).

Highly selective vagotomy
Only the nerves to the fundus and body (the acid-secreting areas) are cut. The nerves to the antrum (nerves of Latarget) are preserved. Dumping is avoided. Although gastrin levels in the blood during meals are higher than normal after this operation, gastrin is no longer effective in eliciting acid secretion. This may be because the oxyntic cells undergo considerable involution when deprived of vagal stimulation.

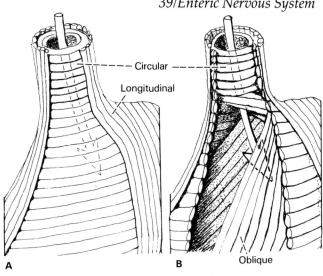

Fig. 39-6 Gastroesophageal junction. A, window cut in longitudinal muscle; B, window cut in circular muscle.

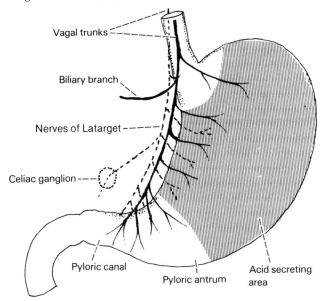

Fig. 39-7 Vagal innervation of the stomach. The acid-secreting area is shaded.

Readings

Bayliss, W. and Starling, E.H. (1899) The movements and innervation of the small intestine. *J. Physiol.*, 24: 99–143.

Burnstock, G. (1979) Interactions of cholinergic, adrenergic, purinergic and peptidergic neurons in the gut. In *Integrative Functions of the Autonomic Nervous System* (Brooks, C.M., Koizumi, K. and Sato, A., eds.), pp. 145–158. Tokyo: University Press; Amsterdam: Elsevier/North Holland Biomedical Press.

Furness, J.B. and Costa, M. (1980) Types of nerves in the enteric nervous system. *Neuroscience*, 5: 1–20.

Gershon, M.D. (1981) The enteric nervous system. *Annu. Rev. Neurosci.*, 4: 227–272.

Gordon-Weeks, P.R. (1981) Are there noradrenergic synapses in Auerbach's plexus? *Scand. J. Gastrol.*, 16, Suppl. 70: 181–182.

Hollender, L.F., Marrie, A., Meyer, Ch., Begin, C. and Alexiou, D. (1980) Anatomical bases of vagotomy. *Anat. Clin.*, 2: 169–180.

Jackson, A.J. (1978) The spiral constrictor of the gastroesophageal junction. *Am. J. Anat.*, 151: 265–276.

Kyosola, K., Rechardt, L., Veijola, L., Waris, T. and Pentilla, O. (1980) Innervation of the human gastric wall. *J. Anat.*, 131: 453–470.

Misiewicz, J.J. (1984) Human colonic motility. *Scand. J. Gastroenterol.*, 19, Suppl. 93: 43–52.

Romeo, G., Sanfilippo, G., Basile, F., Catania, G., Ianello, A. and Carnazza, M.L.M. (1981) Ultrastructural study of parietal cells before and after vagotomy in patients with duodenal ulcer. *Surg. Gynecol. Obstet.*, 153: 61–64.

Wood, J.D. (1981) Intrinsic neural control of intestinal motility. *Annu. Rev. Physiol.*, 43: 33–51.

40
Pelvic Viscera

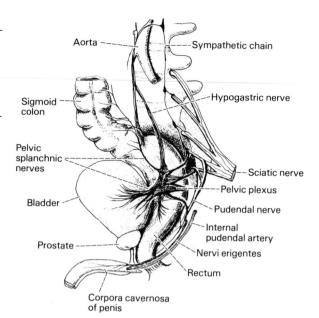

Aorta — Sympathetic chain
Sigmoid colon
Hypogastric nerve
Pelvic splanchnic nerves
Sciatic nerve
Pelvic plexus
Bladder
Pudendal nerve
Internal pudendal artery
Prostate
Nervi erigentes
Rectum
Corpora cavernosa of penis

Fig. 40-1 Pelvic plexus, left side.

The pelvic viscera receive their innervation from the left and right pelvic plexuses, beside the rectum (Fig. 40-1). The nerves contributing to the plexuses are sympathetic, parasympathetic, and afferent. The pelvic splanchnic nerves emerge from the plexuses to supply the hindgut and bladder. The nervi erigentes emerge from the plexuses to supply the erectile tissue of the external genitalia.

Sympathetic system (Fig. 40-2)

Preganglionic fibers emerge from the intermediolateral cell column of the spinal cord at segmental levels T10–L3. The fibers pass through the sympathetic chain and emerge as the *lumbar splanchnic nerves*. These nerves merge in front of the aortic bifurcation, then diverge as the *hypogastric nerves* to reach sympathetic ganglia within the pelvic plexuses. Postganglionic fibers supply the rectum, bladder, and in particular the male genital tract. (For the genital tracts, see Chapter 41.)

Parasympathetic system (Fig. 40-3)

Preganglionic fibers arise in the intermediolateral cell column of sacral segments S2–S4. They descend in the cauda equina and emerge from the sacrum with the corresponding anterior nerve roots. The genitourinary tract is supplied by fibers that synapse in parasympathetic ganglia within the pelvic plexus. The descending colon, sigmoid colon, and rectum are supplied by fibers which pass through the plexus and synapse upon ganglion cells of the myenteric plexus.

Visceral afferents

Afferents from the bladder and rectum traverse the pelvic plexus and synapse in sacral segments S2–S4. Their cell bodies occupy spinal ganglia. From the sacral cord, ascending projections accompany the spinothalamic and spinoreticular tracts.

HINDGUT

The intrinsic nerve supply of the hindgut resembles that of the intestine in general, having myenteric and submucous plexuses with a wide variety of transmitter substances. The sympathetic supply is entirely postganglionic; it terminates in the main upon cholinergic neurons and inhibits them via α_2 receptors. Some fibers probably inhibit the gut directly, via β_2 receptors. The smooth muscle of the internal anal sphincter receives abundant excitatory fibers (α_1 receptors).

About half an hour after the first main meal, the gastrocolic reflex (which may have a hormonal origin)

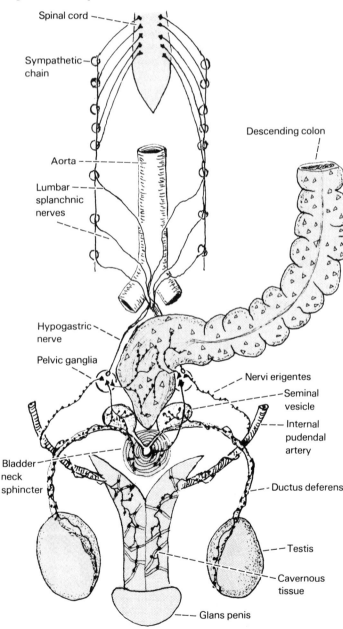

Spinal cord
Sympathetic chain
Descending colon
Aorta
Lumbar splanchnic nerves
Hypogastric nerve
Pelvic ganglia
Nervi erigentes
Seminal vesicle
Internal pudendal artery
Bladder neck sphincter
Ductus deferens
Testis
Cavernous tissue
Glans penis

Fig. 40-2 Sympathetic supply to male pelvic organs and external genitalia.

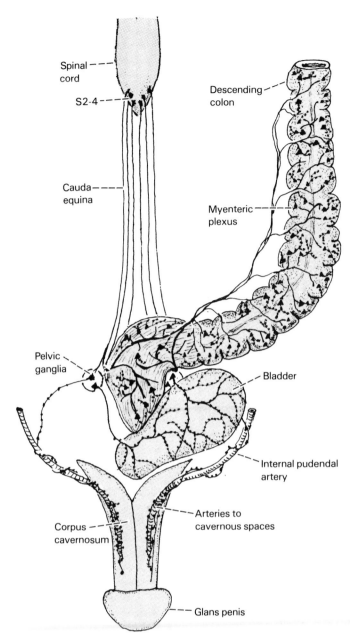

Fig. 40-3 Parasympathetic supply to male pelvic organs, descending colon, and external genitalia.

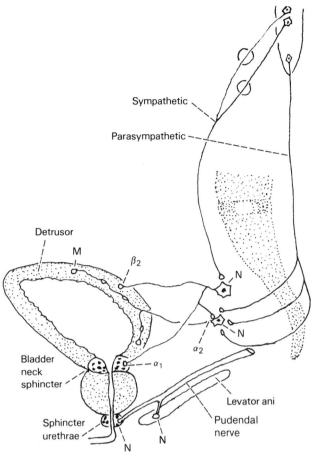

Fig. 40-4 Pelvic visceral receptors. M, muscarinic; N, nicotinic.

BLADDER

Smooth muscle

The detrusor is the same in both sexes. It is composed of interlacing bundles of smooth muscle disposed so as to empty the bladder completely. *The detrusor is intensely supplied with cholinergic nerve fibers and muscarinic receptors.* The cell bodies concerned are in the pelvic ganglia (mainly) and in the bladder wall.

The sympathetic contribution to bladder function is relatively unimportant because the bladder is not significantly affected by resection of the hypogastric nerves. The adrenergic fibers terminate mainly upon cholinergic neurons of the pelvic plexus, which they inhibit via prejunctional α_2 receptors. A small number of adrenergic fibers reach the detrusor, which they inhibit via β_2 receptors (Fig. 40-4).

Males have a smooth muscle sphincter at the bladder neck which is rich in adrenergic nerves; however, this sphincter belongs functionally to the genital tract (Chapter 41).

Non-adrenergic, non-cholinergic nerves

The detrusor muscle contains a variety of peptidergic and other NANC neurons whose somas occupy the pelvic ganglia. Immunohistochemistry and other methods have revealed ATP (adenosine triphosphate), VIP (vasoactive intestinal polypeptide), substance P, somatostatin, and enkephalin. Some of these are

causes feces to be propelled from the sigmoid colon into the rectum. Stretch receptors in the rectal wall activate local myenteric reflexes, as well as signaling rectal distension to higher levels of the CNS. Defecation is less well understood than micturition, but a defecatory control center probably exists in the reticular formation of the pons. Presence of a generator is expected, because defecation requires the integrated action of striated muscle (notably the diaphragm and levator ani) and smooth muscle. Detrusion of rectal contents is under the immediate control of the sacral spinal cord, although integrity of the intrinsic supply is required for smooth peristalsis. The sacral parasympathetic center appears to be controlled by the pontine reticular formation, which may be controlled in turn by higher centers (compare with bladder control, considered next).

271

excitatory; others are inhibitory. The role of NANC nerves in normal bladder function is obscure.

Striated muscles

In men, the urethra just below the prostate is surrounded by the sphincter urethrae. In women a small striated sphincter can be identified at the corresponding level but it is functionally quite negligible. In both sexes the levator ani passes close to the urethra; it exerts a pincer action which can be used at will to interrupt the urinary stream.

The striated muscles are supplied by anterior horn cells in sacral segments 3 and 4. The axons pass above the levator ani and they are unaffected by pudendal block. (The pudendal nerves are often blocked by obstetricians prior to undertaking forceps deliveries.)

Afferents

Afferent fibers from the mucous membrane follow the sympathetic system to reach cord levels T12–L2. From the detrusor, afferents follow the parasympathetic route to reach segments S2–S4. Pain from bladder distension is referred initially to dermatomes T12–L2 (lower abdomen and thighs), and later to dermatomes S2–S4 (sacral pain). From both levels of the cord, impulses travel along the spinothalamic and spinoreticular pathways.

Higher centers (Fig. 40-5)

There is a *detrusor center* in the pontine reticular formation. It receives spinoreticular afferents, and it is played upon by fibers from the cerebral cortex, limbic system, hypothalamus, and cerebellum. Three basic neuronal loops can be identified in the control of bladder function:

Loop 1 links the detrusor center to a 'bladder area' of the motor cortex, located near the upper border of each hemisphere.

Loop 2 connects the detrusor center with the sacral gray matter.

Loop 3 connects the sacral gray matter to the bladder wall. The sacral parasympathetic nucleus is regulated by the detrusor center; it becomes autonomous only if loop 2 is interrupted (by spinal cord injury, for example).

By playing on the detrusor center, the limbic system and hypothalamus are responsible for emotional effects on bladder function such as the desire to micturate in states of excitement or extreme fear.

Micturition

Micturition is initiated by voluntary inhibition of the levator ani. This allows the bladder to descend and its outlet to become funnel-shaped (Fig. 40-6). Urine escapes into the urethra, and mucosal afferents in the urethra relay to the detrusor center, which responds by stimulating the sacral parasympathetic nucleus. Bladder emptying

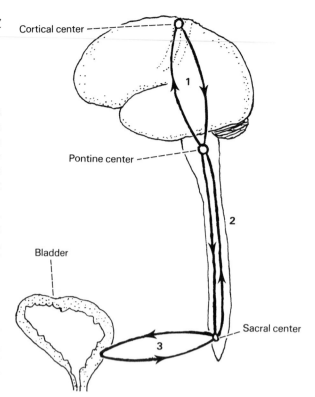

Fig. 40-5 The three principal neuronal loops controlling the bladder: 1, corticoreticular; 2, reticulosacral; 3, sacrovesical.

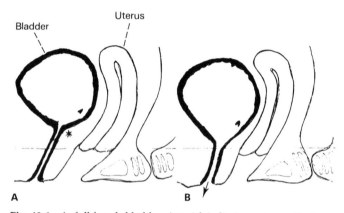

Fig. 40-6 A, full female bladder. Asterisk indicates vesicourethral angle. B, descent of the bladder initiates micturition.

may be assisted by contraction of the abdominal wall, and the urethra is cleared by the bulbospongiosus muscles.

APPLIED ANATOMY

Rectum

If the nervous pathways are intact, fecal continence depends above all else on the integrity of the levator ani. The levator ani (striated muscle) is rich in tonic motor units for its role in supporting all of the pelvic viscera. The external anal sphincter (striated) is mainly composed of phasic motor units, which exert temporary control of flatus and of fluid feces. The internal sphincter ani (smooth) has no supportive action: it responds to rectal filling by relaxation.

Hirschsprung's disease

Hirschsprung's disease, or *megacolon*, is characterized by abdominal distension in infancy, accompanied by inability to defecate. The colon becomes distended with feces. The source of the problem is an *aganglionic segment* of the gut, in which nerve cells are missing from the myenteric and submucous plexuses – always from the rectum, and sometimes from the descending colon as well. Peristaltic activity is irregular in the affected region, and the internal anal sphincter does not relax in response to rectal distension. The aganglionic segment itself is constricted; it contains abundant *preganglionic* cholinergic nerve endings.

One view of the etiology is that ganglion cells fail to migrate to the hindgut from the neural crest. This view is difficult to sustain since the descending colon is farther removed from the sacral cord but is seldom involved. Another view is that the intrinsic neurons are normally delivered to the entire gut by the vagus nerves in embryonic life, and that in Hirschsprung's disease neurons destined for the hindgut fail to complete their migration.

The usual treatment is to remove the rectum and sigmoid and to anastomose the descending colon to the anorectal junction. A wedge of internal anal sphincter must be removed to overcome its inability to relax.

Bladder

Stress incontinence

In women urinary continence depends upon the tone of levator ani. The entire urethra may be removed (because of cancer) without affecting continence. On the other hand, weakness of the levator ani is a common cause of incontinence. In multiparous women repeated stretching of the pubococcygeal muscle during childbirth causes the muscle to sag, unless appropriate exercises (such as voluntary interruption of the urinary stream) are undertaken. Sagging allows the uterus to descend (to *prolapse*), and the bladder descends as well. Descent of the bladder causes obliteration of the urethrovesical angle (Fig. 40-6), and the outlet becomes funnel-shaped at rest. In this condition a momentary increase in pressure (caused by sneezing or coughing, for instance) may cause a jet of urine to be expelled (*stress incontinence*). Stress incontinence can be cured surgically by restoring the normal urethrovesical angle.

In men, incontinence is not produced by local disorders other than gross pathologies of the bladder neck or prostate.

Neurological disorders

Interruption of loop 1 (corticoreticular loop)

Cortical control of the detrusor center is not established until early in the second postnatal year. Until then, the detrusor center empties the bladder every two to four hours, as the bladder fills. *Nocturnal enuresis* (bedwetting) may occur in older children from loss of cortical control of the detrusor center during sleep.

In adults, loop 1 may be interrupted bilaterally by enlargement of the lateral ventricles associated with internal

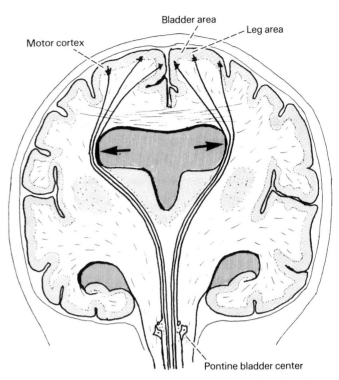

Fig. 40-7 Normotensive hydrocephalus. Expansion of the lateral ventricles (arrows) stretches corticospinal fibers supplying leg motoneurons and corticopontine fibers controlling the bladder.

hydrocephalus (see later), by disease of the anterior cerebral arteries (they supply the pelvic and lower limb areas of the sensorimotor cortex), or by a meningioma of the falx cerebri. Such patients have frequent spontaneous emptying of the bladder – in this sense, a reversion to infantile behavior.

Closely akin is *urge incontinence*. The term embraces a variety of neurological disorders having in common a frequent desire to micturate: including multiple sclerosis, Parkinson's disease, and disease of the frontal lobes of the brain. The evidence from pharmacology indicates hyperactivity of the detrusor center in these patients, implying that the frontal cortex, basal ganglia, and cerebellum normally exert inhibitory control.

Normotensive hydrocephalus occasionally occurs in men some weeks or months after a head injury. The patients develop a triad of symptoms – intellectual deterioration, spastic gait, and urinary incontinence – in that order. The symptoms are caused by expansion of the lateral ventricles, resulting in atrophy of the frontal cortex and in compression of corticospinal and corticopontine fibers skirting the ventricles (Fig. 40-7).

The hydrocephalus is presumed to be initiated by minor obstruction to CSF circulation at the time of injury. Once initiated, ventricular expansion is progressive. CSF pressure is normal at the time of diagnosis, but the enlarged ventricles exert greater pressure on the surrounding white matter merely because they *are* enlarged, in accordance with the Laplace principle.

Withdrawal of 20 ml CSF through a spinal tap produces immediate improvement in the patient's mental state. A cure may be effected by shunting the CSF from the lateral ventricle to the internal jugular vein by means of a catheter. If the correct diagnosis is not made the patient may be mistakenly treated for premature senility.

Interruption of loop 2 (reticulosacral loop)
Transection of the spinal cord interrupts the normal detrusor reflex. An *automatic bladder* develops, as described in Chapter 11. Automatic bladder is usually ascribed to the independent operation of loop 3.

Interruption of loop 3 (sacrovesical loop)
This loop may be damaged anywhere between vertebra T12 or L1 and the bladder – a reminder that the sacral segments

of the cord do *not* occupy the sacral canal. The result is an *atonic bladder:* the organ is flaccid and constantly distended with urine, which dribbles away (overflow incontinence).

Drug therapy
Mild stress incontinence may be treated by alpha agonist drugs: although there is no sphincter at the female bladder neck, the smooth muscle here and in the urethra contains α receptors.

Urge incontinence and *nocturnal enuresis* are treated by drugs that block M receptors. Such drugs are not purely bladder-specific, however, and dryness of the mouth, weakness of ocular accommodation, increased heart rate, and constipation may occur as side-effects (Chapter 6). Beta agonist drugs are only moderately useful because of the scarcity of β receptors in the bladder wall.

Outflow obstruction caused by prostatic hypertrophy may be treated initially either by M receptor agonists (to strengthen the detrusor) or by α receptor blockers (to relax the bladder neck sphincter).

Readings

Andersson, K.-E. and Sjögren, C. (1982) Aspects of the physiology and pharmacology of the bladder and urethra. *Prog. Neurobiol., 19:* 71–89.

Applebaum, A.E., Vance, W.H. and Coggeshall, R.E. (1980) Segmental localization of sensory cells that innervate the bladder. *J. Comp. Neurol., 192:* 203–210.

Bradley, W.E. and Sundin, T. (1982) The physiology and pharmacology of urinary tract dysfunction. *Clin. Neuropharmacol., 5:* 131–158.

Davis, P.W. and Foster, D.B.E. (1972) Hirschsprung's disease: a clinical review. *Br. J. Surg., 59:* 19–26.

Fletcher, T.F. and Bradley, W.E. (1978) Neuroanatomy of the bladder–urethra. *J. Urol., 119:* 153–160.

Gosling, J. (1979) The structure of the bladder and urethra in relation to function. *Urol. Clin. North Am., 6:* 31–38.

Gosling, J.A., Dixon, J.S., Critchley, O.D. and Thompson, S. (1981) A comparative study of the human external sphincter and periurethral levator ani muscles. *Br. J. Urol., 53:* 35–41.

de Groat, W.C., Booth, A.M., Milne, R.J. and Roppolo, J.R. (1982) Parasympathetic preganglionic neurons in the sacral spinal cord. *J. Auton. Nerv. Syst., 3:* 135–160.

Howard, E.R. (1972) Hirschsprung's disease: a review of the morphology and physiology. *Postgrad. Med. J., 48:* 471–477.

Huisman, A.B. (1983) Aspects of the anatomy of the female urethra with special relation to urinary continence. *Contrib. Gynecol. Obstet., 10:* 1–31.

Jensen, D. (1981) Pharmacological studies of the uninhibited neurogenic bladder. *J. Oslo City Hosp., 31:* 97–114.

Juskiewenski, S., Vayasse, P., Gvitard, J., Moscovici, J. and Fourtanier, G. (1981) Innervation of the bladder and urethra. *Anatomia Clinica, 2:* 243–263.

Kluck, Y. (1980) The autonomic innervation of the human urinary bladder, bladder neck and urethra: a histochemical study. *Anat. Rec., 198:* 439–447.

Lowey, A.D. (1981) Descending control of the bladder. *Exp. Neurol., 71:* 19–22.

Maresca, C. and Ghafar, W. (1980) The presacral nerve (plexus hypogastricus superior). *Anatomia Clinica, 2:* 5–12.

Milne, R.J., Foreman, R.D., Giesler, G.J. and Willis, W.D. (1983) Viscerosomatic convergence onto primate spinothalamic neurons: an explanation for referral of pelvic visceral pain. In *Advances in Pain Research and Therapy*, Vol. 5 (Bonica, J.J., Lindblom, U., Iggo, A., Jones, L.E. and Benedetti, C., eds.), pp. 131–138. New York: Raven Press.

Okamoto, E., Satani, M. and Kiwata, K. (1982) Histologic and embryologic studies on the innervation of the pelvic viscera in patients with Hirschsprung's disease. *Surg. Gynecol. Obstet., 155:* 823–828.

Petras, J.M. and Cummings, J.F. (1978) Sympathetic and parasympathetic innervation of the urinary bladder and urethra. *Brain Res., 153:* 363–369.

41
Coital Reflexes

MALE RESPONSES

In men coitus involves three components or stages: *erection* of the penis, *emission* of semen into the urethra, and *ejaculation* of semen into the vagina. Sympathetic, parasympathetic and somatic components of the nervous system are involved (Table 14-1).

Table 41-1 Stages of coitus in man

Stage	Nervous component	Specific nerves	Tissue
Erection	Parasympathetic, sympathetic	Nervi erigentes	Pudendal arteries, cavernous tissue
Emission	Sympathetic	Pelvic splanchnic	Vas deferens, prostate, seminal vesicles, bladder neck
Ejaculation	Somatic	Pudendal	Bulbospongiosus

Erection (Figs. 41-1, 41-2)

The corpora cavernosa contain a spongework of fibromuscular septa, enclosing labyrinthine cavernous

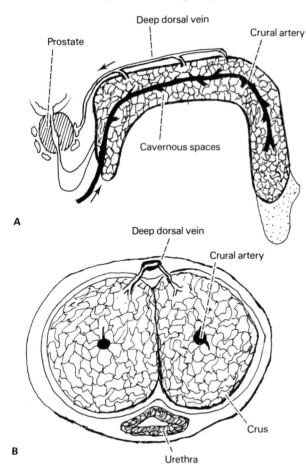

Fig. 41-1 A, sagittal section of corpus cavernosum. (Arrows indicate direction of blood flow.) B, cross-section of penis.

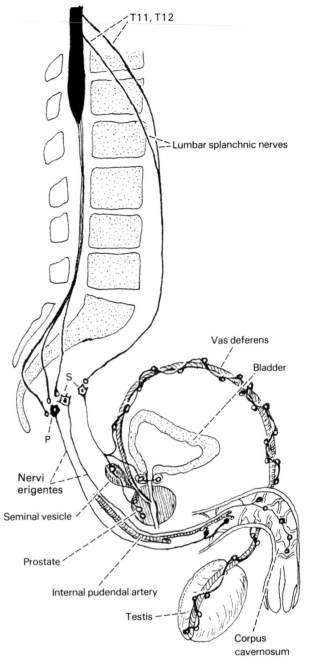

Fig. 41-2 Innervation of male genital tract. P, S, parasympathetic and sympathetic neurons in pelvic ganglia.

spaces. The spaces are fed by crural branches of the internal pudendal artery. The crural arteries have resting sympathetic tone and the spaces are empty.

The *nervi erigentes* (L., erecting nerves) are postganglionic, both sympathetic and parasympathetic. They arise in ganglion cells of the pelvic plexus and they join the internal pudendal artery prior to its entry to the ischiorectal fossa. The sympathetic fibers supply the crural arteries, providing them with resting tone; they also supply smooth muscle – rich in α receptors – in the cavernous tissue septa. The parasympathetic fibers are vasodilator to the crural arteries (Fig. 41-3). Some of these fibers use acetylcholine as transmitter, others use vasoactive intestinal polypeptide (VIP).

Generator

Erection appears to be controlled by a generator located in the caudal pontine reticular formation. In monkeys the generator can be activated by stimulation of the septal area, or of the medial forebrain bundle carrying fibers from it to the brainstem. Stimulation of the human septal area sometimes produces an erection. The motor cortex is not concerned, but the anterior temporal cortex may be important, perhaps because of a projection from the cortical amygdala to the septum (Chapter 22).

From the pontine generator, reticulospinal fibers descend to T12–L1 and S2–S4 segments, to activate both elements of the nervi erigentes. Under normal conditions erection can be produced either by *psychogenic stimulation* alone, or by *reflexogenic stimulation* from the penis. The glans contains encapsulated nerve endings called *genital corpuscles* (Fig. 41-4), whose fibers synapse centrally in the sacral cord. Sexual sensation is mediated by the spinoreticulothalamic pathway, which causes reflex stimulation of the pontine generator as well as activating the septal area via the thalamus. Sexual sensation, including orgasm, is lost after bilateral cordotomy (Chapter 11). Orgasmic sensation may be elicited by stimulation of the septal area.

Mechanism of erection

The mechanism of erection is somewhat speculative, because the detailed anatomy of the fibromuscular cavernosal septa has yet to be worked out. A major contributor to tumescence is flooding of the cavernous spaces following dilatation of the crural arteries. Contraction of smooth muscle in the cavernosal septa evidently provides a moderate obstruction to outflow of blood into the deep dorsal vein. The venous drainage itself does not seem to be blocked, because the penis remains pink. The small amount of cavernous tissue (corpus spongiosum) surrounding the urethra also becomes engorged, perhaps to maintain patency.

Emission (Fig. 41-2)

The mature sperm are stored in the lower end of the ductus (vas) deferens and tail of epididymis. The entire length of the ductus is intensely rich in adrenergic nerve endings and α receptors. So too is the smooth muscle of the bladder neck, prostate, and seminal vesicles. The fibers are distributed by sympathetic ganglion cells in the pelvic plexuses.

At the male climax, peristaltic waves milk the sperm rapidly into the prostatic urethra. The secretions of prostate and seminal vesicles are added by local muscular contraction to complete the semen. Simultaneous closure of the bladder-neck sphincter forces the semen into the penile urethra. Should the bladder neck fail to close properly, an 'internal emission' ('retrograde ejaculation') into the bladder may occur.

Ejaculation

Entry of the semen into the penile urethra stimulates mucosal nerve endings of the pudendal nerve. The

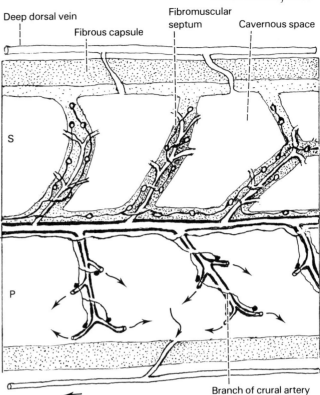

Fig. 41-3 Scheme to show sympathetic (S) and parasympathetic (P) innervation of corpus cavernosum.

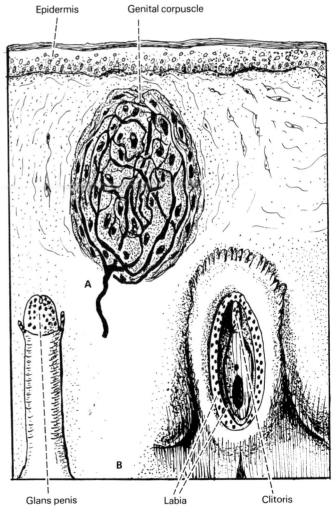

Fig. 41-4 Genital corpuscles. A, structure; B, location (dots).

central ends of these afferents synapse upon pudendal alpha motor neurons in sacral segments of the cord, eliciting contractions of the bulbospongiosus muscle, in particular. The bulbospongiosus empties the urethra.

FEMALE RESPONSES

Erection of the clitoris is comparable to penile erection. VIP seems to be particularly important in providing relaxation of the crural arteries. VIP also relaxes arteries in the vaginal wall, and capillary engorgement causes the vaginal mucous membrane to be moistened by transudate. The cell bodies of the VIP-containing neurons lie beside the cervix.

Clitoral erection is reinforced by tactile stimulation of genital corpuscles in the skin covering the clitoris and inner surfaces of the labia (Fig. 41-4). Corpuscles are absent from the vagina, and vaginal stimulation is relatively ineffective (at least in Western cultures) in producing erection and climax.

At climax, rhythmic contractions of the periurethral muscles take place, comparable to those of the male.

Sperm transport

Although the human uterus and tubes receive a sympathetic innervation, neuromuscular activity seems to be unimportant in sperm transport. The uterus may contract to aid transport, but this contraction is induced by prostaglandins absorbed from the semen.

APPLIED ANATOMY

Impotence is the inability to achieve and maintain the male erection. In the vast majority, impotence is psychogenic, being produced by psychological conditioning. The commonest organic cause is *diabetes*: 50% of men with insulin-dependent diabetes cannot achieve erections. (In the United States alone this accounts for impotence in more than half a million men.) The norepinephrine content of the erectile tissue is greatly reduced in diabetics, presumably because of neuropathy of sympathetic fibers. Thoracolumbar *sympathectomy* (for vascular disease in the lower limbs) is often followed by impotence, for the same reason.

Spinal cord lesions above T10 interrupt reticulospinal pathways to the sympathetic and parasympathetic centers in the cord. However, emission and ejaculation are often achieved by penile manipulation alone (through the sacral reflex arc). Lesions below T10 are likely to include the conus medullaris and/or the cauda equina, and to cause irreversible impotence.

Readings

Benson, G.S., McConnell, J. and Lipshultz, L.I. (1980) Neuromorphology and neuropharmacology of the human penis. *J. Clin. Invest.*, 65: 506–513.

Johnson, M.H. and Everitt, B.J. (1980) *Essential Reproduction.* Oxford: Blackwell.

Karacan, I., Aslan, C. and Hirshkowitz, M. (1983) Erectile mechanisms in man. *Science*, 220: 1080–1082.

Melman, A. and Henry, D. (1979) The possible role of catecholamine of the corpora cavernosa in penile erection. *J. Urol.*, 121: 419–421.

Ottesen, B. (1983) Vasoactive intestinal polypeptide as a neurotransmitter in the female genital tract. *Am. J. Obstet. Gynecol.*, 147: 208–221.

Weiss, H.D. (1972) The physiology of human penile erection. *Ann. Intern. Med.*, 76: 793–799.

Whitelaw, G.P. and Smithwick, R.H. (1951) Some secondary effects of sympathectomy with particular reference to disturbance of sexual function. *New Engl. J. Med.*, 245: 121–130.

X
APPENDIX AND INDEX

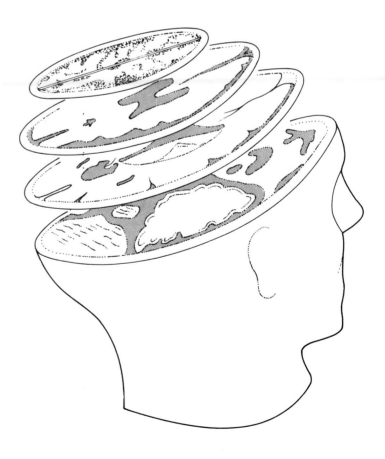

Appendix
Computed Tomographic Scanning

Computed tomographic scanning (CT scanning) of the brain has revolutionized neurological diagnosis and management. It is a safe, non-invasive radiological technique whereby the brain can be visualized in serial sections about a centimeter thick. An X-ray source is rotated around the patient while detectors record the number of X-ray photons emerging from the patient. A computer integrates the information and presents the successive 'cuts' on a monitor as gray-scale images. Contrast can be enhanced, and blood vessels displayed, by prior intravenous injection of an iodinated medium.

The standard plane of brain scans is shown in Figs. A1 and A2. Selected pictures from a normal adult are presented in Figs. A3 to A8.

Readings

Ascherl, G.F., Ganti, S.R. and Hilal, S.K. (1980) Neuroradiology for the clinician. In *Neurology* (Rosenberg, R.N., ed.), pp. 634–718. New York: Grune and Stratton.

Gado, M. and Yousef, S.J.E. (1983) Normal functional anatomy of the brain. In *Computed Tomography of the Whole Brain* (Haaga, J.R. and Alfida, R.J., eds.), pp. 23–43. St Louis: Mosby.

Husband, J.E. and Fry, I.K. (1981) *Computed Tomography of the Body*. London: Macmillan.

Koritki, J.G. and Sick, H. (1983) *Atlas of Sectional Human Anatomy*, Vol. 1, Head, Neck, Thorax. Baltimore & Munich: Urban & Schwarzenberg.

Kretschmann, H.-J. and Weinrich, W. (1984) *Neuroanatomie der kraniellen Computero-tomographie*. Stuttgart & New York: Georg Thieme Verlag (English translation in press).

Pevsner, P.H. (1979) Computed tomographic anatomy – brain, orbits, skull base. In *Medical Imaging: A Basic Course* (Kreel, L., ed.), pp. 47–51. Aylesbury: Wheaton & Co.

Wegener, O.H. (1983) *Whole Body Computerized Tomography* (Long, J.H., trans.). Basel: Karger.

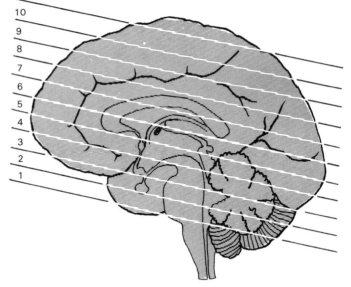

Fig. A1 Standard planes of CT scans, medial view.

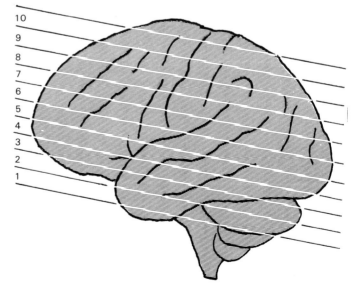

Fig. A2 Standard planes of CT scans, lateral view.

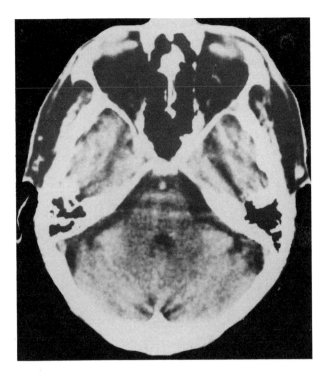

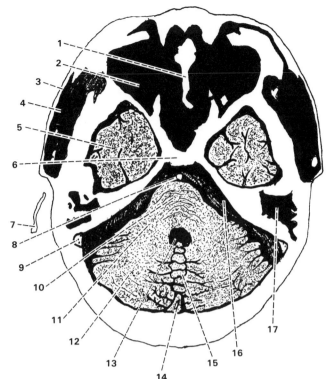

Fig. A3   CT scan in plane 3:

1 Nasal septum
2 Maxillary air sinus
3 Zygomatic arch
4 Temporal fossa
5 Temporal lobe
6 Clivus of sphenoid
7 Pinna
8 Basilar artery
9 Sigmoid sinus
10 Pons
11 Middle cerebellar peduncle
12 Cerebellar hemisphere
13 Fourth ventricle
14 Occipital sinus
15 Cerebellar vermis
16 Subarachnoid space
17 Middle ear cavity

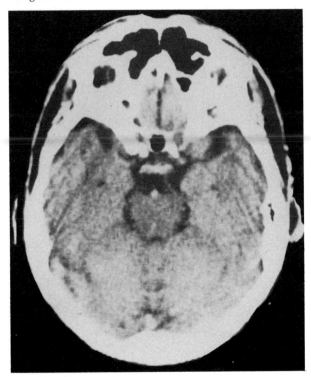

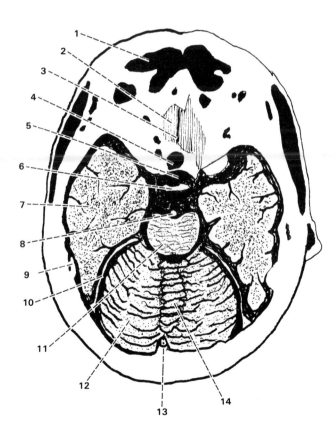

Fig. A4   CT scan in plane 4:

1 Frontal air sinus
2 Frontal lobe
3 Longitudinal fissure
4 Sphenoidal air sinus
5 Pituitary fossa
6 Clivus of sphenoid
7 Temporal lobe
8 Basilar artery
9 Sigmoid sinus
10 Tentorium cerebelli
11 Pons
12 Cerebellar hemisphere
13 Occipital sinus
14 Cerebellar vermis

281

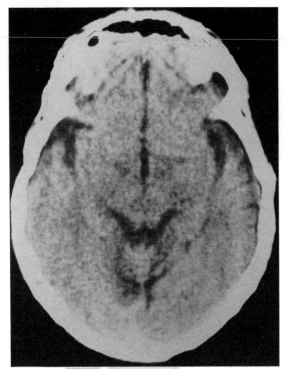

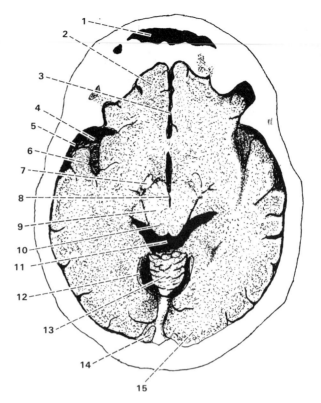

Fig. A5 CT scan in plane 5:

1 Frontal air sinus	9 Midbrain
2 Frontal lobe	10 Superior colliculus
3 Longitudinal fissure	11 Cisterna ambiens
4 Stem of lateral fissure	12 Tentorium cerebelli
5 Subarachnoid space	13 Cerebellar vermis
6 Temporal lobe	14 Superior sagittal sinus
7 Optic nerve	15 Occipital lobe
8 Interpeduncular space	

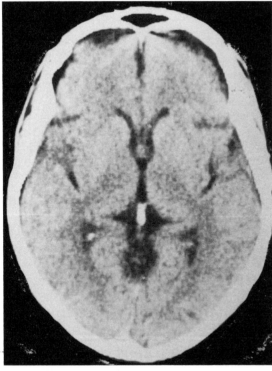

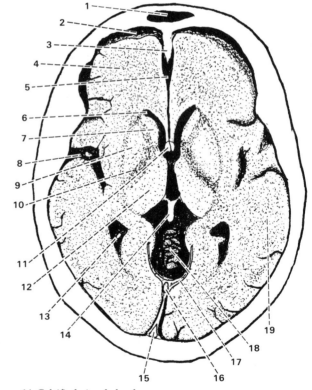

Fig. A6 CT scan in plane 6:

1 Frontal air sinus	8 Stem of lateral sulcus	14 Calcified pineal gland
2 Subarachnoid space	9 Lentiform nucleus	15 Superior sagittal sinus
3 Falx cerebri	10 Internal capsule	16 Straight sinus
4 Frontal lobe	11 Fornix	17 Tentorium cerebelli
5 Longitudinal fissure	12 Thalamus	18 Cerebellar vermis
6 Lateral ventricle	13 Choroidal vessel in	19 Temporal lobe
7 Head of caudate nucleus	lateral ventricle	

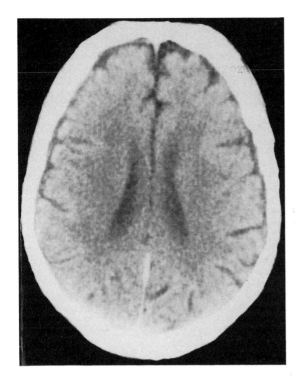
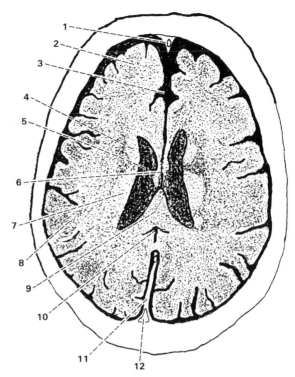

Fig. A7   CT scan in plane 8:

1 Superior sagittal sinus
2 Frontal lobe
3 Longitudinal fissure
4 Head of caudate nucleus
5 Lateral ventricle
6 Fornix
7 Thalamus
8 Parietal lobe
9 Splenium of corpus callosum
10 Subarachnoid space
11 Falx cerebri
12 Superior sagittal sinus

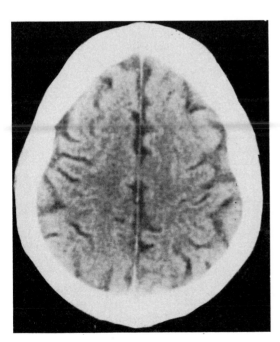
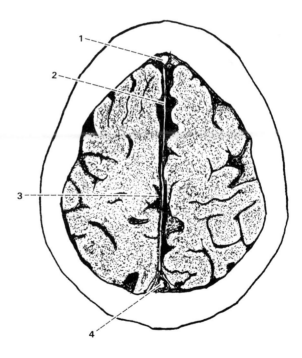

Fig. A8   CT scan in plane 10:

1 Superior sagittal sinus
2 Falx cerebri
3 Subarachnoid space
4 Superior sagittal sinus

Index